Shearer's Manual of Human Dissection

Shearer's Manual of Human Dissection

Sixth Edition

Edited by

Charles E. Tobin, Ph.D.
Professor Emeritus of Human Anatomy
School of Dentistry and School of Medicine and
Assistant Clinical Professor of Otolaryngology
School of Medicine
University of Colorado Health Sciences Center, Denver

John J. Jacobs, Ph.D.
Associate Professor of Anatomy
School of Medicine
Louisiana State University Medical Center, New Orleans

McGraw-Hill Book Company

New York St. Louis San Francisco Auckland Bogotá Guatemala Hamburg
Johannesburg Lisbon London Madrid Mexico Montreal New Delhi
Panama Paris San Juan São Paulo Singapore Sydney Tokyo Toronto

This book was set in Times Roman by Waldman Graphics, Inc.
The editors were Richard W. Mixter and Timothy Armstrong;
the production supervisor was Jeanne Skahan.
New drawings were done by Don Alvarado.
Kingsport Press, Inc., was printer and binder.

SHEARER'S MANUAL OF HUMAN DISSECTION

3 4 5 6 7 8 9 0 KPKP 8 9 8 7 6 5 4 3 2 1

Library of Congress Cataloging in Publication Data

Shearer, Edwin Morrill, date
Shearer's Manual of human dissection.

Includes index.
1. Human dissection—Handbooks, manuals, etc.
I. Tobin, Charles Emil, date II. Jacobs, John J.
III. Title. IV. Title: Manual of human dissection.
QM34.S56 1981 611'.0028 80-15573
ISBN 0-07-064926-X

Contents

Preface

This manual was originally conceived as a source of concise and specific detail in dissection procedures on a regional basis for the novice dissector. The new, revised edition continues to pursue those goals. The style and format of the preceding editions, which have proved to be so successful for teaching and learning human anatomy, have been preserved. As stated in the preface of the fifth edition, the manual is ''planned to achieve a workable balance between the amount of procedure for dissection and the descriptive text'' and ''is a compromise between the classic, lengthy manuals and the very brief guides for dissection.''

Some conspicuous changes and additions have been made that will enhance the manual's instructional value in the contemporary health science community. New figures have been added where needed to clarify dissection procedures or the anatomy. A number of the previously published figures have been replaced with simpler, more explicit ones, and other figures have been enlarged in order to augment their usefulness.

As a means of stimulating the dissector's interest and comprehension, practical and clinical correlates of the anatomy, where readily demonstrable on the dissected cadaver (or on laboratory partners), are presented in the text to show reasons for doing dissections and to whet the dissector's appetite for more.

The clinical correlates and the directions for skin incisions are distinguished at a glance from each other and from the rest of the text by the former being set in indented blocks of type separated from the rest of the text and the latter being set in italics. This feature, combined with the larger figures and the spiral binding, which allows the pages to lie flat on the book stand, should make the manual easy to handle and to use in the laboratory.

Three sections—brain, pelvis, and perineum—have been rewritten. The chapter on the brain bridges the gap between neuroscience courses, in which the brain specimens are usually preserved separately and are not related to the skull, and those gross anatomy programs that omit a study of the brain and its relationships. This manual emphasizes how the brain's surface relates to the bony cranial vault. The chapters on the pelvis and perineum present a complete dissection guide for studying the male and female anatomy separately.

The fourth edition of the *Nomina Anatomica* (1977) was used to update the terminology and nomenclature throughout the text and figures. Where appropriate, more descriptive vernacular terms replace the classic forms. The metric system of measurement is used throughout.

Aside from a few minor alterations, the sequential presentation of regional dissections is the same as that of the fifth edition. Persons involved with organizing anatomy courses can relatively easily rearrange the chapters into an order of dissection that suits the plans and needs of their own curriculum.

A statement from the preface of the fifth edition is equally pertinent to this edition:

> Since the manual is designed as an autonomous unit, it does not have to be used in conjunction with, or with reference to, any specific descriptive text on human anatomy. The dissector should use this book for the purpose for which it was written—as a guide for human dissection. If the student is to obtain a thorough understanding of human anatomy, he should supplement the information gained from the dissection and from the brief descriptions and illustrations in this manual with collateral reading in one of the standard descriptive texts. Frequent reference to one of the standard medical dictionaries will also help to familiarize the dissector with the meaning, origin, and pronunciation of the numerous terms he will encounter.

Too often in recent years, human gross anatomy courses have been reduced to a mere exercise of cutting the human body apart, with the learning of anatomy unfortunately postponed to a later time. The time to learn is while doing; dissectors must therefore be encouraged to learn as they dissect. Inasmuch as human anatomy is usually the first major course in the medical or dental school curriculum, the staff teaching human anatomy are entrusted with the responsibility of guiding students in the formation of efficient and effective learning habits—habits that train the mind to observe accurately, to assimilate, to recall, and to express concisely what is learned. Used properly, this manual, which presents anatomy as clearly as possible, can assist in the learning process because it requires that the dissector read directions carefully, dissect accordingly, and then observe. We hope that the mental process required and the skills acquired to learn anatomy in this manner will reward students again and again with an enthusiasm to learn and the confidence to do so, long after the course in anatomy is over.

My good friend and colleague William J. Swartz deserves to be mentioned and thanked for his advice, time, and criticism. I also received a good deal of editorial assistance from Virginia Howard, to whom I am grateful. Don Alvarado did the new illustrations; his work, which adds greatly to the worth of the manual, speaks for itself.

John J. Jacobs

Introduction

The right to dissect the human body was won after centuries of struggle against the prejudice of the unenlightened. Today's medical and dental students are apt to forget that having at their disposal, legally and without effort on their own part, a well-preserved body for dissection is a privilege for which the anatomist of 300 years ago would have given much. The body on the dissecting table is all the corporeal remains of what was once a human being, and it should be regarded with respect at all times.

The early anatomists—if they were so fortunate as to procure a body—were frequently confronted with the need to work secretly and in stealth; their work had to be done hurriedly because of the rapidity of decay. Modern methods of embalming and preservation eliminate the problem of decay. Your only responsibility, as the dissector, for the preservation of the body in the dissecting room is to prevent it from becoming too dry by keeping it wrapped in cloths dampened with preserving fluid when it is not being dissected or studied.

The technique of human dissection is acquired only by practice. Fortunately, you will develop an adequate technique usually in a relatively short time. It is a different technique from the one you may already be familiar with from studies of comparative anatomy, chiefly because of the vastly larger size of the body. For this reason, the technique of human dissection is less difficult than that used by the comparative anatomist, and often requires patience rather than great skill.

The essential instruments for the dissection of the human body are a strong pair of blunt-pointed forceps and a sharp scalpel with a broad blade of medium to large size. A flexible probe, a medium size hemostat, and a pair of scissors of medium size with one rounded and one pointed end are occasionally needed. Small, sharp-pointed forceps, narrow-bladed, sharp-pointed knives, and various elaborate surgical instruments are not essential for dissecting. The number and kinds of instruments selected need not conform to this list but may vary according to the needs and plan of study in various medical schools.

The method of dissecting the body is a regional one, in which the design is to see everything that is to be seen in a single area of the body at one time, as opposed to the systemic method more commonly followed in studies of comparative anatomy. In approaching any region of the body, first identify the surface landmarks (bones, muscles, vessels, etc.) that can be seen or palpated through the skin. Then you will be instructed to reflect the skin from that region. Skin should be removed only when that region is to be studied, as skin is the best protection against drying of the underlying parts. The actual technique of skin reflection is best learned by practice, but remember that the incisions that mark out a flap of skin for reflection must be made completely through the skin and along its entire length before reflection is begun, and that the skin alone must always be reflected cleanly from the underlying fascia.

The structures to be exposed and studied after the skin is reflected are embedded in various types of connective tissue that come under the generic term ''fascia.'' Before you remove the fascia, its form, extent, and connections should be studied. Not only does this tissue form the framework for (and enclose) the various structures, it is also important in limiting and directing the spread of infections. The dissection of the body consists, to a very great extent, in removing the fascia without injuring the structures it contains. This process—the cleaning of the embedded muscles, nerves, arteries, and other structures—is a tedious business, and you will often be tempted to leave it incomplete and pass on to other things once you have partially cleaned the particular structure you are seeking. This, however, is a bad practice, not only because careless work is, in itself, detrimental to proper observation, but also because of its cumulative effect on the dissection as a whole. Clean each structure in its entirety. The more thoroughly you clean a particular region, the more easily and satisfactorily can you clean and observe ensuing and deeper structures.

When you have cleaned all the structures in a particular region, you should take time to review and study them as they appear in the body. A definite plan of study should be followed for each structure dissected. This plan should include the plane or part of the body in which it is located, the form, size, and shape of the structure, its origin, course, and distribution, and its function. If at any time you wish to test your knowledge of any structure or region, you can write in exact terms a brief description of the part or parts of the body being studied or you can make a drawing or diagram and discuss it with your fellow students. Although function will be studied in more detail in other courses, gross anatomy can be more dynamic and interesting if you have some knowledge of the function of the structure you are dissecting.

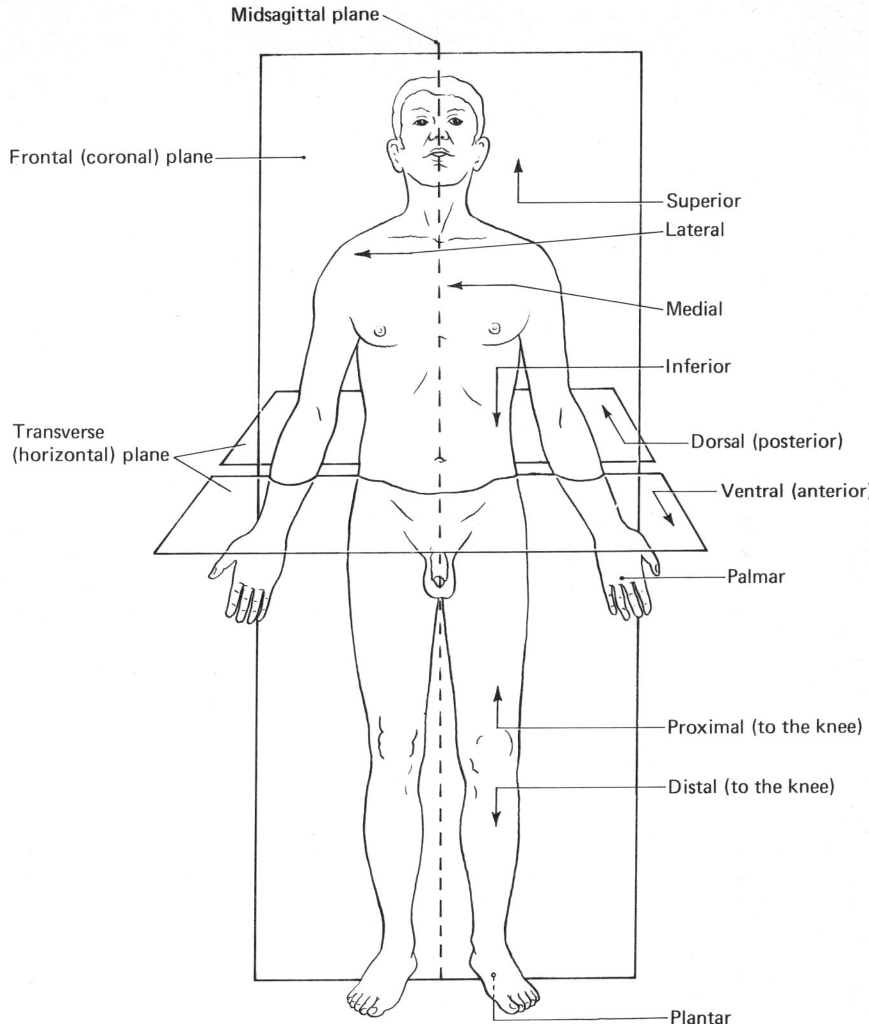

Figure I.1 Anterior view of **planes** and **directions of reference** for the human body in the anatomical position.

Occasionally, a source of pardonable distress to you will be the realization that from a regional study you are expected to acquire a systemic knowledge of human anatomy. The only consolation that can be offered is that here is an opportunity for you to exercise the integrative intellectual powers that those who embark on the study of anatomy may be assumed to possess. Although it is a practical necessity to dissect a series of separate regions, it is by no means a necessity to keep the observations made in separate compartments of your mind. As the dissection proceeds, associate in your mind the knowledge acquired region by region so that you will eventually see

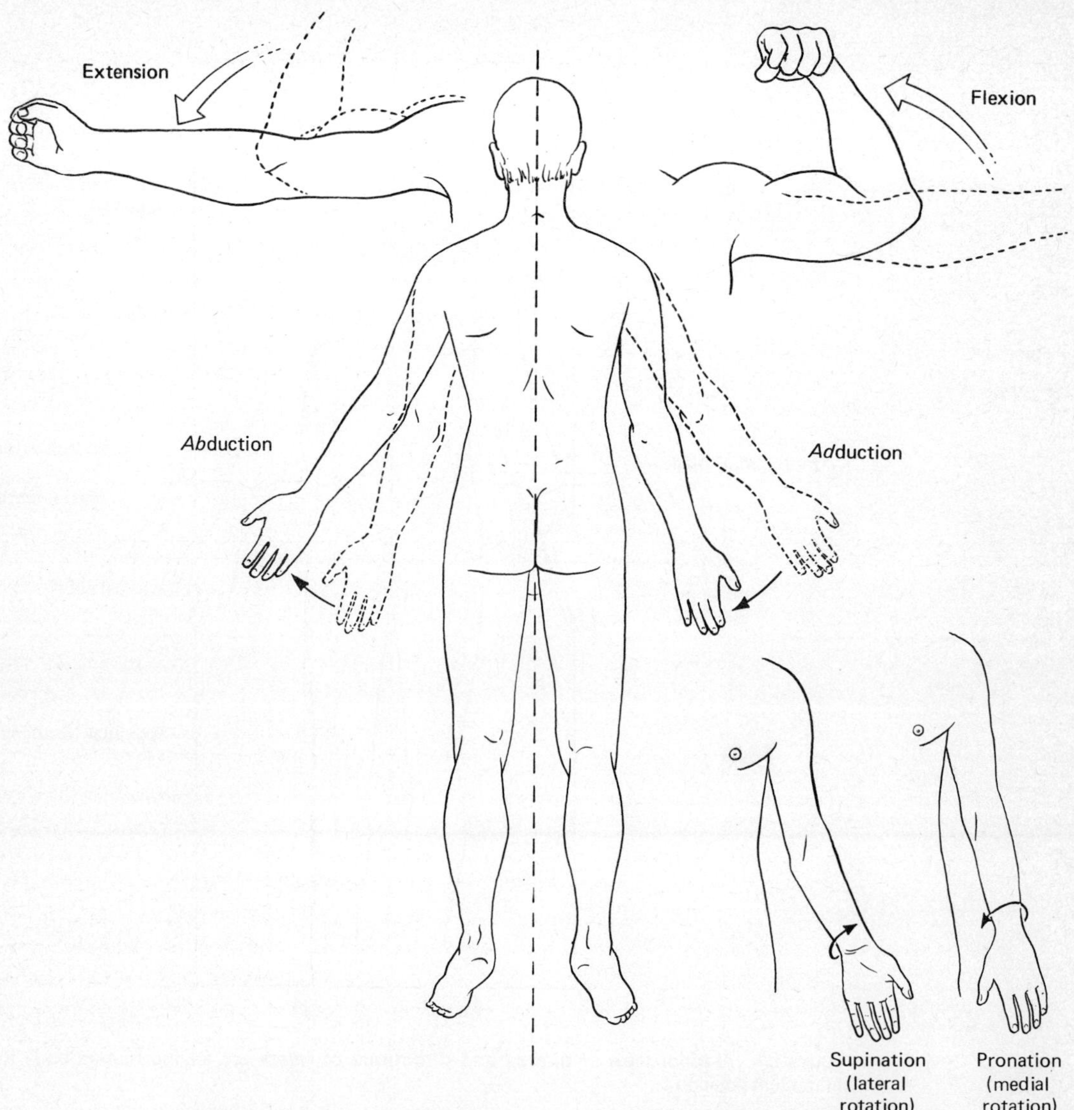

Figure I.2 Terms of movement used in speaking of the human body: **abduction** means to move away from the midline; **adduction,** to move toward the midline; **lateral rotation,** to rotate outward; **medial rotation,** to rotate inward; **flexion,** to bend (decrease the angle of) a joint; and **extension,** to straighten (increase the angle of) a joint.

the body as a whole and be able to reproduce this knowledge in systemic form—even though, for example, you may never actually see the entire arterial system or the entire nervous system at one time.

The order of dissection starts with the back for the following reasons: (1) For those who are not accustomed to human dissection, dissecting the back causes less emotional trauma than dissecting areas of the body that are visible and more familiar, e.g., face, hand. (2) Because the skin on the back is relatively thick, the technique of skinning can be learned faster than with the thinner skin over the ventral areas of the body. (3) The amount of fat in the subcutaneous tissue of the back is usually less than that found in other areas of the body, permitting easier dissection of the superficial vessels and nerves. (4) In this subcutaneous tissue there are no large secretory parts or glands, such as the mammary gland, that require additional dissection skill. (5) The superficial muscles are large, extend over a fairly large area, and are, therefore, easy to clean. (6) The dissector is also introduced to the concept of the smaller, shorter muscles of the deeper sacrospinalis group. (7) The dissection of the vertebral column initiates the concept of the skeleton at an early stage of dissection. (8) The spinal nerves and their component parts are studied at the beginning of the dissection of the total body, facilitating a better understanding of these nerves when they are encountered in subsequent work.

The terms for location and movement are usually described for the body in the ''anatomical position''—that is, standing erect with the arms straight down by the sides and with the forearm and hand in supination (Figs. I.1 and I.2). Although this is not the position of the cadaver on the dissecting table, keep in mind that all descriptions, whether of planes, positions, or relationships, are referred to the anatomical position. Some adjectives and adverbs are used in this manual that do not conform to *Nomina Anatomica* (NA) terminology. These terms are used for the convenience of the dissector—in keeping with the NA policy of translating terms into the vernacular for the sake of clarity. Among these terms are back, backward, below, deeply, down, downward, first, front, highest, lower, lowermost, outward, superior, upper, upward, uppermost. The meaning of these terms should be clear. In applying the terms ''first'' and ''lowermost'' to a number of structures (e.g., ribs, vertebrae), it is assumed that you will count them from the cranial toward the caudal region of the body and therefore will use these terms for the upper and lower structures, respectively.

Shearer's Manual of Human Dissection

Chapter 1

Back

For the dissection of the back, the body lies prone with a block elevating the thorax and the head hanging freely, so that the back of the neck is stretched. Certain surface points should be identified before the skin is reflected. In the midline at the base of the skull is the **external occipital protuberance.** Laterally, behind the lower part of the external ear, is the **mastoid process.** Arching between the external occipital protuberance and the mastoid on each side is the **superior nuchal line.** In the median line of the back, the **spinous processes** of most of the vertebrae may be palpated. The most superior vertebral spine that is ordinarily palpable is that of the seventh cervical vertebra (**vertebra prominens**). The upper cervical spines are separated from the skin by the **ligamentum nuchae,** a strong fibrous band that stretches in the median plane from the external occipital protuberance to the seventh cervical spine and is attached to the spinous processes of all the cervical vertebrae. Inferior to the last lumbar spine, the posterior surface of the **sacrum** is subcutaneous, and below it, between the buttocks, is the **coccyx.** Identify the **crest of** the **ilium** arching laterally from the **posterior superior iliac spine.** The posterior part of the iliac crest is often covered by a fairly thick layer of subcutaneous fat.

Locate the **vertebral border of** the **scapula.** Running laterally and upward from this border at the level of the third thoracic vertebral spine is the **spine of** the **scapula.** It is subcutaneous throughout its length and ends as the broad **acromion process,** the bony prominence of the shoulder.

After these points have been observed, make the following incisions through the skin as shown in Fig. 1.1: (1) a median longitudinal incision from the external occipital protuberance to the tip of the coccyx; (2) from the upper end of the first

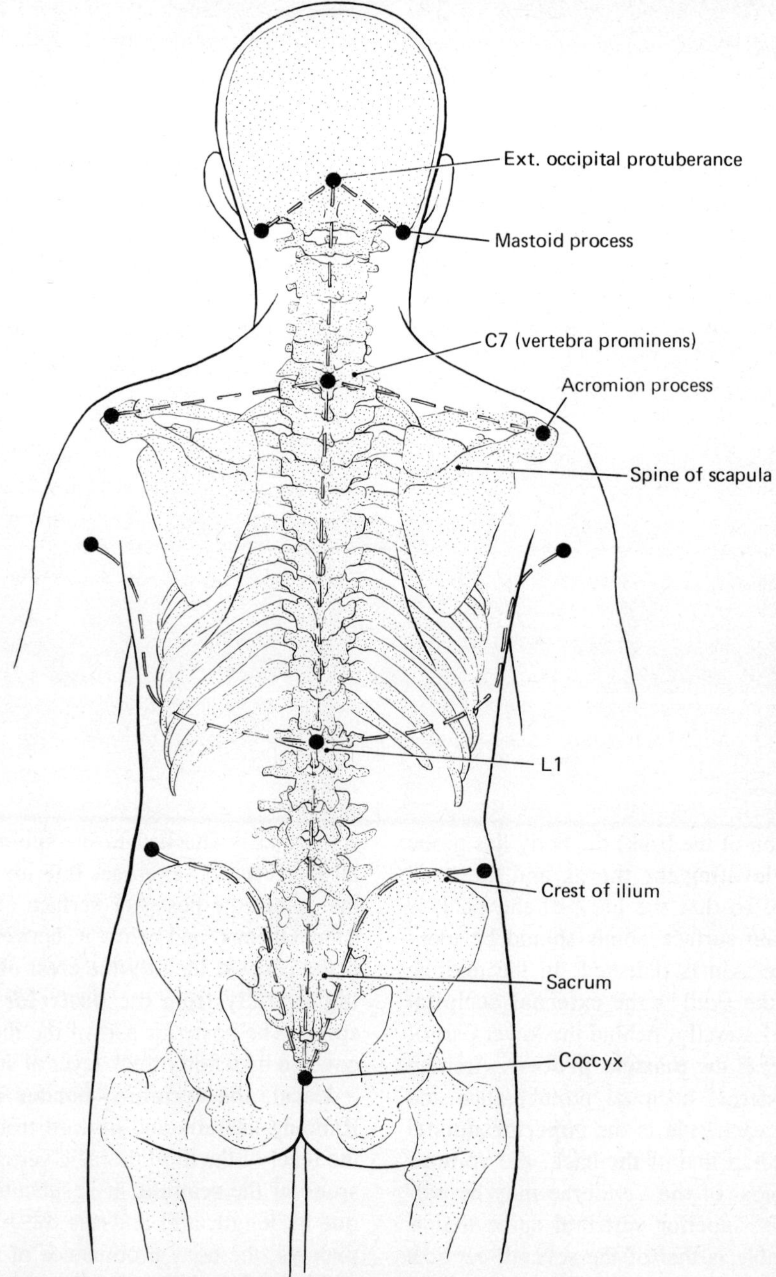

Figure 1.1 Surface landmarks and skin incisions on the back.

incision, one laterally and downward across the back of the skull behind the ears to the mastoid process; (3) from the first incision, one at the level of the first lumbar spine upward and laterally to the posterior axillary fold and then along this fold to the back of the arm; (4) from the first incision, one at the level of the seventh cervical spine straight laterally to the tip of the acromion; and (5) from the lower end of the first incision, one upward and laterally to the posterior superior iliac spine and then along the iliac crest to the posterior axillary line. The three large flaps of skin marked out on each side should be reflected laterally.

Reflection of the skin will expose the **superficial fascia** of the back. Before removing the superficial fascia, dissect some of the **cutaneous nerves** of the back to observe their segmental arrangement. They are derived from **dorsal rami of** cervical, thoracic, and lumbar **spinal nerves.** With the exception of the **greater occipital nerve,** they are small and are usually accompanied by an artery and a vein. They pierce the superficial fascia and muscles of the back just lateral to the median line in the cervical and upper thoracic areas and more laterally in the lower thoracic region.

SUPERFICIAL MUSCLES OF THE BACK

The most superficial muscles of the back are the **trapezius** and the **latissimus dorsi** (Fig. 1.2). Clean the trapezius by removing the superficial and deep fasciae that cover its entire external surface. As the uppermost part of the muscle is being cleaned, secure the **greater occipital nerve.** This large cutaneous nerve is the terminal part of the dorsal ramus of the second cervical nerve. It pierces the trapezius a little below and lateral to the external occipital protuberance and runs upward in the fascia to be distributed to the back of the scalp. It is accompanied in its distribution by the terminal branches of the **occipital artery** (Fig. 1.3). *When cleaning the upper lateral border of the muscle, be careful to preserve structures in the posterior region of the neck.* The **trapezius** is a flat triangular muscle that arises from the medial third of the **superior nuchal line,** the entire length of the **ligamentum nuchae,** and the **spinous processes of** all 12 **thoracic vertebrae.** Its fibers converge laterally to a V-shaped insertion on the posterior border of the lateral third of the **clavicle,** the medial border of the **acromion,** and the upper border of the **scapular spine.**

Clean the **latissimus dorsi.** In removing the superficial fascia from the region just lateral to the lumbar vertebral spines, carefully avoid cutting through or removing the deep fascia, here known as the **thoracolumbar fascia.** It is recognized by the glistening aponeurotic appearance of its external surface. It is attached medially to the lumbar and sacral spines and stretches laterally as a broad aponeurotic sheet. The thoracolumbar fascia differs from the deep fascia that is ordinarily found surrounding muscles in that it is very dense. In the lumbar region of the back, it is arranged in two **lamellae** between which the deep muscles of the back are enclosed. The glistening sheet is the more superficial of these layers (**posterior lamella**) and must be cleaned at the same time as the latissimus dorsi, since the muscle takes origin in part from it.

The latissimus dorsi is a broad, flat muscle that covers the lower lateral part of the back. The lowest part of the trapezius slightly overlaps it. It has a wide origin from the **spinous processes of** the lower five or six **thoracic vertebrae,** the **posterior lamella of** the **thoracolumbar fascia,** the **outer lip of** the posterior half of the **iliac crest,** and small pointed slips from the outer surfaces of the **lower** three or four **ribs,** where it is in close relation to the lower slips of origin of the external oblique muscle of the abdomen. It sometimes also attaches to the inferior angle of the scapula. The fibers converge upward and laterally to a flat tendon that winds around the lower border of the **teres major muscle** to be inserted into the **intertubercular sulcus of** the **humerus.** Its insertion cannot be investigated at present. The upper part of the lateral border of the latissimus dorsi forms the posterior fold of the axilla.

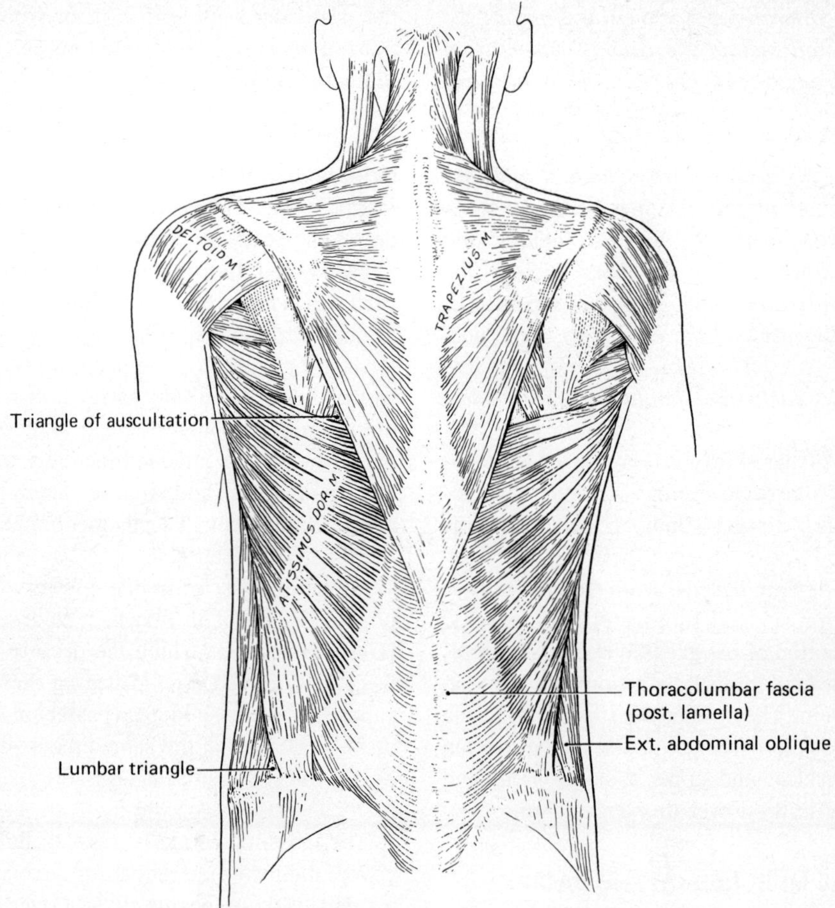

Figure 1.2 Superficial **muscles of** the **back.**

The relationship of the trapezius and latissimus dorsi muscles to other structures on the back creates two clinically important triangles. The upper, the **triangle of auscultation,** is that space bounded by the trapezius muscle, the latissimus dorsi, and the vertebral border of the scapula. This space, on each side of the back, may be enlarged over the sixth and seventh ribs and their interspace when the arms are folded over the chest and the trunk is bent forward. It is used for clearer diagnostic listening to the structures within the thoracic cavity. A lower triangular area on each side, the **lumbar triangle,** is formed by the lower lateral border of the latissimus dorsi, the posterior edge of the external oblique muscle, and the ilium. The internal oblique muscle forms the floor of this triangle, which is a point of potential weakness in the posterior abdominal wall.

The trapezius should now be reflected, but *before the trapezius (or any other muscle) is reflected, insert a finger beneath the muscle and, by palpation, ascertain its bony attachments, relationships to other structures, and nerve and blood supply*. This procedure is done to avoid cutting through adjacent structures, since the thickness of the muscle to be reflected cannot be fully appreciated until it is palpated. *It is also essential to*

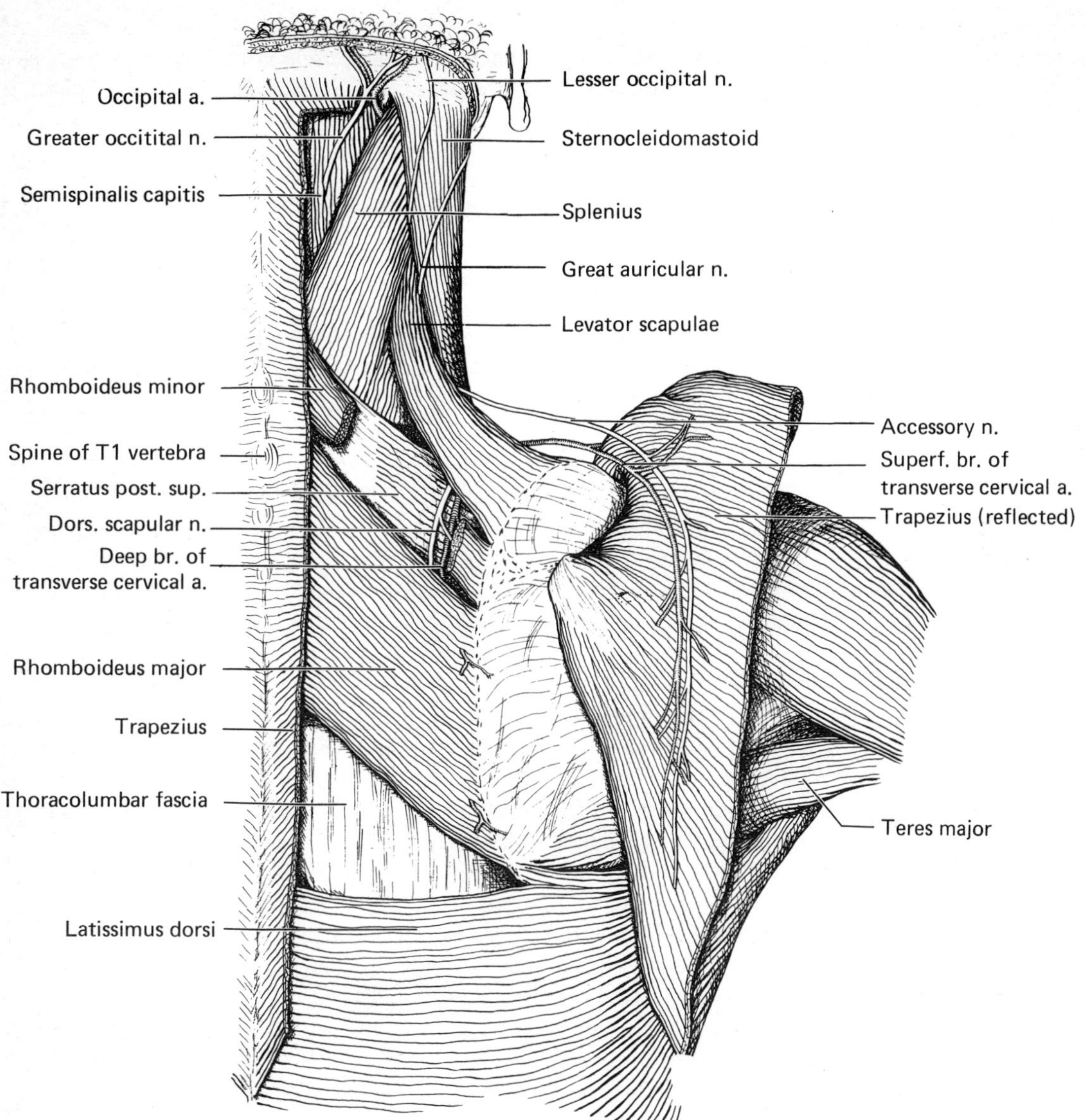

Figure 1.3 The upper part of the **back** after reflection of the trapezius. A segment of the rhomboideus minor has been removed.

always reflect muscles completely to their bony attachments. Now, detach the uppermost fibers of the trapezius from the occipital bone and make a longitudinal incision through the trapezius parallel and about 1 cm lateral to the median line of the body. Reflect the muscle laterally to its insertion. As it is turned laterally, the nerves and vessels that supply the trapezius will be found ramifying on its deep surface.

As a rule, nearly all muscles receive their nerve and blood supply on their deep surface.

The **trapezius** is supplied by the **spinal accessory nerve,** cranial nerve XI (CN XI), supplemented by twigs from the third and fourth **cervical nerves.** These reach the deep surface of the muscle by passing across the posterior triangle of the neck. They are accompanied by the **superficial (ascending) branch of** the **transverse cervical artery** (Fig. 1.3).

Clean the two **rhomboid muscles;** they are sometimes more or less fused. The **rhomboideus minor** is a narrow, flat muscle taking origin from the lower part of the **ligamentum nuchae** and the **spinous process of** the seventh **cervical vertebra.** Its fibers run downward and laterally to be inserted into the **vertebral border of** the **scapula** opposite the scapular spine. The **rhomboideus major** is a much wider, flat muscle immediately inferior to the minor. It takes origin from the upper four or five **thoracic spines** and is inserted into the **vertebral border of** the **scapula** below the scapular spine.

Clean the **levator scapulae.** This is a long, flat muscle that arises by four pointed slips from the posterior tubercles of the **transverse processes of** the upper four **cervical vertebrae.** It is inserted into the **vertebral border of** the **scapula** above the scapular spine. Its origin is covered by the upper part of the sternocleidomastoid and its insertion by the trapezius.

Detach the scapular insertion of the levator scapulae muscle and reflect it upward. Make a vertical incision through both rhomboid muscles about 1.5 cm lateral to their origins and reflect them. As the muscles are being reflected, clean the **dorsal scapular nerve** (nerve to the rhomboids) and **deep branch of** the **transverse cervical artery.** This nerve and artery leave the posterior triangle at the anterior border of the levator scapulae and descend slightly medial to the vertebral border of the scapula and deep to the levator scapulae and the two rhomboids. The **dorsal scapular nerve** is the nerve supply to both rhomboids and sometimes to the levator scapulae, which is supplied chiefly by the third and fourth cervical nerves.

Cut the latissimus dorsi about 2.5 cm from its origin on the thoracolumbar fascia and reflect it laterally. This muscle is much thicker toward its insertion than at its origin.

Clean the posterior serrate muscles. These are two thin, flat muscles that are often more tendinous than muscular. The **serratus posterior superior** is deep to the rhomboids, and its fibers run in the same direction. It arises from the lower part of the **ligamentum nuchae** and the **spines of** the seventh **cervical** and upper two or three **thoracic vertebrae**; it inserts by four slips into the external surfaces of the second through the fifth **ribs.** The **serratus posterior inferior** is covered externally by the latissimus dorsi. It arises from the posterior lamella of the **thoracolumbar fascia** in the region of the lower thoracic and upper lumbar vertebrae. Its fibers run upward and laterally to insert into the external surfaces of the lower four **ribs.** When the posterior serrate muscles have been studied, detach them from their origin and reflect them laterally. As this is done, attempt to identify the small branches of the **intercostal nerves** that emerge from the intercostal spaces to supply them.

As has been seen, the **trapezius** derives its main nerve supply from a **cranial nerve,** the **spinal accessory.** The other muscles of the back that have been studied so far derive their nerve supply from the **ventral rami of spinal nerves.** The **deep muscles** of the back, yet to be displayed, are all supplied by **dorsal rami of spinal nerves.** Remember that they are the only muscles in the body that are so supplied.

Note also that, owing to their attachments, the superficial muscles of the back (except the serrate muscles) are functionally related to movement of the superior extremity.

DEEP MUSCLES OF THE BACK

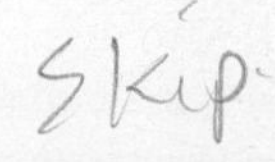

Clean the **splenius muscle.** This is a flat muscle that takes origin from the lower half of the **ligamentum nuchae** and the **spines of** the seventh **cervical** and the first to the sixth **thoracic vertebrae.** Running upward and laterally, the muscle separates into two parts. The large upper portion, the **splenius capitis,** has a linear insertion on the **mastoid process** and the lateral part of the **superior nuchal line.** The lower portion, the **splenius cervicis,** is inserted by two or three tendinous slips into the **posterior tubercles of** the **transverse processes of** the upper two or three **cervical vertebrae,** where it is in close relation to the slips of origin of the levator scapulae. The insertion of the splenius is for the most part covered by the sternocleidomastoid. Detach the splenius from its origin and reflect both parts to their insertions.

In the **vertebral groove** is a thick, elongated mass of muscle known collectively as the **erector spinae.** This muscle mass is thickest in the lower thoracic and lumbar regions, where it is enclosed between the two lamellae of the thoracolumbar fascia. The **posterior lamella** of the fascia has already been exposed. It is attached medially to the lumbar and sacral spines and stretches laterally across the external surface of the erector spinae to become continuous with the fascial sheaths of the internal oblique and transversus muscles of the anterior abdominal wall. Superiorly, it gradually thins out and in the upper thoracic region is hard to recognize as a distinct membranous layer.

Make a longitudinal incision through the posterior lamella, parallel and about 1.5 cm lateral to the median line, from the level of the first to the fourth lumbar spine. From each end of this incision, make a horizontal incision laterally for about 4 cm. The rectangular flap of fascia thus marked out should be turned laterally to expose the posterior surface of the lumbar part of the erector spinae muscles. If the muscle mass is pushed medially, the **anterior lamella of** the **thoracolumbar fascia** will be exposed (Fig. 1.4). Place your fingers anterior to the erector spinae, push medially across the exposed surface of the anterior lamella, and observe that this layer of the fascia is attached medially to the **transverse processes of** the **lumbar vertebrae,** which also lie anterior to the erector spinae. Observe also that the anterior and posterior lamellae of the fascia fuse with one another along the lateral border of the erector spinae. It is this lateral, fused portion of the thoracolumbar fascia that comes into relation with the muscles of the anterior abdominal wall. Finally, make a short longitudinal incision through the exposed portion of the anterior lamella. If the lips of this incision are spread open, the posterior surface of the **quadratus lumborum muscle** will be exposed. This is a muscle in the posterior wall of the abdominal cavity.

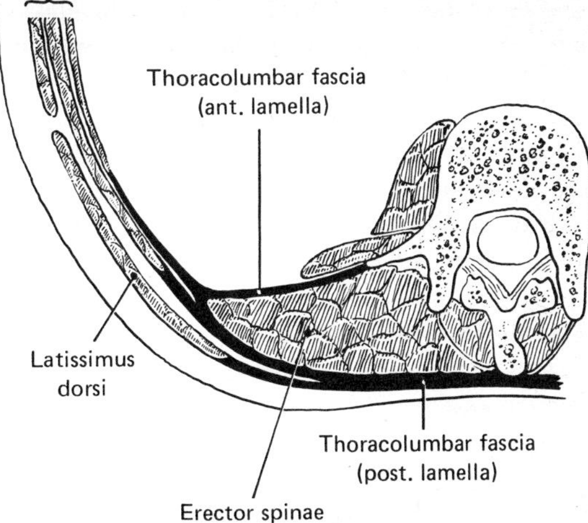

Figure 1.4 Cross section in the lower back region showing the **lamellae of** the **thoracolumbar fascia.**

Clean and study the erector spinae muscles. Inferiorly, the entire mass has a common, large, fleshy origin from the **spines of** all **lumbar vertebrae,** the dorsum of the **sacrum,** the posterior **sacroiliac ligament,** the most posterior part of the **iliac crest,** and the deep surface of the inferior part of the posterior lamella of the **thoracolumbar fascia.** As the fibers pass upward from their origin, the muscle separates into three parallel longitudinal columns. The most lateral column is known as the **iliocostalis,** the middle one as the **longissimus,** and the smallest and most medial as the **spinalis.** A detailed dissection of each slip and subdivision of the erector spinae is not essential, but sufficient cleaning and study should be done to demonstrate the following facts.

The division between the iliocostalis and the longissimus is indicated by the line along which the cutaneous branches of the dorsal rami emerge. The **iliocostalis** is subdivided from below upward into three parts: the **iliocostalis lumborum,** the **iliocostalis thoracis,** and the **iliocostalis cervicis.** The **iliocostalis lumborum** arises from the common origin and is inserted by a series of slips into the lower six or seven **ribs** at their angles. The **iliocostalis thoracis** receives additional slips from the lower six ribs just medial to their angles and is inserted into the angles of the upper six **ribs.** The **iliocostalis cervicis** receives muscle slips from the upper ribs and is inserted into the **transverse processes of** the lower three or four **cervical vertebrae.** The slips of insertion of the iliocostalis can be seen while the muscle is in position, but the slips of origin are covered by the main mass of the muscle. They may be exposed by rolling the entire muscle laterally. Note that the three parts of the iliocostalis are not actually separated structurally; the subdivision is an arbitrary matter of anatomical nomenclature.

For purposes of anatomical description, the **longissimus** is similarly subdivided into three parts—the **longissimus thoracis,** the **longissimus cervicis,** and the **longissimus capitis.** The **longissimus thoracis** arises at the common origin of the erector spinae and is inserted by means of two long series of muscular slips. The more lateral series is inserted into the **transverse processes of** the **lumbar vertebrae** and into the lower ten **ribs** lateral to their tubercles; the more medial series is inserted into the **accessory tubercles of** the **lumbar vertebrae** and the tips of the transverse processes of the thoracic vertebrae. The **longissimus cervicis** receives slips of origin from the transverse processes of the upper thoracic vertebrae and is inserted into the **posterior tubercles of** the transverse processes of the second to the sixth **cervical vertebrae.** The **longissimus capitis** arises from the transverse processes of the upper three or four thoracic vertebrae and the articular processes of the lower cervical vertebrae. As its fibers pass upward, they form a narrow bandlike muscle that is inserted into the posterior part of the **mastoid process** under cover of the splenius capitis and sternocleidomastoid muscles.

The **spinalis** is the smallest of the three parts of the erector spinae. Its fibers run upward from the upper **lumbar** and lower **thoracic spinous processes** to be inserted into the **spinous processes** of a variable number of the upper thoracic vertebrae. The **spinalis thoracis** is usually the only subdivision demonstrable. The **spinalis cervicis** is frequently absent or insignificant, and the **spinalis capitis** is fused with and considered part of the **semispinalis capitis muscle.**

Free and elevate the longissimus capitis laterally to identify the **occipital artery.** The origin of the occipital artery from the external carotid will be seen in a later dissection. Emerging from the deep surface of the mastoid process, the occipital artery ordinarily passes deep to the longissimus capitis just inferior to its insertion. Occasionally it crosses the longissimus superficially. It will now be seen running medially and upward in the interval between the splenius and semispinalis muscles. Near the medial border of the upper part of the splenius, it becomes superficial by piercing the trapezius or by winding around the lateral border of that muscle. It is distributed to the back of the scalp, in company with the **greater occipital nerve.**

Deep to the erector spinae are the **transversospinalis muscles.** The largest of this group is the **semispinalis capitis,** which has been exposed by the reflection of the trapezius and the splenius. This large muscle takes origin by a series of tendinous slips from the **articular processes of** the fourth, fifth, and sixth **cervical vertebrae** and the **transverse processes of** the first five or six **thoracic vertebrae.** It has a thick, fleshy insertion into the occipital bone between the **superior** and **inferior nuchal lines** just lateral to the external occipital crest. Observe that the semispinalis is pierced by the **greater occipital nerve** and that in the cervical region the semispinales of the two sides are separated only by the **ligamentum nuchae.**

The remainder of the transversospinales consists of several groups of small muscular slips that connect individual vertebrae. They are the **semispinalis cervicis, semispinalis thoracis, multifidi, rotatores, levatores costarum, interspinales,** and **intertransversarii.** In view of the large number of back problems that patients present, you should be familiar with the anatomy and function of these muscles. Do not dissect them in detail, but with the aid of a text, clean and identify a few when the vertebral canal is opened.

SUBOCCIPITAL TRIANGLE

Use the handle of a forceps and by blunt dissection retract the **semispinalis capitis** muscle laterally from the **ligamentum nuchae.** Identify the course of the **greater occipital nerve** and the dorsal ramus of the **third cervical nerve** medial to, or occasionally passing through, the substance of this muscle. Transect this muscle at the level of the spine of the third cervical vertebra. Reflect the cut ends upward and downward to expose the **rectus capitis major** and **minor** and the **obliquus capitis superior** and **inferior muscles.** Follow the greater occipital nerve proximally toward its origin, and you will find that it winds directly around the inferior border of the inferior oblique muscle. This will aid in identifying the small **suboccipital triangle,** which is made up of the inferior and superior oblique and the rectus major muscles (Fig. 1.5). These muscles, in addition to the rectus minor, extend from the axis to the atlas, and from the atlas and axis to the base of the occipital bone. As you clean the fascia and veins (suboccipital venous plexus) from the triangle, look for the branches of the dorsal ramus of the first cervical nerve, which supplies these four small muscles. Insert probe or sharp end of a forceps through the fascia and ligaments in the floor of the upper part of this triangle. A potential space will be felt between the base of the **occipital bone** and the **arch of** the **atlas.** Clean away the fascia and ligaments and identify the course of the **vertebral artery** over the arch of the atlas. Review the attachments and the relationships of the ligaments of the atlas, axis, and occipital bone from a descriptive text.

VERTEBRAL CANAL AND SPINAL CORD

Preparatory to opening the vertebral canal (a **laminectomy**), clean the **laminae** and **spinous processes** of the vertebrae as completely as possible. This is done by retracting the larger, longer muscles laterally and by removing the smaller ones that fill the vertebral groove on each side. Retain a few dorsal rami of the thoracic nerves, so that they may later be traced to the main trunk of the nerves from which they arise. Now open the **vertebral canal** by removing the entire series of laminae and spinous processes from the level of the

Figure 1.5 The **suboccipital region.**

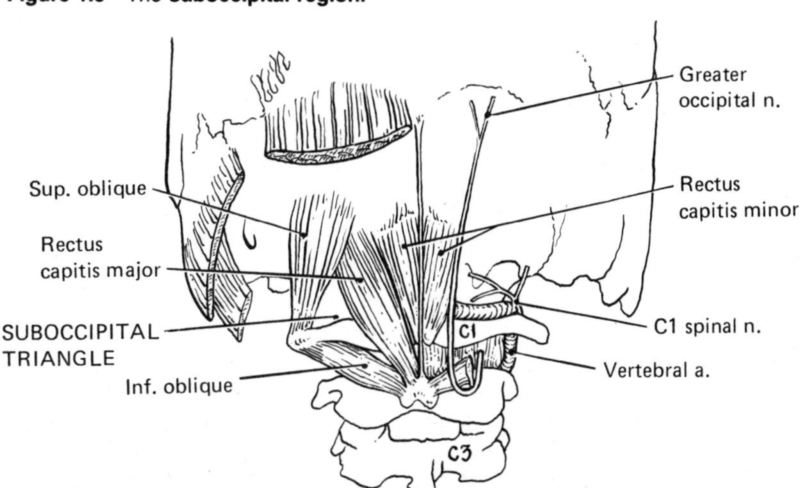

second cervical vertebra down to the middle of the sacrum. Successive laminae and spines are held together by the **ligamenta flava** and the **interspinous ligaments** and may be removed in one piece. Cut through the **laminae** as far laterally as possible on each side. In dealing with the sacrum, remember that the posterior wall of the sacral canal is very thin and that it is important to remove only this wall, and *not* to cut through the body of the sacrum.

When the vertebral canal is opened, a narrow space filled with fat will be exposed lying between the periosteum of the vertebrae and the dura mater of the spinal cord. This is the **epidural space.** In the fat are the **spinal arteries** and the **internal vertebral venous plexus.** The spinal arteries are a paired series of vessels that enter the canal through the **intervertebral foramina.** At certain vertebral levels, the arteries supplying the cord and the meninges are larger than at other levels. The venous plexus is drained by spinal veins that leave the canal through the intervertebral foramina.

Since these veins do not contain valves, blood can flow through them in either direction, depending on the intrathoracic and abdominal pressures. Clinically, therefore, they are very important when the metastasis of tumor cells or viruses is considered.

Clean the external surface of the **spinal dura mater** by removing the epidural fat and venous plexus. The dura mater is the most external and the strongest of the three coverings (**meninges**) of the spinal cord. At the foramen magnum, it is firmly bound to the occipital bone and becomes continuous with the inner layer of the **cranial dura mater.** In the vertebral canal, now exposed, it lies loosely and takes the form of a fibrous tube. At about the level of the second sacral vertebral segment, it contracts to a filament, the **filum of the dura mater (coccygeal ligament),** which extends downward through the sacral canal and hiatus to attach to the dorsum of the coccyx. Observe the series of lateral prolongations of the dura, which pass into the intervertebral foramina; within these are enclosed the **roots of** the **spinal nerves.**

Open the dura by a longitudinal incision along its entire length; reflect the cut edges laterally and pin them to the sides of the vertebral canal to expose the **spinal arachnoid,** the second of the spinal coverings. It is a thin, delicate, gauzy membrane. At the foramen magnum it is continuous with the cranial arachnoid; inferiorly, it extends as far as the dura and ends by blending with the filum of the dura. The arachnoid also has a series of lateral prolongations, which surround the roots of the spinal nerves and blend with the dura in the intervertebral foramina. Between the dura and the arachnoid is the **subdural space,** an interval of capillary thickness. In life, it contains a lymphlike fluid.

Slit the arachnoid longitudinally to expose the **spinal pia mater,** the **spinal cord,** and the **roots of** the **spinal nerves.** The pia is the innermost of the three meninges. It is a delicate membrane that so closely invests the outer surface of the spinal cord and the roots of the nerves that it is best regarded as an integral part of the spinal cord. The **subarachnoid space** lies between the pia and the arachnoid. It is much larger than the subdural space, particularly in the lower lumbar region. The space contains cerebrospinal fluid (CSF), which bathes and cushions the cord. Numerous **arachnoid trabeculae** traverse the subarachnoid space to attach to the pia.

Study the external form of the spinal cord. It is directly continuous with the medulla oblongata of the brain, beginning at the **foramen magnum** and ending at about the level of the lower border of the **first lumbar vertebra.** The tapering inferior end of the spinal cord, from which the sacral nerve roots arise, is known as the **conus medullaris.** From the tip of the conus a threadlike structure, the **filum terminale,** continues downward through the subarachnoid space; below the termination of the dura, the filum terminale is enclosed within the filum of the dura. Observe that the diameter of the spinal cord is greater in the lower cervical region, the **cervical enlargement,** and in the lower thoracic region, the **lumbar enlargement.** This is because of the large size of the lower cervical and the lumbar spinal nerves, which arise from these two regions to supply the extremities.

Arising from the spinal cord, each by two roots, are eight pairs of cervical nerves, twelve pairs of thoracic nerves, five pairs of lumbar nerves, five pairs of sacral nerves, and one pair of coccygeal nerves. Transect the spinal cord and its meningeal coverings at the level of the second and sixth thoracic vertebrae. Cut the spinal nerves on each side, about 2.5 cm lateral to this segment, and remove the segment of spinal cord, its meningeal coverings, and the attached nerve roots from the spinal canal. Open the meningeal coverings by a longitudinal incision along the length of the ventral surface of this segment. The **dorsal roots** are made up of **afferent** (sensory) **nerve fibers** and arise from the posterolateral sulcus on the posterior aspect of the cord. The **ventral roots** are made up of **efferent** (motor) **nerve fibers** and arise from the anterolateral sulcus on the anterior aspect of the cord. Each root arises not as a single structure but as a linear series of **rootlets,** which unite to form a single root. The dorsal and ventral roots of each nerve remain distinct within the vertebral canal and unite to form a **spinal nerve** only upon reaching the intervertebral foramina.

The length of the spinal nerve roots increases steadily from above downward, since the length of the cord is so much less than that of the vertebral canal. Observe that the cervical roots pass almost directly laterally to reach the intervertebral foramina, while in the thoracic region the roots take a course of constantly increasing obliquity, downward and laterally. The lumbar and sacral roots, which arise in close succession from the lower part of the cord, pass almost vertically downward through the subarachnoid space in a brushlike aggregation of filaments known as the **cauda equina.**

Owing to the large space between the fourth and fifth lumbar vertebrae, the horizontally positioned lumbar spines, the absence of the spinal cord in the lower lumbar area, and the freely floating cauda equina, clinicians can easily and safely pass a needle into the subarachnoid space (lumbar puncture) to withdraw CSF for laboratory evaluation or to administer anesthetics (spinal anesthesia) and diagnostic media. The iliac crests lie at the level of the fourth lumbar vertebral spine and thus guide the clinician in this procedure.

Laterally, between the dorsal and ventral roots, the pia is thickened along the length of the cord to form the **denticulate ligament.** The ligament has a serrate or toothlike appearance created by 20 to 22 processes that traverse the subarachnoid space and arachnoid to fuse with the dura.

The denticulate ligaments serve to anchor the spinal cord, and they aid the neurosurgeon in distinguishing the dorsal from the ventral roots.

In the upper part of the spinal cord, above the level of the fifth cervical nerve roots, note the rootlets forming the **spinal part of** the **accessory nerve** (CN XI). These fibers arise from the lateral part of the spinal cord and form a single trunk that ascends between the denticulate ligament and the dorsal roots of the spinal nerves to enter the skull through the foramen magnum.

With the bone forceps, chip away the articular processes forming the posterior boundary of one or two of the intervertebral foramina in the lower thoracic region to expose the **dorsal root** (spinal) **ganglion** and the trunk of the spinal nerve. The ganglion, one on each dorsal root, is a slight swelling just proximal to the point of union with the ventral root. The nerve trunk and the ganglion are enclosed in a prolongation of the dura mater and arachnoid, which must be carefully cleared away. Observe that the **trunk of** the **spinal nerve** is very short, as each divides almost at once into a **ventral** and a **dorsal ramus.** The dorsal ramus passes directly backward through the deep muscles of the back. The ventral ramus passes laterally to be distributed to the body wall and extremities; it is usually larger than the dorsal ramus. The ventral rami of the thoracic nerves are the **intercostal nerves;** those of the cervical, lumbar, and sacral nerves take part in the formation of the **cervical, brachial, lumbar,** and **sacral plexuses.**

Chapter 2

Pectoral Region

Before dissecting the **pectoral region,** identify the bony points that may be felt through the skin. In the midline at the base of the neck is the **jugular (suprasternal) notch,** which marks the superior border of the manubrium. At each side of the jugular notch the prominent medial end of the **clavicle** may be felt; it takes part in the sternoclavicular articulation, which is the only bony articulation between the superior extremity and the axial skeleton. The clavicle is palpable along its entire length. At its lateral end, it articulates with the **acromion process of** the **scapula,** which also is subcutaneous and which forms the bony prominence of the shoulder. The **sternum** may be felt through the skin in the midline along the entire length of the **manubrium** and **body of** the **sternum.** At the lower end of the body is a depression in the anterior body wall corresponding to the **xiphoid process** of the sternum. About 4 cm below the jugular notch is a prominent transverse bony ridge. This is the **sternal angle,** the junction of the manubrium and body. It is on the same horizontal plane as the lower border of the fourth thoracic vertebra.

The sternal angle is an important landmark in that it indicates the level at which the second rib joins the sternum and may be used as a starting point for counting the ribs on the surface of the body.

The position of the **nipple** in men and young, undeveloped women is generally over the fourth intercostal space about 10 cm lateral to the sternum. It is a rounded pigmented elevation of the **areola,** which is the thickened, pigmented skin over the center of the **breast** (**mammary gland**).

Usually paired, there may be more (supernumerary) than two nipples (polythelia), or more than two breasts (polymastia) located anywhere along the "milk line," which extends from the axilla to the groin region. Absence of the breasts is called "amastia."

Abduct the arms and observe the **axillary folds.** These are folds of skin, fascia, and muscle that bound the **axilla** or armpit. The **anterior axillary fold** is formed by the pectoralis major and minor muscles. The **posterior axillary fold,** which extends farther inferiorly, is formed principally by the latissimus dorsi. Between the two folds, the skin, covered with hair, is indented to form the arched floor of the axilla.

For the dissection of the pectoral region and axilla, the arms should be abducted and tied in this position to a long board placed under the shoulders and extending outward on each side. Abduct the arms only until they resist further movement; full abduction will tear the muscles. During later dissections, gradually abduct the arms until the axilla is fully exposed. *With the body so placed, the following skin incisions should be made as shown in Fig. 2.1: (1) in the midline from the jugular notch to the middle of the xiphoid process; (2) from the upper end of the first incision, one laterally on each side along the full length of the clavicle to the tip of the acromion; (3) from the lower end of the first incision, one laterally and somewhat inferiorly across the thoracic wall to the posterior axillary fold; and (4) from the lower end of the first incision, one upward and laterally to the nipple, which is encircled, then upward and laterally along the line of the anterior axillary fold and down the front of the arm for about 15 cm. Transverse incisions should then be made across the front of the arm for about 5 cm. The large flaps of skin thus marked out should be reflected laterally. Some difficulty may be met in reflecting the skin of the axilla, since this skin, which is quite thin, is firmly attached to strands of axillary fascia.*

The **superficial fascia** of the pectoral and axillary regions has no specific characteristics, except that in its uppermost part are the fibers of origin of the **platysma,** a superficial muscle of the neck. In the female, however, it contains the **breast (mammary gland),** which should now be

Figure 2.1 Surface landmarks and skin incisions on the thorax.

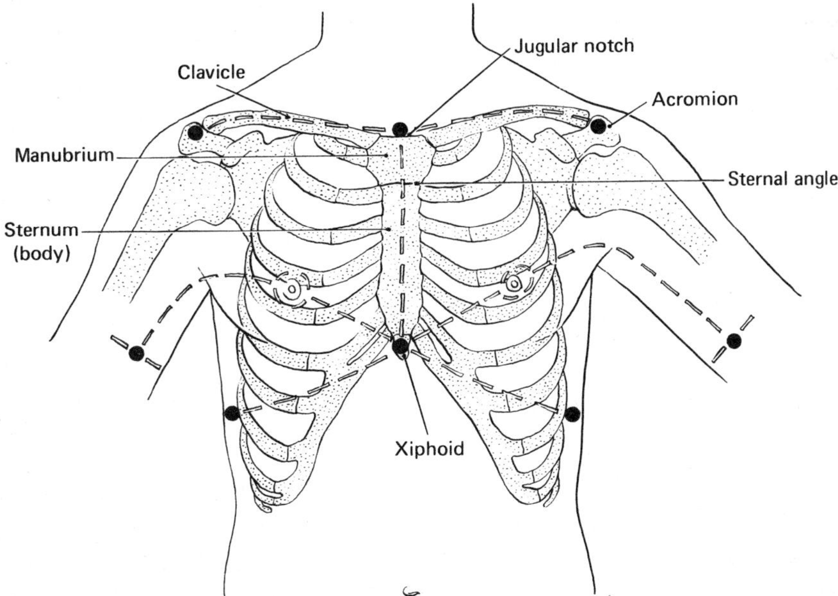

studied. Dissect the cutaneous vessels and nerves, paying attention to those related to the breast.

The **breast** does not have a distinct connective tissue capsule. It is embedded in the general subcutaneous fatty tissue overlying the pectoralis major and serratus anterior muscles and is separated from the deep muscular fascia by the **retromammary space.** The body of the gland is partitioned radially around the nipple into 15 to 20 lobes by dense, fibrous connective tissue septa. Each lobe contains fat, glandular elements and a single **lactiferous duct** that opens separately into a depression on the nipple. In older women, the glandular tissue is atrophied and replaced by fat. Sagittally section the breast through the nipple and locate, by gently picking out the fat, a lactiferous duct. Look also for the **lactiferous sinus,** a dilation of the duct just proximal to its opening on the nipple. Note that some of the dense connective tissue is arranged in strands that extend to the skin; these are the **suspensory ligaments.**

A tumorous growth within the substance of the breast will often invade, push against, and shorten the suspensory ligaments, causing the skin to dimple where the ligaments attach to the dermis. Dimpling is a first alert to breast cancer, the most common type of cancer in women.

Breast tumor metastases to the central nervous system, lungs, and other parts of the body occur via its lymphatic and venous drainage systems. It is important that you learn both from a descriptive text.

The **pectoralis major muscle** should now be cleaned. On one side, remove the superficial fascia (including the breast and nipple) and the deep fascia covering the muscle. Cut through the fascia (until the muscle fibers are exposed) in a transverse line running from the lower border of the medial end of the clavicle outward to the anterior aspect of the arm and in a vertical line along the lateral aspect of the sternum. This will mark out a triangular flap of fascia that can be reflected laterally and downward to expose the sternocostal portion of the muscle. Move the blade of the scalpel in the direction in which the muscle fibers run. When the lower border of the muscle is reached, the flap of fascia removed from its surface may be cut away and discarded. Next remove the fascia from the upper or clavicular portion of the muscle in the same manner by reflecting it upward and laterally.

On the other side, leave the breast as a landmark, and for observation of its blood supply from vessels supplying the pectoral muscles. The pectoralis major muscle on this side can be cleaned by reflecting the fascia from the peripheral borders of the breast.

The **pectoralis major** is a large triangular muscle consisting of a small **clavicular portion** and a larger **sternocostal portion.** The clavicular portion arises from the anterior surface of the medial half of the **clavicle.** The superficial fibers of the sternocostal portion arise from the lateral part of the entire length of the anterior surface of the **manubrium** and **body of** the **sternum.** Its deeper fibers arise from the anterior surfaces of the second to the sixth **costal cartilages,** which cannot be seen until the muscle is reflected. Laterally, the fibers converge to insert into the **crest of** the **greater tubercle of** the **humerus,** which is now under cover of the deltoid muscle.

Attempt to find some of the small **anterior cutaneous nerves** and **vessels** that pierce the pectoralis major in longitudinal series slightly lateral to the sternum. These are the terminal portions of the upper intercostal nerves and vessels; they supply the skin over the anterior part of the chest.

Clean the terminal part of the **cephalic vein.** It is a large superficial vein of the superior extremity, sometimes reduced in size or lacking, which is found in the groove between the upper border of the pectoralis major and the **deltoid** muscles. It disappears from view in the **deltopectoral triangle,** a small triangular depression bounded by the anterior border of the deltoid, the upper border of the pectoralis major, and the lower border of the middle portion of the clavicle. Remove the fat from it and look for the small **deltopectoral lymph nodes** that are often present. Emerging through the fat is also the **deltoid branch of** the **thoracoacromial artery,** which accompanies the

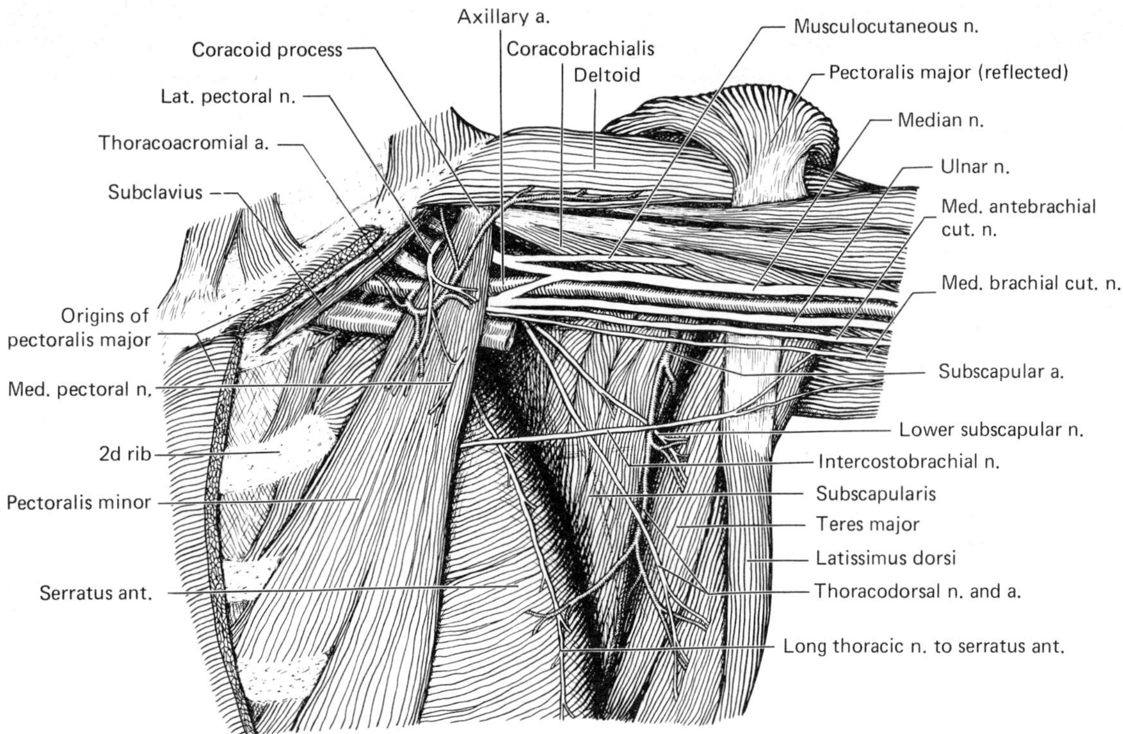

Figure 2.2 The **axilla,** opened anteriorly by reflection of the pectoralis major.

cephalic vein laterally and supplies the anterior border of the deltoid.

The **anterior wall** of the axilla is formed by the pectoralis major and minor muscles. On one side detach the clavicular portion of the pectoralis major near its origin, and cut through the sternocostal portion by an incision running parallel and about 2.5 cm lateral to the sternum (Fig. 2.2). The detached segment of muscle can then be turned laterally toward its insertion. As this is done, the subjacent pectoralis minor muscle is exposed, and the nerves and vessels that supply the pectoralis major are seen entering its deep surface. Clean the nerves and arteries. The nerves are branches of the **medial** and **lateral pectoral nerves.** The lateral pectoral nerve is derived from the lateral cord of the brachial plexus, and it reaches the deep surface of the pectoralis major by winding around the medial border of the pectoralis minor. The medial pectoral nerve, from the medial cord of the brachial plexus, usually pierces the pectoralis minor but may appear at its lateral border. The arteries entering the deep surface of the pectoralis major are the **pectoral branches of** the **thoracoacromial artery;** they also appear at the medial border of the pectoralis minor. The pectoralis major cannot usually be reflected properly without dissecting these vessels and nerves from its undersurface. Cut them, but retain a cube of muscle attached to the vessels and nerves for easier identification later.

Observe the **clavipectoral fascia.** This fascia occupies the triangular gap between the medial border of the pectoralis minor muscle, the lower border of the clavicle, and the anterior thoracic wall. It is pierced by the cephalic vein, the lateral pectoral nerve, and the deltoid and pectoral branches of the thoracoacromial artery. Superiorly, it splits to enclose the **subclavius muscle.** Cut through the clavipectoral fascia just below the clavicle to expose this muscle. The small **subclavius** arises from the **first rib** and its **cartilage** near their junction and runs upward and laterally to be inserted into a groove on the undersurface of the middle third of the **clavicle.** Splitting again to enclose the pectoralis minor muscle, the clavipectoral fascia passes laterally from the inferior lateral border of the muscle as the **suspensory ligament of** the **axilla** to fuse to the axillary fascia.

Study the **pectoralis minor muscle** (Fig. 2.2). It arises from the anterior surfaces of the second to the fifth **ribs** near their cartilages; the fibers run upward and converge to a tendinous insertion on the **coracoid process of** the **scapula.**

The axilla may now be completely opened from the front by removal of the clavipectoral fascia and reflection of the pectoralis minor. Detach the pectoralis minor near its origin and turn it upward to its insertion. As this is done, the **medial pectoral nerve,** whose terminal portion has been seen entering the pectoralis major, is seen entering the deep surface of the pectoralis minor, which it also supplies. This nerve should be preserved for future reference.

Chapter 3

Axilla

The **axilla** is a potential space, roughly pyramidal, lying between the upper part of the arm and the upper lateral thoracic wall (Fig. 3.1). Its **anterior wall** was studied in Chapter 2. The **medial wall** of the axilla is formed by the upper ribs and intercostal muscles, covered externally by the **serratus anterior muscle.** Its narrow **lateral wall** is formed by the medial surface of the upper part of the humerus, covered by the **coracobrachialis muscle.** Its **posterior wall,** which extends farther inferiorly than does the anterior wall, is formed from above downward and laterally by the **subscapularis, teres major,** and **latissimus dorsi muscles.** The **apex of** the **axilla** is a triangular opening, the **cervicoaxillary canal,** bounded by the first rib, the upper border of the scapula, and the posterior border of the clavicle. Through it, major nerves and vessels pass from the neck into the axilla and then into the superior extremity.

Abnormal narrowing of the canal can severely affect the vascular and nerve supply to the superior extremity, resulting in one of the many neurovascular compression syndromes.

The **base** or **floor of** the **axilla** is formed by the **axillary fascia** and skin.

Dissection of the axilla consists of removing the axillary fascia and fat without injuring the structures embedded in them. As the fat is removed, numerous lymph nodes will be found. Their form and position should be noted, but they need not be retained. The axillary lymph nodes are numerous and are subdivided into groups. They receive the efferent lymph vessels from the superior extremity, the breast, and the area of the trunk above the umbilicus.

Swollen nodes (lymphadenitis) are frequently palpable in the axilla, which becomes tender and painful.

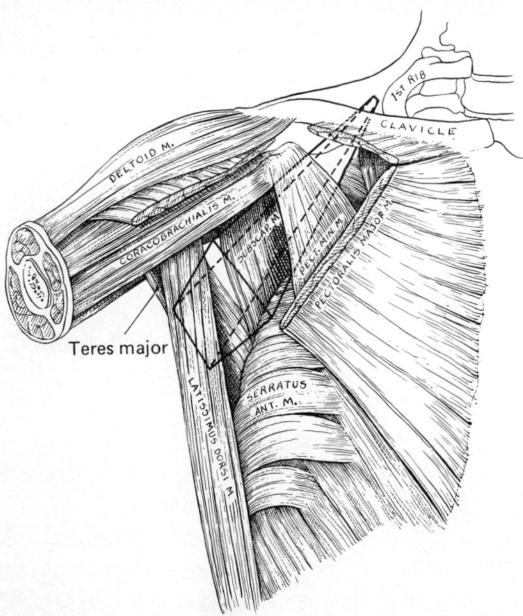

Figure 3.1 The **axilla,** shaped like a **pyramid,** has four walls, a base, and an apex.

Since the nodes are often involved in the metastases of breast cancers, they are routinely removed as part of a mastectomy.

Those parts of the latissimus dorsi, teres major, and subscapularis muscles, forming the posterior wall of the axilla, should be cleaned at this time to aid in identifying their nerve and blood supply. Retract the ventral part of the latissimus dorsi muscle from the chest wall. The **lateral cutaneous branches** of the intercostal nerves in this area should also be cleaned and studied.

Expose the nerves and vessels entering the arm from the lateral part of the axilla (Fig. 3.2). Start by removing the deep fascia from the upper part of the arm, where it forms the lateral wall of the axilla. This will expose the **coracobrachialis muscle** and the **short head of** the **biceps brachii muscle,** which arise together from the **coracoid process of** the **scapula.** Descending along the medial border of the coracobrachialis is the large **median nerve.** Medial to it, the distal part of the **axillary artery** should be exposed and cleaned. Medial to the artery is the **ulnar nerve;** it may be overlapped by the **axillary vein,** whose general position is medial and somewhat anterior to the artery. Also medial to the axillary artery and closely related to the axillary vein are the **medial antebrachial cutaneous** and **medial brachial cutaneous nerves.** The latter usually communicates with the **intercostobrachial nerve,** the lateral cutaneous branch of the second intercostal nerve. Emerging from the second intercostal space, it crosses the floor of the axilla to reach the medial aspect of the arm. Now push the coracobrachialis laterally and expose the **musculocutaneous nerve.** This nerve lies lateral to the median nerve in the upper part of the arm and disappears from view where it enters the substance of the coracobrachialis. Trace the median nerve proximally, and observe that it is formed at about the level of the outer margin of the pectoralis minor by the junction of two smaller nerves, the **lateral** and **medial heads of** the **median nerve.** The medial head crosses in front of the axillary artery. If the distal part of the axillary artery is now drawn forward and medially, a large nerve lying immediately behind it in the lateral part of the axilla will be exposed. This is the **radial nerve.**

The various nerves that have been exposed are the **terminal branches of** the **brachial plexus.** Their distribution cannot be studied until the arm is dissected, but they can be traced to their origins in the medial part of the axilla. Before doing this, however, you should have a general idea of the plan of the brachial plexus and its relation to the axillary artery.

The **brachial plexus** is derived from the ventral rami of the fifth, sixth, seventh, and eighth cervical and the first thoracic nerves (Fig. 3.3). These nerves, which are known as the **roots of** the **plexus,** are situated in the posterior triangle of the neck. Here they combine to form the **trunks** of the plexus as follows: the **fifth** and **sixth cervical roots** form the **upper trunk,** the **seventh cervical** alone forms the **middle trunk,** and the **eighth cervical** and **first thoracic** form the **lower trunk.**

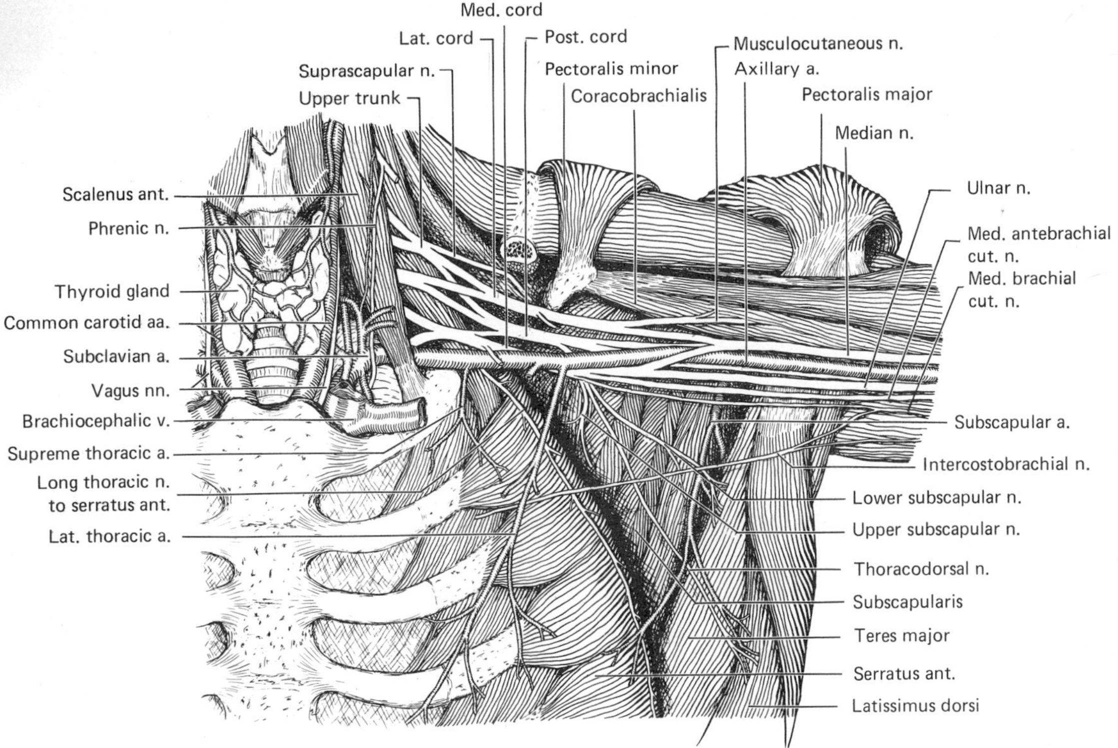

Figure 3.2 Complete dissection of the **brachial plexus.** The clavicle has been removed and both pectoral muscles reflected.

The three trunks enter the upper medial part of the axilla through the cervicoaxillary canal, and each breaks into an **anterior** and a **posterior division,** which are recombined to form the **cords** of the plexus. The **lateral cord** is formed by the anterior divisions of the upper and middle trunks, the **medial cord** is a direct continuation of the anterior division of the lower trunk, and the **posterior cord** is formed by the junction of all three posterior divisions. The three cords are arranged about the second part of the axillary artery in positions corresponding to their names. The nerves already exposed in the lateral part of the axilla are the **terminal branches** derived from the three cords.

The **axillary vein,** usually described as a single channel, often consists of two or more parallel anastomosing vessels. Its tributaries correspond to and accompany the branches of the axillary artery. Having observed the important fact that throughout its course the axillary vein lies medial and somewhat anterior to the artery, remove the veins to facilitate cleaning and studying the arteries and nerves.

Clean the **axillary artery** and its branches. The axillary artery is an anatomical subdivision of the great arterial channel that supplies the superior extremity. It begins at the lateral border of the **first rib** as a direct continuation of the **subclavian artery** and ends at the lateral border of the **teres major muscle** (which corresponds roughly to the lateral part of the posterior axillary fold), beyond which its continuation is known as the **brachial artery.** The axillary artery is further divided for descriptive purposes into **three parts.** The **first** is **medial** to the pectoralis minor muscle and, consequently, posterior to the clavipectoral

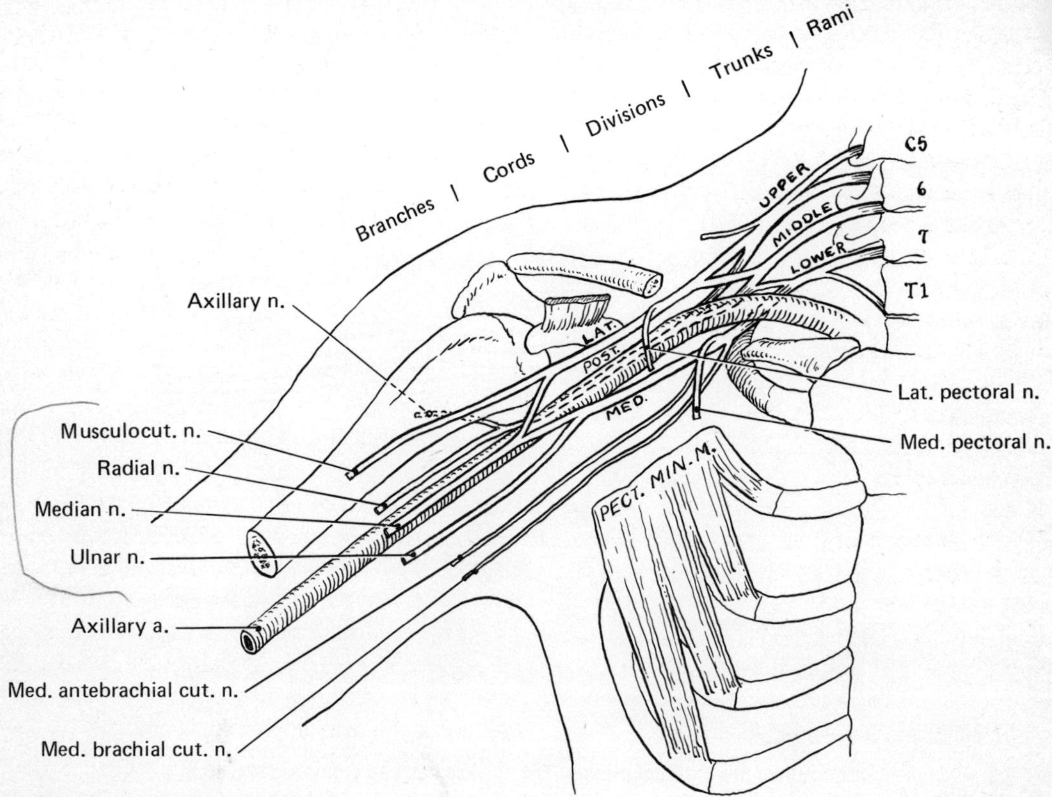

Figure 3.3 The **brachial plexus**—its axillary relationships.

fascia. The **second** lies **posterior** to the pectoralis minor, and the **third** and longest part is **lateral** to the pectoralis minor. Observe that where the distal half of the third part extends beyond the lower border of the pectoralis major, it is covered only by the fascia and skin.

The branches of the axillary artery vary, but most are as follows. From the **first part** arises one small branch, the **supreme thoracic artery,** distributed to the upper part of the thoracic wall. From the **second part,** near its beginning, arises the **thoracoacromial artery.** This short, thick trunk pierces the clavipectoral fascia and divides into a group of radiating branches, which are described from the regions they supply as **deltoid, pectoral, acromial,** and **clavicular.** The **lateral thoracic artery** arises from the middle of the **second part** of the axillary artery and runs downward under cover of the pectoralis minor to be distributed to the lateral thoracic wall, the pectoral muscles, and the breast.

The **third part** of the axillary artery has three branches: the subscapular and the anterior and posterior humeral circumflex arteries. The **subscapular artery** runs downward from the axillary artery, close to the posterior wall of the axilla. About 2.5 cm below its origin it ends by dividing into the **thoracodorsal** and **scapular circumflex arteries.** The scapular circumflex leaves the axilla by passing backward into the groove between the subscapularis and the teres major. The thoracodorsal continues its descent on the posterior wall of the axilla and is distributed chiefly to the latissimus dorsi, serratus anterior, and teres major muscles. Secure the **thoracodorsal nerve,** which accompanies the thoracodorsal artery downward and laterally on the posterior axillary wall to be distributed to the latissimus dorsi muscle. The **anterior humeral circumflex artery** is a small branch that arises separately or from a common trunk with the **posterior humeral circumflex artery** from the anterolateral aspect of the axillary, and runs laterally across the front of the arm to disappear behind the coracobrachialis muscle. The **posterior humeral circumflex artery** is considerably larger. It arises from the posterior aspect of the axillary artery and runs backward and downward to disappear almost at once into a groove in the posterior wall of the axilla, between the adjacent borders of the subscapularis and teres major muscles. The large **axillary nerve** accompanies the artery into the groove.

Now complete the study of those parts of the brachial plexus that lie in the axilla. Begin with the **lateral cord.** It lies lateral to the second part of the axillary artery and may be identified by tracing proximally the **musculocutaneous nerve** and the **lateral head of** the **median nerve,** which are its terminal branches. Its only other branch is the **lateral pectoral nerve,** which was previously identified and should now be traced to its origin. Trace the lateral cord proximally; identify the anterior divisions of the upper and middle trunks, which join to form it.

The **medial cord** lies medial to the second part of the axillary artery. Its terminal branches are the **ulnar nerve** and the **medial head of** the **median nerve,** which crosses in front of the third part of the axillary artery. Proximal to its termination, the medial cord gives rise to the **medial antebrachial cutaneous nerve,** the **medial brachial cutaneous nerve,** and the **medial pectoral nerve,** all of which have been identified. Traced proximally, the medial cord is a direct continuation of the anterior division of the lower trunk.

The **posterior cord** lies posterior to the second part of the axillary artery. Its two large terminal branches, the **axillary** and **radial nerves,** have been identified and may now be traced to their origins. Its other branches are three smaller nerves, the **upper** and **lower subscapular nerves** and the **thoracodorsal nerve.** The latter has already been seen as the nerve of supply to the latissimus dorsi. Find the subscapular nerves by dissecting in the fat close to the posterior wall of the axilla. The **upper subscapular,** often represented by two branches, supplies the subscapularis muscle; the **lower subscapular** supplies the subscapularis and teres major muscles. The two subscapular nerves and the thoracodorsal nerve often arise from the posterior cord by a common trunk and sometimes appear to arise from the axillary nerve rather than directly from the posterior cord. Trace the posterior cord proximally and observe that it is formed by the union of the posterior divisions of all three trunks.

As the final step in the dissection of the axilla, clear away the fascia from its medial wall to expose the **serratus anterior muscle** and its nerve supply. The serratus anterior is a large, flat muscle that arises by a series of pointed slips from the outer surfaces of the first eight **ribs** about 2.5 cm lateral to the costochondral junctions. Its fibers run posteriorly around the thoracic wall to be inserted into the inner aspect of the **vertebral border of** the **scapula** along its entire length. Its nerve supply, the **long thoracic nerve,** runs downward over the external surface of the muscle in about the midaxillary line. It is derived from the fifth, sixth, and seventh cervical nerves.

When the long thoracic nerve is severed or crushed, the vertebral border of the scapula protrudes dorsally, resembling a tiny wing, as the respective arm pushes forward against resistance. This functional loss of the serratus anterior muscle results in what is called "winging of the scapula."

Chapter 4

Triangles of the Neck

The anterior and posterior triangles of the neck are anatomical regions, the delineation of which is dependent principally upon the position of the **sternocleidomastoid muscle.** The **anterior triangle,** its apex directed inferiorly, lies anterior to the sternocleidomastoid, the anterior border of which forms the posterolateral boundary of the triangle. Its superior boundary is formed by the lower border of the mandible, and its medial boundary is formed by the median line of the neck from the **mental symphysis** to the **jugular notch** of the sternum. The anterior triangles of the two sides are separated from each other by the median line only. The **posterior triangle,** its apex directed superiorly, lies posterior to the sternocleidomastoid, the posterior border of which forms the anterior boundary of the triangle. Its inferior boundary is formed by the middle third of the clavicle, and its posterior boundary is formed by the anterior border of the trapezius muscle.

Reflect the skin in a single flap from the surface of both triangles and the sternocleidomastoid muscle as shown in Fig. 4.1. To do this make three skin incisions: (1) a median incision from the mental protuberance downward to the jugular notch; (2) from the upper end of the first incision, one posteriorly and laterally along the inferior border of the mandible to its angle, and then continued posteriorly and superiorly below the ear, across the mastoid process, and for about 2.5 cm along the superior nuchal line; (3) from the lower end of the first incision, one laterally along the clavicle to the acromion. Reflect the skin posteriorly from the anterior median line. Be careful to reflect cleanly the skin alone from the underlying fascia, which is generally quite thin in the neck. The su-

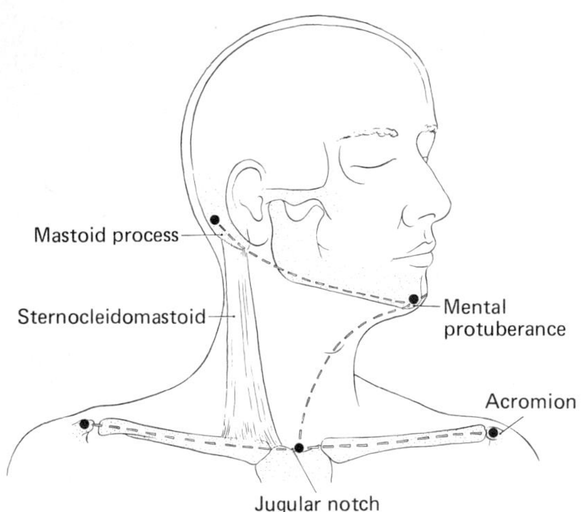

Figure 4.1 Surface landmarks and skin incisions on the neck.

perficial fascia of the neck is not different from the same layer in other regions, except that anteriorly it contains the **platysma muscle,** *which you want to preserve. As you approach the posterior triangle, be careful not to damage the anterior border of the* **trapezius muscle.** *Note and save the cutaneous nerves that enter the dissection field; they will be identified below.*

Clean the **platysma** by removing the superficial fascia that covers it. This thin, sheetlike muscle belongs to the facial expression group of muscles, and is often poorly developed. Do not mistake the fibers of the sternocleidomastoid for those of the platysma; avoid this confusion by observing the direction in which the fibers run. The **platysma** arises from the skin and superficial fascia covering the upper portion of the pectoralis major and anterior deltoid muscles; its fibers pass upward and medially across the clavicle in a broad, flat sheet that covers the lower anterior part of the posterior triangle, the lower two-thirds of the sternocleidomastoid, and the superolateral part of the anterior triangle. It is inserted into the inferior border of the mandible and the skin of the lower part of the cheek and the angle of the mouth, where it also intermingles with some of the muscles about the mouth. The latter part of its insertion cannot be seen at present unless the face has been dissected. Locate the branches of the **supraclavicular nerves** within the superficial fascia at the inferior edge of the platysma muscle (Fig. 4.2); separate the lower fibers of the muscle, if necessary, to identify the nerves. When the platysma has been observed, reflect it from the clavicle upward and medially to the lower border of the mandible; leave it attached to the facial muscles. Do this with care to avoid damaging the nerves and vessels that lie immediately subjacent to the platysma. As the angle of the mandible is approached, attempt to secure the **cervical branch of** the **facial nerve;** it emerges from behind the lower part of the parotid gland to enter the deep surface of the platysma, which it supplies. Observe that the lower tip of the **parotid gland** fills in the narrow interval between the posterior border of the ramus of the mandible and the anterior border of the sternocleidomastoid. The main body of the parotid is covered by the skin of the face.

Now clean the sternocleidomastoid muscle, but retain in position the structures that cross its external surface. They are the **external jugular vein** and the four **cutaneous branches of** the **cervical plexus.** The nerves pierce the deep investing fascia of the posterior triangle at the posterior border of the sternocleidomastoid and turn forward across the muscle (Fig. 4.2). The **lesser occipital nerve** crosses the upper posterior part of the sternocleidomastoid to distribute branches to the skin of the lower lateral part of the scalp posterior to the external ear. The **great auricular nerve** runs upward and slightly forward over the upper half of the sternocleidomastoid to supply the skin of this part of the neck, a small part of the skin of the face in the region of the angle of the mandible, and the posterior part of the ear pinna. The **transverse cutaneous nerve of** the **neck** crosses the sternocleidomastoid transversely at about its middle to supply the skin over the anterior triangle. The **medial supraclavicular nerve** crosses the lower lateral portion of the sternocleidomastoid to distribute to the skin in the region of the sternoclavicular articulation.

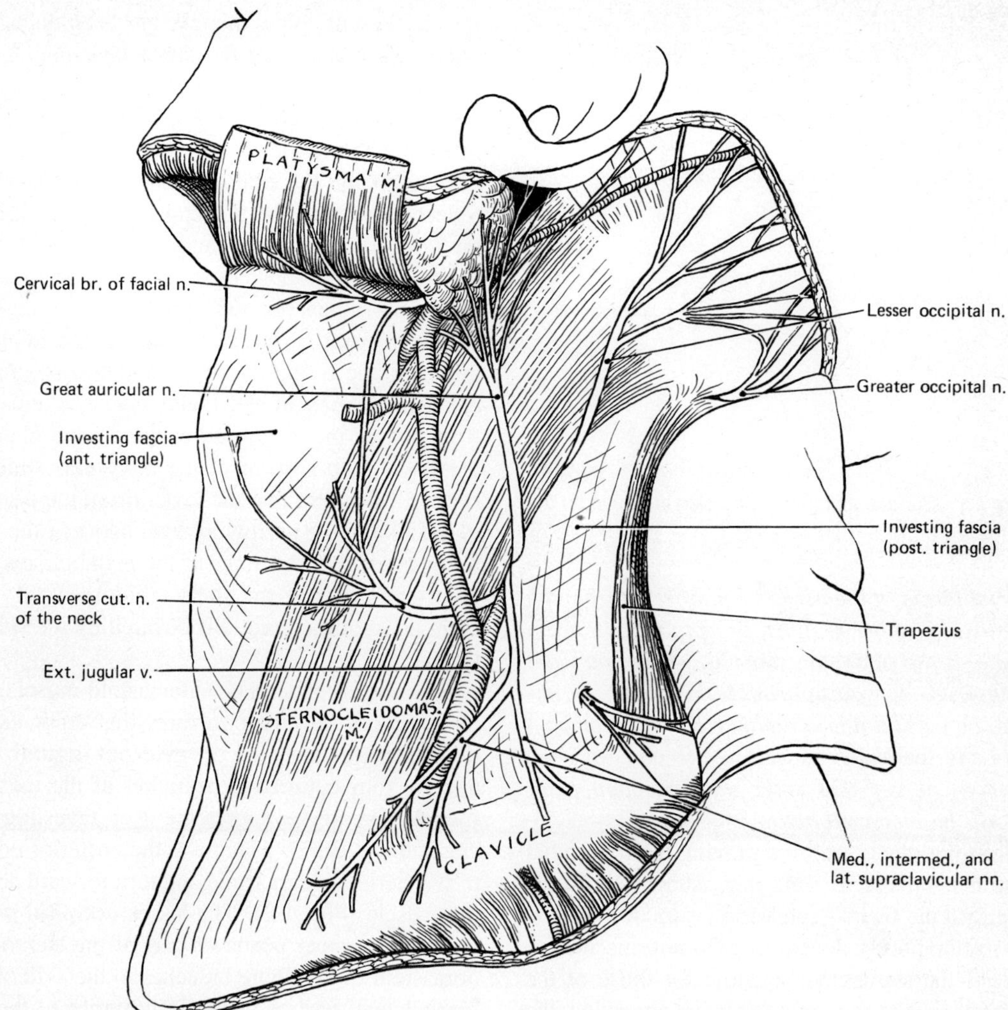

Figure 4.2 Superficial dissection of the anterior and posterior **triangles of** the **neck.**

The **external jugular vein** is somewhat variable in size and occasionally entirely missing. Typically (but with high variability), it is formed on the sternocleidomastoid posterior and inferior to the angle of the mandible by the junction of the **posterior auricular vein** and the **retromandibular vein.** It descends across the sternocleidomastoid and pierces the deep investing fascia just posterior to the muscle, about 1.5 cm superior to the clavicle in the posterior triangle, to terminate in the **subclavian vein.**

The **sternocleidomastoid muscle** arises by two heads: a medial one from the front of the **manubrium sterni** and a more lateral one from the upper border of the medial third of the **clavicle.** It is inserted on the outer surface of the **mastoid process** and the lateral half of the **superior nuchal line.**

POSTERIOR TRIANGLE

When the sternocleidomastoid and the structures crossing it have been cleaned and studied, proceed to the posterior triangle (Fig. 4.3). For this dis-

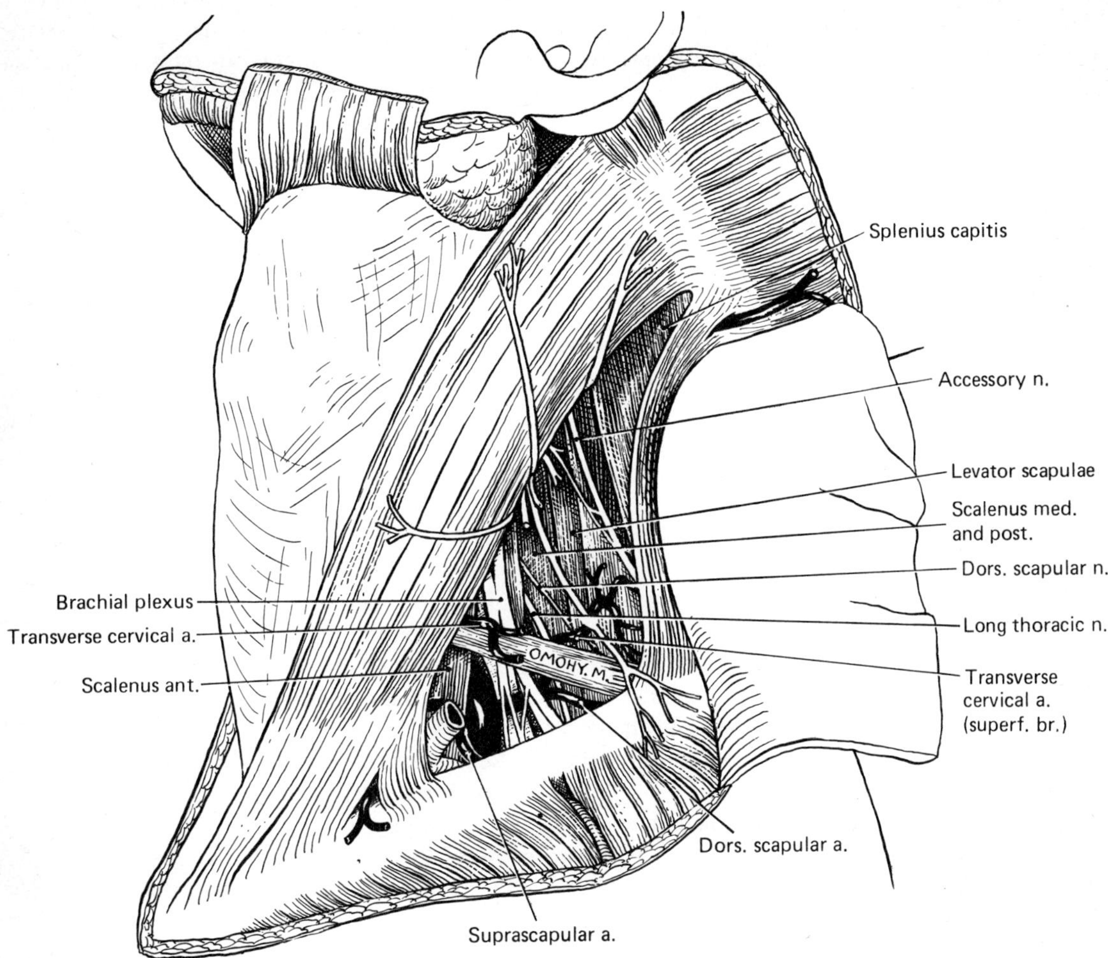

Figure 4.3 Deep dissection of the **posterior triangle of** the **neck.**

section, the shoulder should be depressed and the head turned as far as possible to the opposite side. A large wood block placed under the scapulae will help.

The **trapezius** muscle was studied when the back was dissected (see page 3). Now clean its upper anterior border in order to define completely the boundaries of the posterior triangle. This border runs inferiorly and laterally from about the middle of the superior nuchal line to the upper border of the clavicle at about the junction of its middle and lateral thirds. The roof of the posterior triangle is formed by the **investing layer of** the **deep cervical fascia,** which stretches between the sternocleidomastoid and the trapezius and is attached inferiorly to the clavicle. This fascia is pierced by the structures that have already been seen crossing the sternocleidomastoid and by the remaining supraclavicular nerves, which you should now identify. The **supraclavicular nerves** are all derived, as will be apparent later, from a single trunk that arises from the lowest loop (between the third and fourth cervical spinal nerves) of the cervical plexus. They usually pierce the investing fascia of the posterior triangle as three separate trunks, **medial, intermediate,** and **lateral,** to supply the skin over the lower part of the posterior triangle, over the upper part of the pectoralis major, and over the region of the acromion. Lateral supraclavicular branches cross the trapezius superficially.

The floor of the posterior triangle is formed by the external surfaces of several of the deep muscles of the neck covered by the **prevertebral layer of cervical fascia.** The muscles, from above down, are the **splenius capitis,** the **levator scapulae,** and the **scalenus medius** and **posterior** (Fig. 4.3). Only a portion of each of these muscles appears in the triangle, but they should be identified as the dissection proceeds. The **scalenus anterior** sometimes appears in the lower anterior corner of the triangle but is usually completely covered by the sternocleidomastoid. The actual extent of the triangle is the potential space, much deeper below than above, between the musculofascial floor and the fascial roof. Clean the structures contained within it and the muscles that make up its floor by carefully removing the fascia and fat. Note that inferiorly the posterior triangle is directly continuous with the axilla by means of a triangular aperture known as the **cervicoaxillary canal;** the canal is bounded by the clavicle, the upper border of the scapula, and the first rib.

Trace the **cutaneous nerves** that have already been displayed back to the points at which they emerge from under the posterior border of the sternocleidomastoid. The cervical plexus, from which all these nerves arise, is under cover of the sternocleidomastoid and will be displayed later, when that muscle is reflected. Next identify and clean the **accessory nerve;** it is the eleventh cranial nerve (spinal root of). It emerges from under the sternocleidomastoid closely related to the **lesser occipital nerve,** and runs downward and posteriorly on the levator scapulae to disappear under the trapezius, which it supplies. Somewhat lower, one or two smaller nerve twigs will be found following a similar course through the triangle; they are **muscular branches** (C3 and C4) **of** the **cervical plexus,** which provide additional supply to the trapezius.

Clean the **inferior belly of** the **omohyoid muscle** and locate its nerve supply. This muscle subdivides the posterior triangle into an upper **occipital** and a lower **subclavian (supraclavicular) triangle,** as it courses from the posterior border of the sternocleidomastoid, anterior to the anterior scalene, toward its attachment to the superior border of the scapula.

On a slightly deeper plane, the **transverse cervical artery,** usually a branch of the **thyrocervical trunk of** the **subclavian artery,** emerges from behind the sternocleidomastoid and crosses the posterior triangle about 1.5 cm above, and roughly parallel to, the clavicle. It divides into two branches: the **superficial branch** passes laterally under cover of the trapezius and the **deep branch** enters the floor of the triangle in the interval between the scalenus medius and the levator scapulae to distribute smaller branches deep to the rhomboids. The origin and course of these arteries are variable; often only the superficial branch (**superficial cervical artery**) arises off the thyrocervical trunk, while the deep branch (**dorsal scapular artery**) arises directly off the subclavian artery (Fig. 4.3).

Next direct your attention to the roots and trunks of the **brachial plexus,** which lies deep in the lower anterior part of the posterior triangle. The **roots of** the **plexus** are the ventral rami of the fifth, sixth, seventh, and eighth cervical and the first thoracic nerves. They pass downward and laterally into the triangle from the interval between the scalenus anterior and the scalenus medius muscles. The roots combine to form the upper, middle, and lower **trunks,** which continue their course downward and laterally, resting against the scalenus medius, to enter the axilla through the cervicoaxillary canal.

The brachial plexus or the subclavian artery may be compressed as it passes between the scalene muscles or the cervicoaxillary canal, resulting in some manifestation of the "neurovascular compression syndrome." Symptoms include pain and dysfunction of the superior extremity.

Clean the **upper trunk** first. It is formed by the junction of the ventral rami of the fifth and sixth cervical nerves and gives rise to two branches in the posterior triangle: the **suprascapular nerve** and the **nerve to** the **subclavius.** The latter is a small twig that passes downward and forward through the areolar tissue of the lower part of the triangle, and then behind the clavicle to supply the subclavius muscle. The suprascapular nerve is a much larger branch that passes laterally toward the upper border of the scapula. The **middle trunk** of the plexus lies below the upper trunk and is a direct continuation of the ventral ramus of the seventh cervical nerve; it has no branches in the posterior triangle. The **lower trunk** is formed by the junction of the ventral rami of the eighth cervical and first thoracic nerves; its course in the posterior triangle is very short, and it also is devoid of branches in this area.

Identify and clean the **dorsal scapular** and the **long thoracic nerves** (Fig. 4.3). Both are derived from the upper roots of the plexus, but their origin is too far medial to be seen at present. They enter the triangle through the scalenus medius muscle and pass downward on the surface of that muscle, inclining somewhat posteriorly. The **dorsal scapular nerve** is the higher of the two; it leaves the triangle by entering the floor in the interval between the scalenus medius and the levator scapulae in close relation to the deep branch of the transverse cervical artery. The **long thoracic nerve (nerve to serratus anterior)** takes a more vertical course and passes posterior to the trunks of the plexus into the axilla.

Clean the portions of the **subclavian vein** and the **subclavian artery** that are presently available. The subclavian vein lies immediately posterior to the clavicle in the lower anterior corner of the posterior (subclavian) triangle and passes medially behind the sternocleidomastoid and anterior to the scalenus anterior. In this region it receives the termination of the external jugular vein. Posterior to the subclavian vein, the **suprascapular artery** crosses anterior to the scalenus anterior in the lowest part of the posterior triangle and joins the **suprascapular nerve** close to the upper border of the scapula. The second part of the subclavian artery lies posterior to the scalenus anterior, which separates it from the vein. The third part extends from the lateral border of the scalenus anterior to the outer border of the first rib and should now be cleaned. It rests on the upper surface of the first rib and lies below and in front of the lower trunk of the brachial plexus; at the outer border of the first rib, it becomes the **axillary artery.** It typically has no branches, but occasionally either the dorsal scapular or the suprascapular artery, or both, may arise from it.

ANTERIOR TRIANGLE

The **anterior triangle** is also roofed by the **investing layer of deep cervical fascia.** This fascia stretches from the anterior border of the sternocleidomastoid muscle of one side to that of the other. Superiorly, it is attached to the lower border of the mandible and more posteriorly helps form the fascial sheath of the parotid gland. It is firmly attached to the body of the hyoid bone, whose position should be determined by palpation. Inferiorly, it attaches to the clavicle, and in the midline, the fascia splits into anterior and posterior layers that attach to the anterior and posterior borders, respectively, of the jugular notch of the manubrium, thus enclosing between them a potential space known as the **suprasternal space** (of Burns). The space contains a few lymph nodes, areolar connective tissue, and a venous arch that joins the anterior jugular veins. The **anterior jugular veins** are formed on the external surface of the fascia by several small veins in the region of the mental protuberance; each descends just lateral to the median line to enter the suprasternal space. Just above the manubrium, each turns laterally posterior to the sternocleidomastoid to terminate in the external jugular or the subclavian vein. The anterior jugular vein shows variable communications with other veins and is apt to be particularly large if the external jugular is small.

Carefully remove the investing layer of deep cervical fascia. All the layers of the deep cervical fascia should be reviewed from one of the standard descriptive texts.

Clean the **digastric muscle.** The two bellies of this muscle form a wide V. The **anterior belly** arises from the **digastric fossa of** the **mandible**; the **posterior belly** arises from the **mastoid notch of** the **temporal bone.** The latter attachment is at present hidden by the mastoid process and the sternocleidomastoid muscle. The two bellies narrow to an **intermediate tendon** that lies just above the lateral part of the body of the **hyoid bone,** to which it is bound by a slip of the deep cervical fascia. In close relation to the posterior belly, you will find the **stylohyoid muscle.** This slender muscle arises from the base of the **styloid process** and inserts on the **hyoid bone** near the junction of the body and the greater horn (cornu); it is usually pierced near its insertion by the intermediate tendon of the digastric. The **common facial vein** will be found crossing the posterior belly of the digastric and the stylohyoid muscles externally; preserve it.

Identify the **thyroid cartilage,** which forms the prominence of the larynx commonly known as "Adam's apple." It lies a short distance inferior to the hyoid bone, to which it is connected by the thyrohyoid membrane. Both cartilage and membrane are mostly covered by the **infrahyoid muscles,** which you should now clean. The **sternohyoid muscle** arises from the inner surfaces of the **manubrium** and the capsule of the sternoclavicular joint; its fibers run almost vertically upward to insert on the lower border of the **hyoid bone** just lateral to the median line. The **inferior belly of** the **omohyoid** has already been seen in the posterior triangle, where it takes origin from the **scapula.** The intermediate tendon lies posterior to the sternocleidomastoid. The **superior belly** runs upward and forward through the anterior triangle to insert on the **hyoid bone** just lateral to the insertion of the sternohyoid. The sternothyroid and thyrohyoid muscles are partly covered by the two muscles just described. The **sternothyroid** arises from the inner surface of the **manubrium,** below the origin of the sternohyoid, and inserts on an oblique line on the lamina of the **thyroid cartilage.** The **thyrohyoid** arises from the same line on the **thyroid cartilage** and inserts on the lower border of the **hyoid bone** under cover of the insertions of the sternohyoid and omohyoid muscles.

Identify the branches of the **ansa cervicalis** that supply the sternohyoid, sternothyroid, and omohyoid muscles. These nerves enter the sternohyoid and sternothyroid at their posterolateral borders. The branch to the inferior belly of the omohyoid was identified in the previous dissection (see page 26); that to the superior belly of the omohyoid enters its lateral border. You can trace these nerves back to their source later, but it is advisable to identify them now, since the ansa cervicalis may be variable and hard to identify in the subsequent dissection of the neck.

Observe that the **digastric** and the **omohyoid muscles** divide the anterior triangle of the neck into three subsidiary triangular spaces; the submandibular, the carotid, and the muscular triangles. The **muscular triangle** is bounded by the midline of the neck below the hyoid bone, the anterior border of the superior belly of the omohyoid, and the anterior border of the lower half of the sternocleidomastoid; its principal contents are the infrahyoid muscles, which have already been cleaned. The **carotid triangle** is bounded by the posterior border of the superior belly of the omohyoid, the anterior border of the upper half of the sternocleidomastoid, and the lower border of the posterior belly of the digastric; its principal contents are the carotid arteries and their branches. The **submandibular (digastric) triangle** is bounded by the two bellies of the digastric and the lower border of the mandible. Finally, a small space, the **submental triangle,** is common to both sides, being bounded by the anterior bellies of the digastric muscles and the hyoid bone.

Identify the **facial artery** and the **(anterior) facial vein** at the point where they cross the lower border of the mandible. This is about 2 cm anterior to the angle, with the artery usually lying anterior to the vein. Observe that the vein crosses the submandibular triangle superficially and joins a branch (posterior facial vein) of the **retromandibular vein,** which emerges from the parotid gland, to form the **common facial vein.** The common facial vein crosses the submandibular triangle externally and enters the carotid triangle, to terminate, usually, in the **internal jugular vein.** Occasionally, it joins the external jugular vein or, more rarely, the anterior jugular vein. The course of the facial artery in the submandibular triangle is at present hidden by the submandibular gland, which you should now clean.

The facial vein does not have valves. Infections (e.g., from acne) in the region of the nose and mouth are noteworthy in that they may cause a venous thrombosis that can involve the cavernous sinus.

The large superficial portion of the **submandibular gland** occupies most of the space of the submandibular triangle. Displace the gland downward and medially, and observe that a thin-walled duct emerges from the deep surface and passes forward under cover of the posterior border of the mylohyoid muscle. Accompanying the duct is a narrow process of the glandular substance, which is known as the deep portion of the gland.

Clean the portion of the **facial artery** that lies in the submandibular triangle. It arises in the carotid triangle from the **external carotid artery,** and enters the submandibular triangle by passing deep to the stylohyoid and digastric muscles. It passes upward and laterally in a groove on the deep surface of the submandibular gland and then courses downward on the inner surface of the mandible to its lower border, around which it turns to reach the face. In the submandibular triangle, it gives rise to **glandular branches** and to a **submental branch,** which passes forward to be distributed to the digastric and mylohyoid muscles. The submental artery is closely related to the terminal part of the **mylohyoid nerve,** a branch of the mandibular nerve that will be seen when the infratemporal fossa is dissected. The nerve descends along the inner surface of the mandible to the submandibular triangle, where it supplies the mylohyoid muscle and the anterior belly of the digastric.

Clean the **mylohyoid muscle,** a flat sheet of muscle that forms the floor of the submandibular and submental triangles. Arising from the **mylohyoid line** on the inner surface of the mandible, its fibers pass downward and medially to insert on the body of the **hyoid bone** and into a **median raphe** that extends from the hyoid bone to the lower end of the mental symphysis.

Direct attention now to the **carotid triangle** (Fig. 4.4). Dissect the fascia about 1 cm above the greater horn of the hyoid bone and expose the **hypoglossal nerve** where it rests against the hyoglossus muscle. Trace it forward and notice that it passes deep to the stylohyoid muscle and then disappears under the mylohyoid muscle. Trace it backward and notice that it bends superiorly to disappear under the posterior belly of the digastric. Just below the digastric, it is crossed externally by the occipital artery. The **hyoglossus muscle** is one of the extrinsic muscles of the tongue. Its fibers run upward from the greater horn of the hyoid bone; a portion of them help form the floor of the carotid triangle, but most are presently hidden by the digastric and mylohyoid muscles. Close to the posterior border of the muscle, the hypoglossal nerve appears to give rise to a small branch, the **nerve to** the **thyrohyoid muscle,** which runs downward and forward to supply the thyrohyoid muscle (Fig. 4.4). It actually arises from the first cervical nerve and accompanies the hypoglossal nerve along its course.

Further dissection of the carotid triangle consists largely of removing a portion of the **carotid sheath.** It is the fascial sheath that encloses the **common** and **internal carotid arteries,** the **internal jugular vein,** and the **vagus nerve.** It is not a distinct membranous sheath but a condensation of fascia in which the structures are embedded.

The **internal jugular vein,** unless it is unusually large and filled with blood, will appear only in the upper angle of the carotid triangle, since the lower part of its course is completely overlapped by the sternocleidomastoid. The lower part of the **common carotid artery** is also covered by the

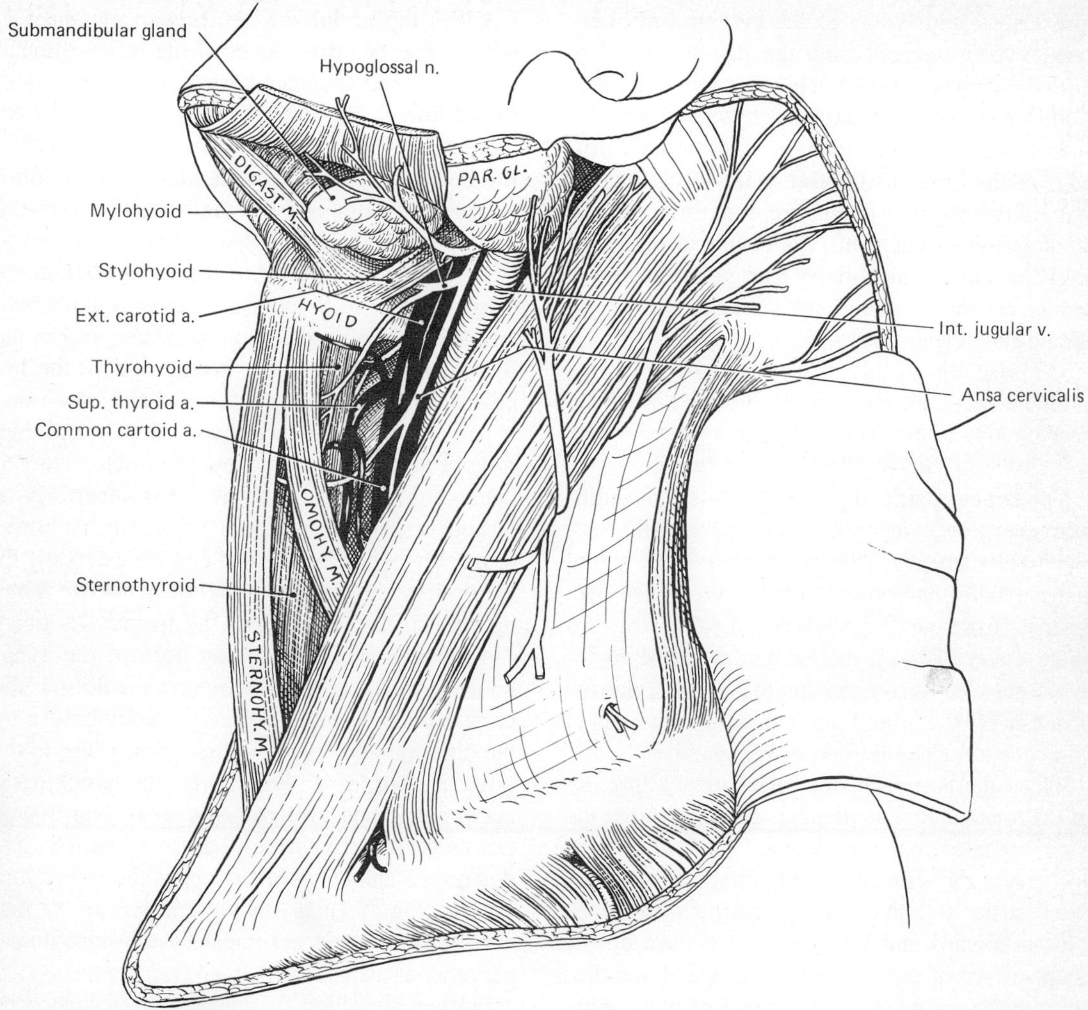

Figure 4.4 Deep dissection of the **anterior triangle of** the **neck.**

sternocleidomastoid, but its terminal portion can now be exposed just anterior to the sternocleidomastoid and posterior to the thyroid cartilage. The common carotid ends at about the level of the upper border of the thyroid cartilage (vertebral level C4) by dividing into **internal** and **external carotids.** Clean the external carotid and its branches in so far as they lie within the carotid triangle. Note the **carotid sinus** (and the nerves to it), a dilatation at the termination of the common carotid or the beginning of the internal carotid; it is important in the regulation of systemic blood pressure.

At its origin, the **external carotid artery** lies anterior to the internal carotid. It ascends in the neck, inclines somewhat posteriorly, so that it comes to lie lateral to the internal carotid, and then passes from view under the posterior belly of the digastric. The first branch of the external carotid is usually the **ascending pharyngeal,** a small vessel that arises from the medial surface of the external carotid and ascends deeply on the pharyngeal wall; it will be seen again in a later dissection (see page 69).

The **superior thyroid artery** arises a short distance above the origin of the external carotid and runs anteriorly, medially, and then inferiorly under cover of the omohyoid muscle to reach the thyroid gland. Near its origin it gives rise to a small **hyoid branch** and, shortly after it bends inferiorly to a larger **superior laryngeal branch** that runs anteriorly and pierces the thyrohyoid membrane to enter the larynx.

The **lingual artery** arises at the level of the greater horn of the hyoid bone and runs forward, usually with a slight upward bend, to disappear under the hyoglossus muscle.

The **facial artery** arises either slightly above the lingual or by a common stem with it. Running forward and upward, it passes deep to the posterior belly of the digastric to reach the submandibular triangle, where its further course has already been seen.

The external carotid gives rise to the **occipital artery** from its posterior aspect, close to the lower border of the digastric muscle. This vessel runs posteriorly and upward, crossing the internal jugular vein laterally; you will expose its further course later.

Attempt to display the **internal** and **external laryngeal nerves** (Fig. 5.2). They are terminal branches of the **superior laryngeal branch of** the **vagus,** but this cannot be demonstrated at present. Both run downward and forward deep to the internal and external carotid arteries. The **internal laryngeal nerve** passes deep to the lingual artery, near the origin of the artery, and pierces the thyrohyoid membrane in company with the superior laryngeal artery. The **external laryngeal nerve** is considerably smaller. Find it at a slightly lower level, crossing deep to the superior thyroid artery and passing under cover of the sternothyroid muscle to supply the cricothyroid muscle, one of the intrinsic muscles of the larynx.

Chapter 5

Structures under the Sternocleidomastoid

Review the attachments of the **sternocleidomastoid;** then, by flexing the head and neck forward and rotating the head from side to side, free and elevate the sternocleidomastoid so that the underlying structures can be cleaned and studied without cutting the muscle.

Clean the **subclavius muscle.** It extends from the first rib to the inferior surface of the lateral part of the clavicle. Attempt to locate the **nerve to the subclavius,** a branch off the upper trunk of the brachial plexus.

If you need to remove a segment of the clavicle, as some people like to do when dissecting the posterior triangle in conjunction with the axilla, make a cut through the periosteum along the ventral surface of the clavicle, extending from the medial border of the deltoid through the lower fibers of the clavicular and the sternocostal attachments of the sternocleidomastoid. By blunt dissection, reflect the periosteum from the surfaces of the clavicle between the deltoid and the sternocleidomastoid. Insert the handle of a forceps between the periosteum and the lateral edge of the clavicle and, while depressing the subjacent structures, saw through the clavicle at the medial border of the deltoid. Dissect free and elevate the lower fibers of the sternocleidomastoid to expose the sternoclavicular articulation. Be sure to leave the clavicular attachment of the muscle intact.

The **sternoclavicular articulation** is the synovial joint between the medial end of the clavicle, and the clavicular notch of the manubrium sterni and the upper border of the first costal cartilage (Fig. 5.1). It is surrounded by a strong fibrous capsule; clean its anterior surface, known as the **anterior sternoclavicular ligament.** Note the **costoclavicular ligament,** a strong band of fibers extending laterally from the cartilage of the first rib to the periosteum over the costal tubercle on the inferior surface of the clavicle. Cut through

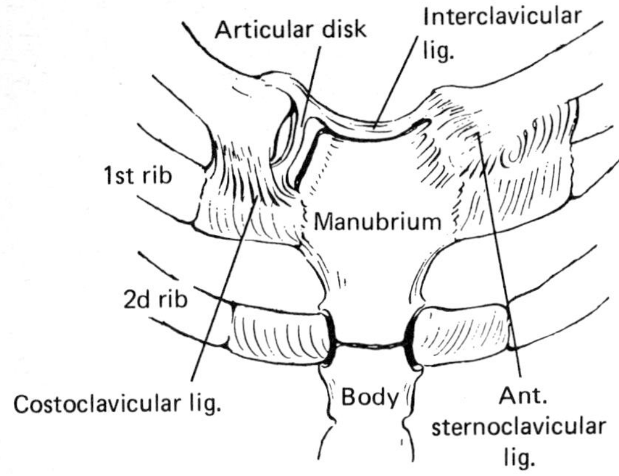

Figure 5.1 The **sternoclavicular joint.**

the entire circumference of the **capsule** close to the manubrium and detach the clavicle. Observe that the fibers forming the posterior part of the capsule **(posterior sternoclavicular ligament)** are thicker and tougher than the anterior ones, and that posteriorly the capsule is closely related to the origins of the sternohyoid and sternothyroid muscles. This can be seen by elevating and reflecting the clavicle and attached sternocleidomastoid superiorly. Note also that the joint is separated into two distinct cavities by a fibrocartilaginous **articular disk** that intervenes between the clavicle and the first rib and manubrium.

The success of the following dissection of the neck depends largely on the completeness with which you free the sternocleidomastoid from its surrounding structures as far as its attachment to the skull. As you elevate the muscle, observe that there may be, in relation to its deep surface in the region below and behind the angle of the mandible, a considerable aggregation of large **deep cervical lymph nodes.** After you observe them, carefully but completely remove them, together with the mass of fatty areolar tissue in which they are embedded. Secure the **accessory nerve.** It emerges from under the posterior belly of the digastric, behind the internal jugular vein, and runs downward and posteriorly across the deep surface of the sternocleidomastoid, which it innervates, to enter the posterior triangle. Also entering the deep surface of the sternocleidomastoid, in close relation to the accessory nerve, is the **sternocleidomastoid branch of** the **occipital artery.** It occasionally arises as a direct branch of the external carotid artery, in which case it, as well as the occipital artery, will cross the hypoglossal nerve laterally.

Clean the **internal jugular vein** as it emerges from under the posterior belly of the digastric muscle and descends through the neck deep to the sternocleidomastoid. It terminates posterior to the sternoclavicular articulation by joining the subclavian vein to form the brachiocephalic vein. It is crossed laterally by the intermediate tendon of the omohyoid muscle and often by the **descending cervical root of** the **ansa cervicalis.** The internal jugular vein is enclosed in the carotid sheath, where it lies lateral to the internal carotid artery superiorly and the common carotid inferiorly. The tributaries of the internal jugular vein, with the exception of the common facial vein, correspond roughly to the lower branches of the external carotid artery.

Display the **ansa cervicalis** (Fig. 5.2). This portion of the cervical plexus, which supplies the infrahyoid muscles, is a nerve loop formed by a branch **(superior root)** of the first cervical nerve (called the **descendens hypoglossi** since it accompanies the hypoglossal nerve in part of its course), and a branch **(inferior root)** derived from a loop between the second and third cervical nerves **(descendens cervicalis).** The superior root leaves the hypoglossal nerve and emerges from under the posterior belly of the digastric and descends in close relation to the lateral aspect of the carotid sheath. The inferior root runs downward and forward, passing either lateral or medial to the internal jugular vein; it joins the superior root at an extremely variable level to form the **loop of** the **ansa cervicalis.** Branches from the lower end of the loop supply the **sternohyoid,** the **sternothyroid,** and **both bellies of** the **omohyoid** (Fig. 5.2). (To find the ansa more easily, first isolate a nerve

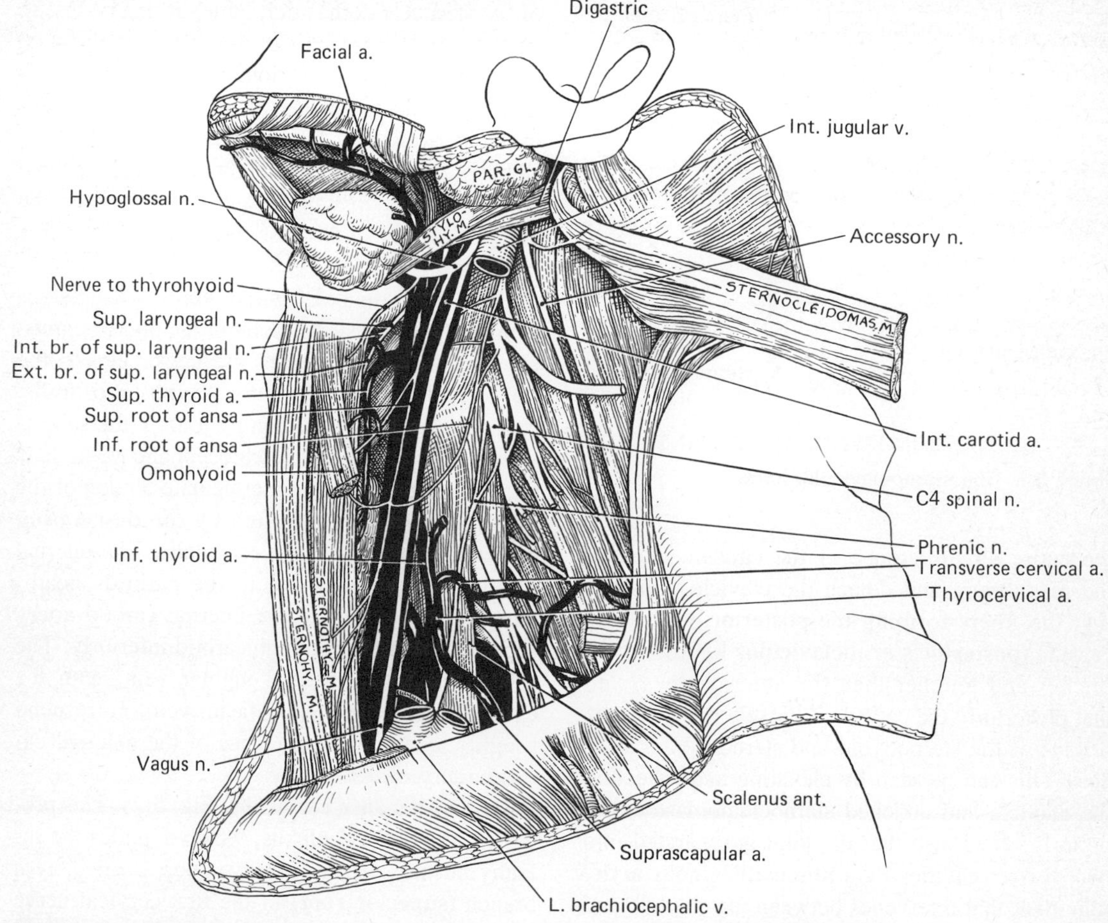

Figure 5.2 Dissection of the **structures under** the **sternocleidomastoid muscle.** The internal jugular vein has been removed.

supplying one of the muscles and then follow it proximally to the loop.)

Direct attention next to the derivation of the **cervical plexus,** a looped nerve plexus composed of cutaneous nerves, ansa cervicalis, muscular nerves, and phrenic nerve and derived from ventral rami of the first four cervical nerves. It lies deep to the upper part of the sternocleidomastoid. The first cervical nerve is small and will be exposed in a later dissection. It emerges above the transverse process of the atlas and turns downward in front of that process to join the second cervical nerve. The second, third, and fourth cervical nerves are each successively larger and enter the present area of dissection by passing laterally and downward from between the anterior and posterior tubercles of the transverse processes of the corresponding cervical vertebrae. The plexus takes the form of **three loops.** The **first** is that noted above between the first and second nerves and lies anterior to the transverse process of the atlas. The **second loop** is formed between the second and third nerves, and the **third** between the third and fourth nerves. The **cutaneous branches of** the **plexus,** which have already been seen in the dissection of the posterior triangle, should now be traced back to their origins. The **lesser occipital, great auricular,** and **transverse cervical cutaneous nerves** all arise from the second loop. **Medial, intermediate** and **lateral supraclavicular nerves** arise from the third loop, usually by a common stem.

Muscular branches also arise from the roots of the cervical plexus. The largest is the **phrenic nerve,** derived principally from the fourth cervical nerve; it passes downward and medially on the anterior surface of the **scalenus anterior** to enter the thoracic cavity posterior to the brachiocephalic vein. It usually receives a twig from the fifth cervical nerve, and often one from the third. Muscular twigs, derived from the second and third loops, cross the posterior triangle to reach the deep surface of the sternocleidomastoid and the trapezius, respectively. Muscular branches of the cervical plexus pass from the second, third, and fourth nerves directly into the longus colli, longus capitis, and scalene muscles for their supply.

The derivation of the superior and inferior roots of the ansa cervicalis has been given.

Free and elevate the intermediate tendon of the omohyoid and reflect the superior belly upward. Divide the sternohyoid and sternothyroid muscles just above the manubrium and reflect them upward. Then clean and study the common carotid artery and the vagus nerve, both of which are enclosed in the carotid sheath (Fig. 5.2).

On the right side, the **common carotid artery** arises posterior to the sternoclavicular joint as a branch of the brachiocephalic artery. On the left side, it arises in the superior mediastinum of the thorax as a branch of the aortic arch and enters the neck posterior to the left sternoclavicular joint. Its course in the neck is similar on both sides, extending from the sternoclavicular joint upward and somewhat posteriorly to the level of the upper border of the thyroid cartilage, where it terminates by dividing into **internal** and **external carotids.** The common carotid artery has no other branches. Except at its termination, it is covered laterally by the sternocleidomastoid and anteriorly, in the lower part of its course, by the omohyoid, sternothyroid, and sternohyoid muscles. Laterally, it is related to the internal jugular vein. Medially, it is related to the trachea and in the middle portion of its course, to the thyroid gland. Posteriorly, it rests against the prevertebral muscles (longus colli and longus capitis).

The carotid pulse can be felt by sliding your fingers laterally along the thyroid cartilage into the posterior depression between the cartilage and the sternocleidomastoid muscle.

The **vagus nerve** lies in the most posterior part of the carotid sheath. It is medial to the internal jugular vein and lateral to the internal carotid artery above and the common carotid below. It passes into the thorax posterior to the sternoclavicular joint; on the left side, it lies between the common carotid artery and the brachiocephalic vein, and on the right side, between the brachiocephalic artery and the brachiocephalic vein.

You should now review the brachial plexus in its entirety and its relationships to the clavicle; replace the clavicle during the review (Fig. 3.3).

When review of the brachial plexus is completed, the superior extremity, together with its girdle, can be removed, if the extremity is to be taken from the body and studied elsewhere. However, if possible leave it attached to the body so the relationships can be maintained for future study and review. For removal, divide the **serratus anterior** *by a vertical incision at about the midaxillary line. Then sever the three* **trunks of** *the* **brachial plexus,** *the first part of the* **axillary artery,** *and the* **axillary vein.** *The upper trunk of the brachial plexus should be cut proximally to the origin of the* **suprascapular nerve.**

Chapter 6

Root of the Neck

The **subclavian artery** lies deep in the root of the neck. On the right side, it arises posterior to the sternoclavicular joint as one of the terminal branches of the brachiocephalic artery; on the left side, it arises in the thorax as a branch of the aortic arch and enters the root of the neck posterior to the sternoclavicular joint, where it lies posterior and slightly lateral to the common carotid artery. In the root of the neck the subclavian artery is divided, for descriptive purposes, into three parts. Since the subdivision is based on the relationship of the artery to the scalenus anterior muscle, first clean and study the muscle.

The **scalenus anterior** arises by slips from the anterior tubercles of the **transverse processes of** the third through the sixth **cervical vertebrae.** Descending under cover of the sternocleidomastoid, its fibers narrow to a tendinous insertion on the **scalene tubercle on** the upper surface of the first **rib.** Find the **phrenic nerve** crossing its anterior surface from above downward and medially. Parallel, but more medial to the phrenic, you will also find the **ascending cervical artery** on the anterior surface of the muscle. At its insertion, the scalenus anterior is crossed anteriorly by the **subclavian vein** and, at a slightly higher level, by the **transverse cervical** and **suprascapular arteries** (Fig. 6.1).

The **first part of** the **subclavian artery** extends from the sternoclavicular joint upward and laterally to the medial border of the scalenus anterior; the **second part** runs laterally posterior to the scalenus anterior; and the **third part** runs laterally and slightly downward from the lateral border of the scalenus anterior to the outer border of the first rib, where it becomes the axillary artery.

While cleaning the **first part of** the **subclavian artery,** observe that it is covered anteriorly by the

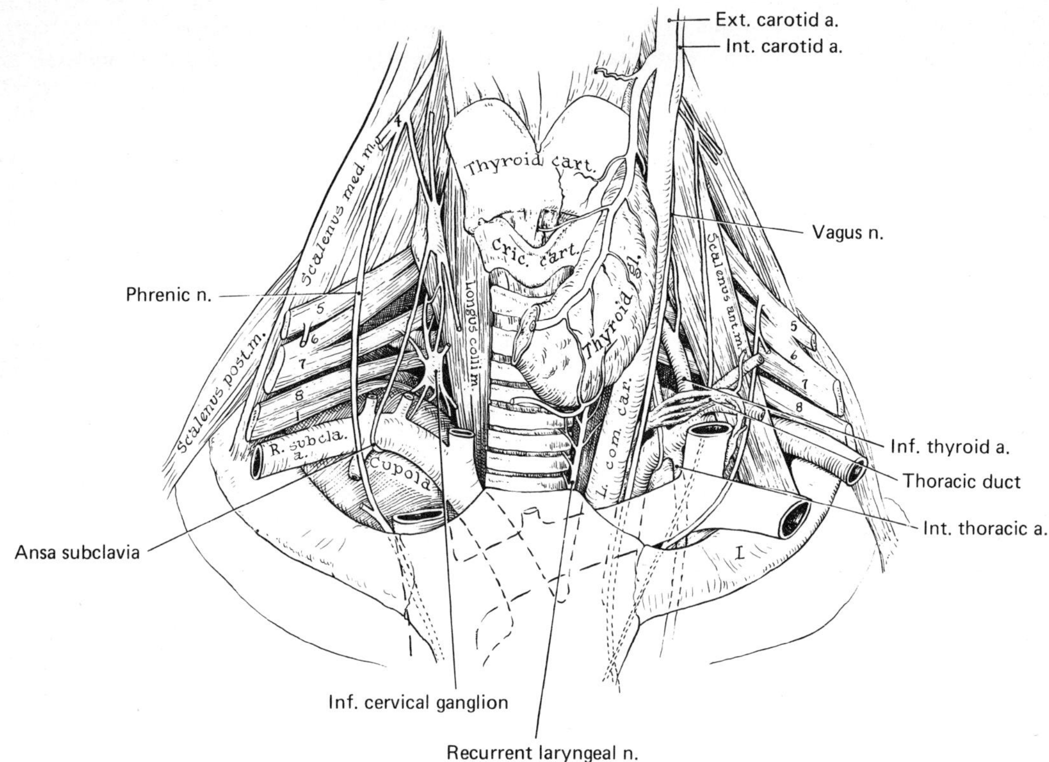

Figure 6.1 The **root of** the **neck.** The dissection on the right side is deeper than that on the left side.

clavicle and the sternocleidomastoid and that it is crossed by the **phrenic** and **vagus nerves,** the **vertebral vein,** and part of the sympathetic chain, the **ansa subclavia** (Fig. 6.1). On the left side, it is also crossed by the terminal part of the **thoracic duct.** The thoracic duct emerges from behind the left common carotid artery at the level of the lower border of the thyroid gland and runs laterally and downward, passing posterior to the vagus nerve and anterior to the subclavian artery, to join the terminal part of the internal jugular vein, the subclavian vein, or the beginning of the brachiocephalic vein.

The first branch of the subclavian is the **vertebral artery.** It ascends almost vertically to enter the transverse foramen of the sixth cervical vertebra behind the most lateral part of the longus colli muscle. The **vertebral vein** descends anterior to the vertebral and subclavian arteries to join the brachiocephalic vein. It is frequently very large and may obscure the dissection of the arteries, in which case you should remove it.

Slightly more laterally, the thyrocervical trunk and the internal thoracic artery arise from the first part of the subclavian. The **thyrocervical trunk** runs superiorly for a short distance and usually divides into the **transverse cervical,** the **suprascapular,** and the **inferior thyroid arteries.** The first two vessels pass laterally across the scalenus anterior. The inferior thyroid may be regarded as the main continuation of the thyrocervical trunk. It ascends and then bends medially and downward, passing in front of the vertebral artery and posterior to the common carotid artery and the vagus nerve to reach the thyroid gland. Near its origin, the inferior thyroid gives rise to the **ascending**

cervical artery, a small branch that you saw ascending on the scalenus anterior. The **internal thoracic artery** runs downward and forward from the subclavian to reach the anterior thoracic wall behind the first costal cartilage. Near its origin, it is related to the phrenic nerve, which it crosses either anteriorly or posteriorly.

Insert a probe posterior to the scalenus anterior muscle and elevate the lower part of it, to observe the **second part of** the **subclavian artery.** Note that the first and second parts of the subclavian rest inferiorly and posteriorly against the **cervical pleura,** by which they are separated from the lung. The **apex of** the **lung** and the cervical pleura (cupola) rise for a considerable distance above the anterior aspect of the first rib into the root of the neck. The only branch of the second part of the subclavian is the **costocervical trunk.** It runs upward and posteriorly across the pleura and terminates by dividing into the **deep cervical** and **supreme intercostal arteries.** The former ascends posterior to the scalenus medius to reach the deep muscles at the back of the neck. The supreme intercostal descends on the posterior thoracic wall to give rise to the first two posterior intercostal arteries.

The **third part of** the **subclavian artery** rests upon the upper surface of the **first rib** and is related posteriorly to the scalenus medius and the lower trunk of the brachial plexus. It usually has no branches but occasionally gives rise to the **dorsal (descending) scapular** or the **suprascapular artery,** or both.

You will have to retract the sternohyoid and sternothyroid muscles laterally to study the thyroid gland, trachea, and esophagus. The **thyroid** is a bilobed gland that lies anterior and lateral to the upper part of the trachea. It consists of two **lateral lobes** connected by a much smaller median portion, the **isthmus,** which crosses the front of tracheal rings two, three, and four. Anterolaterally, the gland is covered by the infrahyoid muscles; posterolaterally, it is related to the common carotid artery. The most superior extent of the lateral lobes is to the oblique attachment of the sternothyroid muscle on the thyroid cartilage. In the median line, the isthmus is covered only by skin and fascia.

The extensive blood supply of the thyroid gland is provided by the **superior** and **inferior thyroid arteries,** which anastomose freely with each other and with similar vessels of the opposite side. The blood is drained from the gland by the **superior** and **inferior thyroid veins.** The inferior thyroid vein does not accompany the artery but descends in front of the trachea to drain into the brachiocephalic vein. It may be single or paired. A **middle thyroid vein,** which passes laterally into the internal jugular vein, is frequently present.

Cut across the isthmus of the thyroid gland and reflect the two halves of the gland laterally. Study its posterior surface and attempt to identify the **parathyroid glands;** there are usually two pairs, a **superior** and an **inferior.** They are small, flattened, oval bodies, closely applied to the posterior surface of the lateral lobes of the thyroid, sometimes embedded within the thyroid substance. They may be distinguished from the thyroid by their lighter color.

The **trachea** is a median tubular organ that begins at the lower border of the **cricoid cartilage** (vertebral level C6). From the cricoid cartilage, the trachea descends through the neck into the thorax. Its lumen is kept permanently open by a series of U-shaped cartilaginous bars in its wall. Observe that posteriorly, where the trachea rests against the anterior surface of the esophagus, the two ends of each bar are joined by muscles.

> Surgical opening of the trachea (tracheostomy), usually through the upper tracheal rings, permits artificial ventilation of the lungs when an obstruction hinders respiration through the airway.

The **esophagus** is a hollow tubular organ that begins at the lower border of the cricoid cartilage as a direct continuation of the **pharynx** and descends into the thorax. You will get only a sketchy view of it while the trachea is in place, since the esophagus lies immediately posterior to the trachea and anterior to the bodies of the vertebrae and the prevertebral muscles. Except when food is passing through, it is closed and flattened anteroposteriorly.

Dissect in the groove between the esophagus and the trachea to expose the **recurrent (inferior) laryngeal nerve,** which ascends in the groove to reach the larynx. The origin of the **left** recurrent laryngeal, a branch of the left vagus, is within the thoracic cavity and cannot be seen at present. The **right** recurrent laryngeal, however, arises from the right vagus as it crosses the subclavian artery. From its origin, the right recurrent turns medially and upward, passing posterior to the beginnings of the right subclavian and common carotid arteries, to reach the interval between the esophagus and the trachea.

Note the intimate relationship of the recurrent laryngeal nerves to the thyroid gland. While performing a thyroidectomy, the surgeon must first preserve the nerves; if they are injured, the patient will suffer serious laryngeal muscular paralysis affecting speech and respiration.

Chapter 7

Head and Neck

FACE

The surface features of the face are those with which you are, for the most part, already familiar. The **mental protuberance,** the lower border and the **angle of** the **mandible** are readily palpable through the skin. The prominence of the cheek is formed by the **zygomatic bone;** extending posteriorly, it joins the zygomatic process of the temporal bone to form the **zygomatic arch.** The lips are covered with a **mucous membrane** that is continuous externally with the skin of the face and internally with the mucous membrane lining the mouth. At the **nostrils,** the skin of the face is continuous with the mucous membrane lining the nasal cavities. The free margins of the upper and lower eyelids together form a slitlike orifice known as the **rima palpebrarum.** At the rima, the skin of the eyelids is continuous with the **conjunctiva,** a delicate membrane that forms the inner linings of both eyelids and is reflected over the anterior part of the eyeball. The conjunctiva as a whole encloses a space, the **conjunctival sac,** that is open to the exterior at the rima palpebrarum. The sac lies between the inner surfaces of the eyelids and the anterior surface of the eyeball. Medially, in the free margin of each eyelid, there is a slight elevation called the **lacrimal papilla.** On the summit of the papilla, notice an opening, the **lacrimal punctum.** The punctum marks the beginning of the **lacrimal canaliculus,** which conveys tears from the conjunctival sac to the **lacrimal sac.**

Begin the dissection by making the following incisions through the skin (Fig. 7.1): (1) a median one running downward from the **bregma** *across the forehead, along the bridge of the nose, to the mental protuberance; (2) a transverse incision*

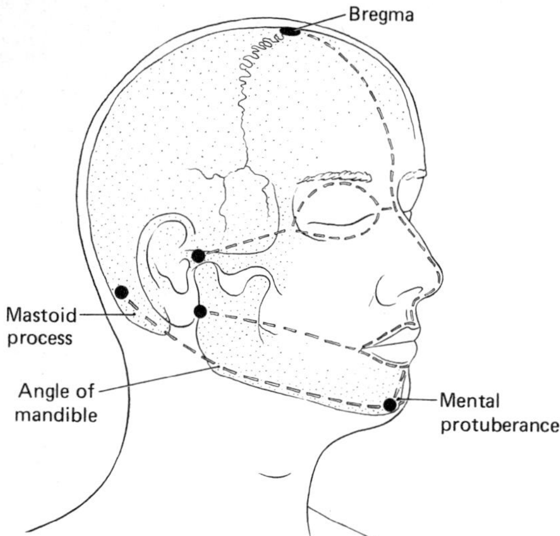

Figure 7.1 Surface landmarks and skin incisions on the face.

starting at the first incision at the level of the rima palpebrarum and running laterally and backward to a point just anterior to the external auditory meatus (this incision must bifurcate in the region of the upper and lower eyelids, so that it will pass through the skin of each lid just above and below the rima); (3) a transverse incision from the angle of the mouth running laterally to the posterior border of the ramus of the mandible (from the angle of the mouth, this incision should be extended medially along the red margins of the upper and lower lips); (4) a transverse incision along the lower border of the mandible from the **mental protuberance** *to a point slightly posterior to the angle. By these incisions, you will map out three flaps of skin that you should reflect laterally from the median line. Note that since the superficial muscles of the face are inserted into the skin, you will encounter some difficulty in reflecting only the skin from the face. Carefully cut the strands of the muscles from the deep surface of the skin and reflect the skin cleanly. In the temporal region, the* **superficial temporal vessels** *lie immediately subjacent to the skin; do not reflect them with the skin. The proper plane for reflecting the skin, particularly in specimens with a large amount of subcutaneous fat, can be achieved by removing the skin and subcutaneous tissue from the outer surface of the upper part of the platysma muscle, which has been exposed, and continuing this plane of dissection upward onto the face.*

In going through this dissection, you may prefer to use one side of the face for concentrating on the muscles and the other side for the nerves and arteries.

The superficial muscles of the face are known as the **muscles of facial expression** (Fig. 7.2). For the most part, these muscles take origin from one of the bones of the face and insert into the skin and superficial fascia. Since they are difficult to demonstrate satisfactorily in the cadaver, only a few of them will be studied.

The **orbicularis oculi** is a circular muscle that surrounds the rima palpebrarum. Its fibers lie just beneath the skin in the upper and lower eyelids and also over the bony rim of the orbit, from which some of its fibers take origin.

The **frontalis** is a thin, flat muscle that lies just under the skin of the forehead. Its fibers arise from the **galea aponeurotica,** the aponeurosis in the scalp that joins the frontalis and the occipitalis muscles. It inserts into the skin of the eyebrows and the root of the nose, blending to some extent with the upper part of the orbicularis oculi.

The **nasalis** is a small muscle that arises at the side of the bridge of the nose and runs downward and laterally to be inserted in the skin at the junction of the wing (ala) of the nose and the cheek.

The **orbicularis oris** surrounds the opening of the mouth and is the main intrinsic muscle of the lips. Its fibers are derived largely from the other superficial muscles yet to be observed and are inserted into the skin covering the lips externally and into the mucous membrane lining the lips internally.

Three muscles converge downward to enter the upper lip. The **zygomaticus minor** arises from the zygomatic bone, the **levator labii superioris** from the infraorbital margin above the infraorbital foramen, and the **levator labii superioris alaeque nasi** from the maxilla near the root of the nose.

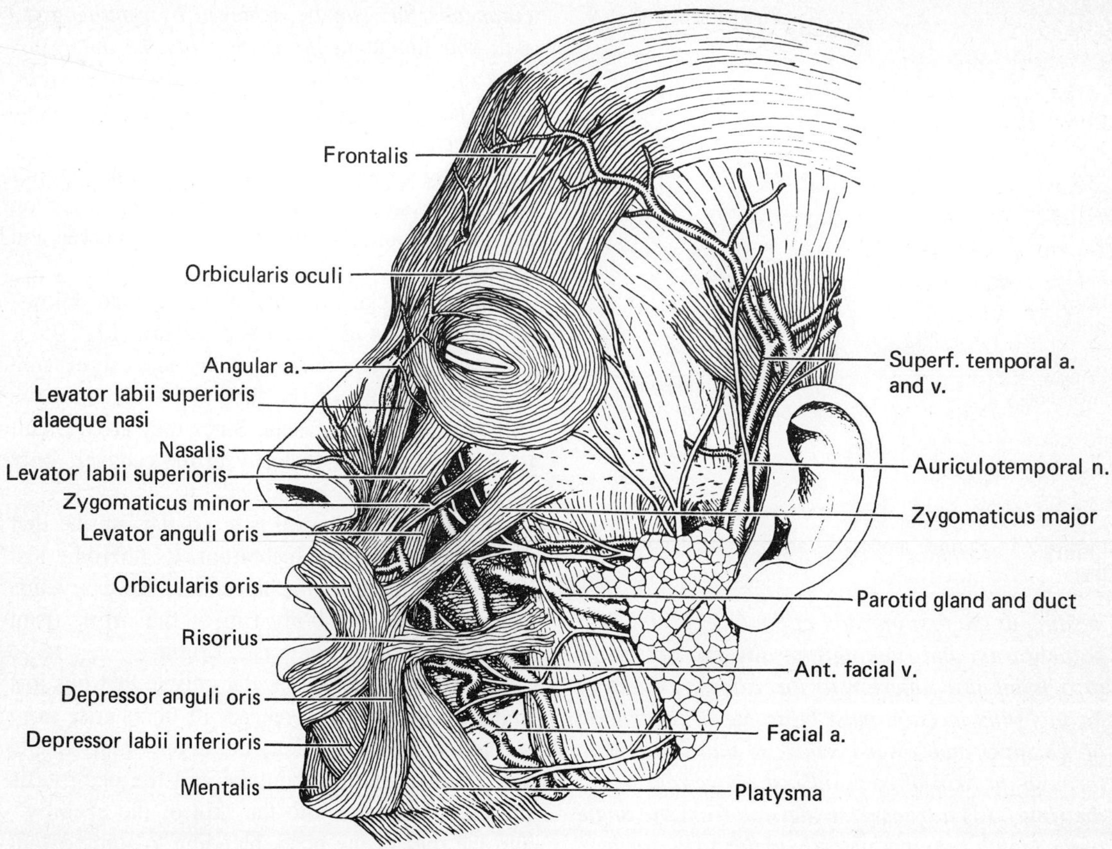

Figure 7.2 **Superficial** dissection of the **face.** The branches of the facial nerve, seen emerging from the borders of the parotid gland, are not labeled.

All three muscles insert into the skin of the upper lip and some blend with the orbicularis oris; the third one has an additional insertion into the ala of the nose, which, as the name implies, it helps to raise and flare.

The **zygomaticus major** is a flat, bandlike muscle arising from the external surface of the zygomatic bone lateral to the origin of the zygomaticus minor; it passes to the angle of the mouth to insert into the skin and orbicularis oris muscle.

The **risorius** is a purely superficial muscle that arises from the superficial fascia over the parotid gland. It passes forward across the cheek to the angle of the mouth, where it blends with the orbicularis oris.

The **depressor anguli oris muscle** arises from the lower part of the anterior half of the mandible and converges upward toward the angle of the mouth, where it partly inserts directly into the skin and partly joins the orbicularis oris.

The **depressor labii inferioris** arises from the external surface of the mandible below the canine and premolar teeth and runs upward and medially into the orbicularis oris.

The **platysma,** a thin muscular sheet, lies mostly in the neck. Its more posterior fibers, however, run upward across the mandible and blend with the depressor anguli oris, the risorius, and the orbicularis oris.

Depending on your requirements, review the

anatomy of the other facial muscles in one of the descriptive texts.

The muscles just described, as well as the deeper muscles of facial expression, are all supplied by branches of the **facial nerve** (CN VII); attempt now to demonstrate them. Since the branches enter the deep surface of the muscles, you should not have disrupted them, if you have done a careful dissection.

As the trunk of the **facial nerve** emerges from the **stylomastoid foramen,** it passes directly into the **parotid gland.** Within the substance of the gland, it divides into two trunks that in turn break up into numerous branches that emerge separately onto the face from under cover of the superior and anterior borders of the parotid. First, carefully clean the external surface of the parotid and identify the branches of the facial nerve as the borders of the gland are cleaned (Fig. 7.2).

The **parotid gland** occupies the interval between the posterior border of the ramus of the mandible and the anterior border of the sternocleidomastoid muscle and mastoid process. A flattened portion is prolonged forward over the external surface of the ramus of the mandible and posterior part of the masseter muscle. The **duct of** the **parotid,** usually of considerable size, emerges from the anterior border of the gland and crosses the cheek anteriorly about 1.5 cm below the zygomatic arch. It pierces the middle of the cheek to open into the **oral cavity** at the **parotid papilla,** which is on the level of the second upper molar tooth. The parotid gland is enclosed in a sheath of dense fascia that is continuous anteriorly with the deep fascia covering the external surface of the masseter muscle.

Find the **temporal** and **zygomatic branches of** the **facial nerve** emerging from under the superior border of the gland. The temporal branch runs upward over the temporal fascia to be distributed to the superior and anterior auricular muscles (two small, unimportant muscles of the external ear) and to the frontalis. The zygomatic branch runs upward and forward across the zygomatic bone to reach the orbicularis oculi.

Emerging from under the anterior border of the parotid, find the **buccal** and **mandibular branches of** the **facial nerve.** The buccal branches, usually two or three, pass forward across the cheek to supply the zygomaticus major and minor, levator labii superioris, levator labii superioris alaeque nasi, nasalis, orbicularis oris, risorius, levator anguli oris, and buccinator. The mandibular branch passes forward just above the lower border of the mandible to reach the depressor anguli oris and depressor labii inferioris. The **cervical branch of** the **facial nerve** descends into the neck below the angle of the mandible to supply the platysma. These branches of the facial nerve, particularly the buccal and mandibular branches, usually communicate with one another on the face by small connecting loops.

Now trace the terminal branches of the facial nerve backward through the substance of the parotid gland by carefully cutting away, a bit at a time, the glandular tissue. In this way, you will expose the structures that are embedded in the gland: the trunk of the **facial nerve** and the beginning of its branches, the terminal part of the **external carotid artery,** and the **retromandibular vein.**

Paralysis of the muscles of facial expression, and of the autonomically regulated cutaneous glands and smooth muscle elements, results from facial nerve damage (Bell's palsy). During the dissection, consider the difficult task of the surgeon who must preserve the nerve when, for example, removing a tumorous parotid gland.

The **facial nerve** will be exposed first, since it winds superficially around the external carotid artery and the retromandibular vein. Shortly after emerging from the stylomastoid foramen, the facial nerve gives rise to a small **posterior auricular branch** that passes upward and backward on the external surface of the mastoid process to supply the posterior auricular and the **occipitalis** muscles. Just below this, the trunk gives off a branch that descends deeply to supply the **stylohyoid** and the **posterior belly of** the **digastric.** The facial nerve,

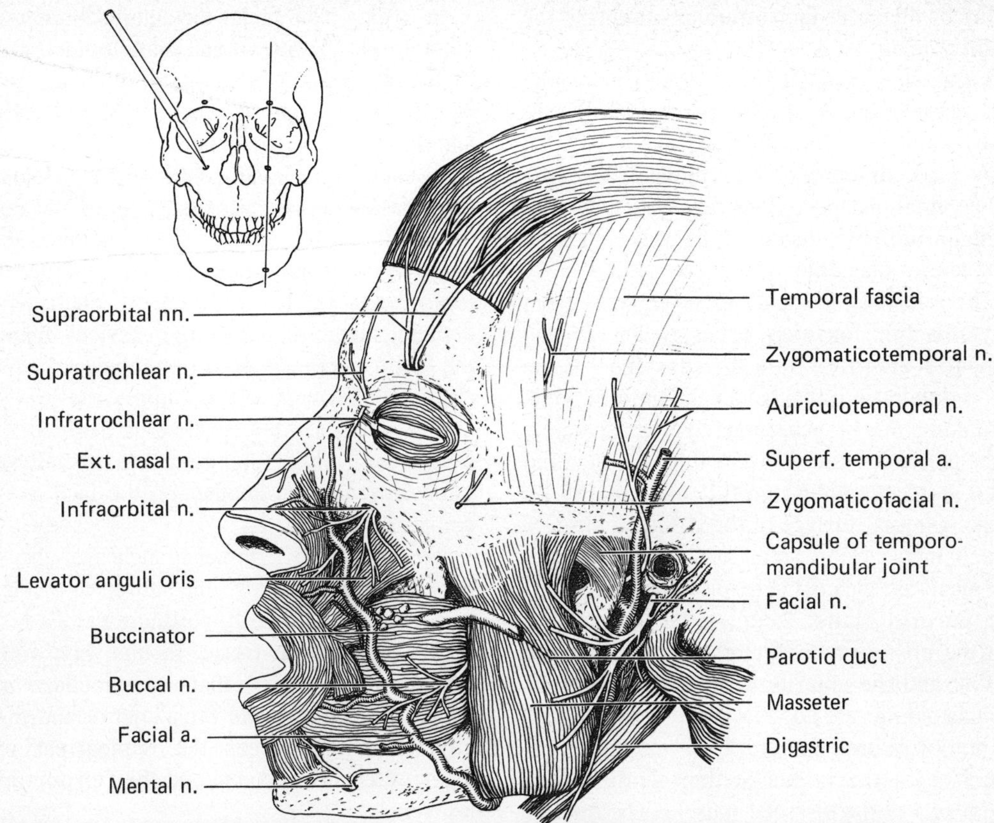

Figure 7.3 Deep dissection of the **face.** The parotid gland has been removed. The inset shows the relationship of the main foramina for superficial nerves and vessels.

still within the parotid, then usually divides into two trunks, an upper and a lower. The **temporal, zygomatic,** and **buccal** branches arise from the **upper trunk;** the **buccal, mandibular,** and **cervical** branches from the **lower trunk** (Fig. 7.3).

The **retromandibular vein** is formed in the region of the root of the zygomatic arch by the union of **superficial temporal** and **maxillary veins.** It descends through the parotid lateral to the external carotid artery, and usually crosses the digastric muscle superficially. At about the level of the angle of the mandible, it divides into two; one branch (posterior facial vein) usually passes forward to join the anterior facial vein to form the common facial vein, which drains into the **internal jugular vein,** and the other branch crosses the sternocleidomastoid to join the **posterior auricular vein** in forming the **external jugular vein.** Since the retromandibular vein lies superficial to the external carotid artery, it may have to be removed in cleaning the artery.

Ascending from the carotid triangle of the neck, deep to the stylohyoid and the posterior belly of the digastric, the **external carotid artery** becomes embedded in the deepest part of the parotid gland, where it is crossed externally by the facial nerve (Fig. 7.3). It ascends behind the posterior border of the ramus of the mandible and terminates posterior to the neck of the mandible by dividing into the **maxillary** and **superficial temporal arteries.** The styloid process is medial to it and separates it from the internal carotid artery. Just above the posterior belly of the digastric, it gives rise to a small **posterior auricular branch,** which accompanies the posterior auricular branch of the facial nerve across the external surface of the mastoid process.

Only the beginning of the maxillary artery can be seen at the present time. It passes forward and medially, deep to the neck of the mandible, to enter the **infratemporal fossa.**

Clean the superficial temporal artery, and at the same time find the auriculotemporal nerve. The **superficial temporal artery** ascends immediately in front of the ear and, at about the level of the upper tip of the auricle, divides into frontal and parietal branches, which ramify in the scalp over the frontal and parietal bones, respectively. Near its origin, it gives rise to the **transverse facial artery,** which passes forward across the face just above the parotid duct. At a slightly higher level, the superficial temporal gives rise to the **middle temporal artery,** which runs forward and pierces the temporal fascia to enter the temporal muscle.

The **auriculotemporal nerve** is a cutaneous nerve derived from the **mandibular division of** the **trigeminal nerve** (CN V). It emerges on the face from behind the condylar process of the mandible and turns upward, in close relation to the superficial temporal artery, to be distributed to the skin of the upper part of the auricle and the greater part of the temporal region (Figs. 7.2 and 7.3).

The **facial artery** reaches the face by winding over the lower border of the mandible at the anterior border of the masseter muscle. It passes upward and forward across the face, pursuing a somewhat tortuous course, to the medial angle of the eye, where its terminal portion is known as the **angular artery.** As it courses across the face, it usually passes deep to the muscles of facial expression, which you should elevate or divide in order to expose the artery. The **superior** and **inferior labial arteries** originate from the anterior aspect of the facial artery and run forward and medially in the upper and lower lips, respectively, to anastomose with similar branches from the opposite side. A **lateral nasal branch** supplies the side of the nose. Numerous irregular branches arise from its posterior aspect to supply the skin and muscles of the cheek.

Clean the **masseter muscle,** one of four muscles belonging to the group known as the **muscles of mastication.** It is a thick quadrilateral muscle that covers the ramus of the mandible externally. It arises from the lower border and internal surface of the **zygomatic arch** and inserts on the external surface of the **ramus** and **body of** the **mandible** near the angle. Its nerve supply, which crosses the **mandibular notch** to enter the deep surface of the muscle, is derived from the **mandibular division of** the **trigeminal nerve;** it will be dissected later.

The **cutaneous nerves** of the face are all derived from the **trigeminal nerve** (CN V). There are three divisions of this nerve, the **ophthalmic, maxillary,** and **mandibular nerves;** each contributes cutaneous branches that appear on the face. Although their terminal ramifications are superficial, the main trunks, which you should now expose, are deep and enter the face by emerging through foramina in the facial bones. To expose the nerves, some of the superficial muscles of facial expression that cover them will have to be separated or retracted (Fig. 7.3).

The cutaneous branches of the **ophthalmic nerve** are the **supraorbital, supratrochlear, infratrochlear, external nasal,** and **lacrimal nerves.** The largest of these is the **supraorbital.** It leaves the orbit at the **supraorbital notch** or **foramen** and passes upward on the frontal bone deep to the frontalis muscle. Its branches pierce the frontalis to supply the skin of the forehead and scalp. The **supratrochlear nerve** is small; it emerges from the upper medial angle of the orbit, under cover of the frontalis and the orbicularis oculi, and supplies the skin in the region of the glabella. The **infratrochlear nerve,** also small, appears on the face just above the medial angle of the eye; it supplies the skin of the upper eyelid and the upper part of the side of the nose. The **external nasal nerve** emerges between the nasal bone and the nasal cartilage and supplies the skin on the bridge of the nose. The **lacrimal nerve** supplies the skin on the lateral part of the upper eyelid but is usually difficult to find.

The cutaneous branches of the **maxillary nerve** are the **infraorbital, zygomaticofacial,** and **zygomaticotemporal nerves.** The **infraorbital** is the terminal part of the maxillary nerve proper. It emerges from the **infraorbital foramen** and branches deep to the infraorbital head of the levator labii superioris to supply the skin of the upper lip, the wing of the nose, the upper part of the cheek, and the lower eyelid. The **zygomaticofacial nerve** emerges through a small foramen in the zygomatic bone to supply the skin over the zygomatic arch. The **zygomaticotemporal** is a minute nerve that emerges through a foramen on the internal aspect of the zygomatic bone and pierces the temporal fascia to supply a small area of skin in the anterior temporal region.

The cutaneous branches of the **mandibular nerve** are the **auriculotemporal,** the **buccal,** and the **mental nerves.** The **auriculotemporal nerve** has already been exposed. The **buccal nerve** emerges from under the anterior border of the masseter and runs downward and forward to supply the skin of the lower part of the cheek. The **mental nerve** emerges from the **mental foramen** of the mandible, under the depressor anguli oris, to supply the skin of the chin and lower lip.

The location of two of the larger nerve trunks can be facilitated by finding the foramina through which they emerge. First note their positions on a skull; then insert the pointed end of a probe through the facial muscles about 1 cm inferior to the midpoint of the inferior orbital ridge. Move the probe around until it enters the **infraorbital foramen.** Similarly, the **mental foramen** can be found by passing the probe through the muscles over the mandible at the level of the root of the second premolar tooth. The **supraorbital foramen** (or notch) lies on the straight line drawn between the other two foramina (Fig. 7.3, inset). When the foramina have been located, separate the fibers of the overlying muscles and secure the nerves emerging through the foramina.

The only deeper muscles of facial expression to which attention need be paid are the levator anguli oris and the buccinator. The **levator anguli oris** arises from the canine fossa of the maxilla under cover of the superficial muscles and descends to the angle of the mouth, where some of its fibers insert directly into the skin and others join the orbicularis oris. The **buccinator** lies in the substance of the cheek. It arises from the molar portion of the alveolar process of the **maxilla,** the external surface of the **mandible** just below the molar teeth, and the **pterygomandibular raphe.** The latter is a fibrous band that extends from the pterygoid hamulus to the upper border of the mandible at the junction of the body and the ramus (see page 74). The muscle fibers pass forward to insert into the mucous membrane near the angle of the mouth and to join the orbicularis oris. Posteriorly, just anterior to the masseter, the buccinator is covered externally by a thick mass of fatty tissue, the **buccal pad;** remove it while cleaning the muscle. The buccinator is pierced by the **parotid duct** and by small branches of the buccal nerve that supply the mucous membrane lining the cheek. The levator anguli oris and the buccinator are both supplied by **buccal branches of** the **facial nerve.**

TEMPORAL AND INFRATEMPORAL REGIONS

The **temporal fascia** is strong and membranous and covers the external surface of the **temporal muscle.** Two thin muscles of the facial group, the superior and anterior auricular muscles, lie superficial to the fascia; remove them. The temporal fascia is attached above to the **superior temporal line,** and below to the upper border of the zygomatic arch and the posterior border of the zygomatic bone. It is thickest inferiorly, where it splits into two layers between which there is a small amount of fatty tissue.

Remove the temporal fascia and clean the external surface of the **temporal muscle,** a muscle of mastication. It arises from the temporal fossa and inserts into the borders and the entire internal surface of the **coronoid process of** the **mandible.**

The masseter muscle must be reflected in order to expose the insertion of the temporal. Insert the handle of a forceps between the zygomatic arch and the outer surface of the temporal muscle. While depressing the temporal muscle, saw through the **zygomatic arch** at its most anterior and posterior ends (Fig. 7.4, cuts A); these cuts should encompass the origin of the masseter. The anterior saw cut must pass posteriorly from below upward to avoid damaging the lateral wall of the orbit. Reflect the arch with the attached masseter downward to the insertion of that muscle by elevating the branches of the facial nerve and passing the masseter muscle and zygomatic arch beneath the nerves. When you reflect the masseter, a small bit of the muscle should be left attached to the nerve that enters its deep surface through the **mandibular notch.** This will aid you later when you are tracing the nerve to its origin. Note the direction of the superficial (downward and backward) and the deep (downward and forward) fibers of the masseter muscle.

When you have thoroughly cleaned the temporal muscle, saw through the **coronoid process** of the mandible at its junction with the ramus (Fig. 7.4, cut B), and reflect the coronoid process with the temporal muscle upward toward the origin of the muscle. This reflection is often complicated by the fact that the deep surface of the temporal muscle is connected by small muscle fasciculi to the deeper muscles of the region (buccinator and lateral pterygoid). Cut the fasciculi if they exist. The temporal muscle is supplied by two or three **deep temporal nerves,** which run upward on the great wing of the sphenoid to enter the deep surface of the muscle; preserve them.

Figure 7.4 Bone cuts needed to open the infratemporal fossa.

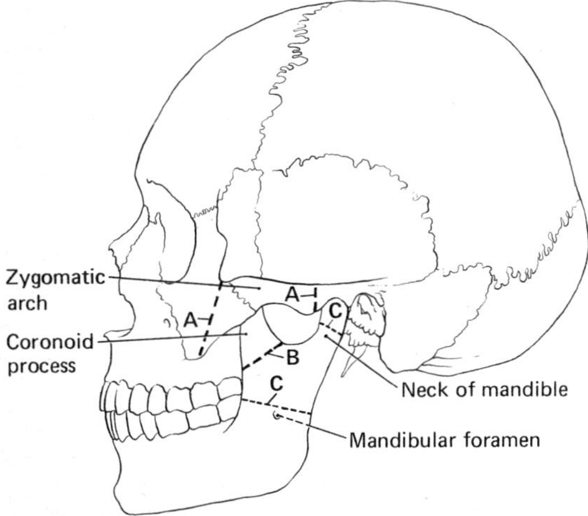

Remove the facial muscles from the area of the mental foramen, being careful to preserve the branches of the **mental nerve** and **artery.** Elevate the facial artery and facial vein from the mandible. Starting at the mental foramen, carefully chip away with a mallet and chisel, aided by bone forceps, the outer table of the mandible to open the **mandibular canal** and expose the course of the **inferior alveolar nerve.** The nerve runs forward through the mandible giving off **dental branches** to the roots of all the lower teeth and **gingival branches** to the mucous membrane of the gum, all of which pass through minute canals in the bone. The **inferior alveolar artery** accompanies the nerve and gives rise to small branches that correspond to those of the nerve.

In order to open the **infratemporal fossa** fully, it is necessary to remove the upper part of the ramus of the mandible. To do this, make two transverse cuts with a saw or bone forceps (Fig. 7.4, cuts C); the superior cut should pass through the neck of the mandible at its junction with the ramus, and the inferior cut must cross the ramus high enough to avoid cutting the **inferior alveolar nerve** and **artery,** which enter the **mandibular foramen** on the inner surface of the ramus.

The **pterygoid plexus of veins** surrounds the maxillary artery and its branches. The plexus usually drains into the deep facial vein, which empties into the facial vein. The plexus also is connected to the cavernous sinus via emissary veins that traverse foramina in the base of the skull.

The latter connections are particularly relevant to the clinician, since infections involving the infratemporal region may pass into the cavernous sinus with the possibility of an ensuing thrombosis.

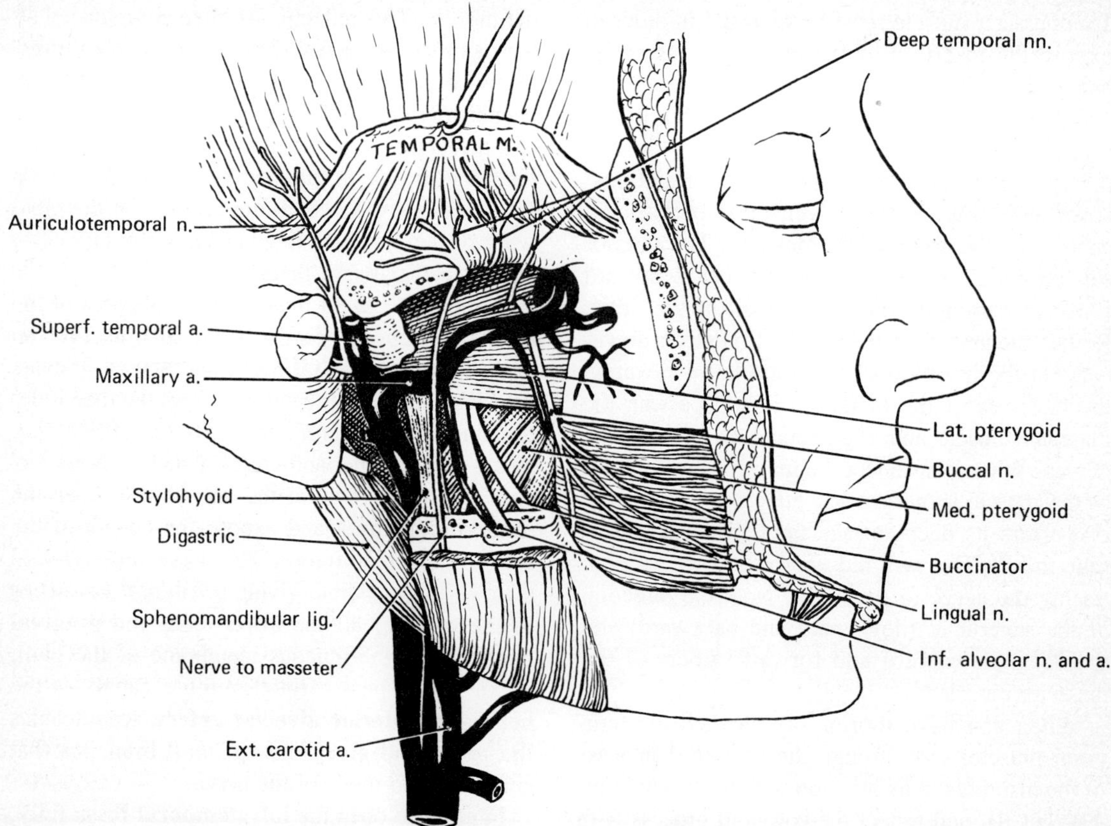

Figure 7.5 Dissection of the **infratemporal fossa.**

Cut away the veins as the other structures are cleaned.

Clean the **lateral pterygoid muscle** first, taking care to preserve any nerves and arteries that may cross its external surface (Fig. 7.5). The lateral pterygoid arises by two heads that are separated by a slight groove. The lower head is the larger one and arises from the external surface of the **lateral pterygoid plate** and from the **tuberosity of** the **maxilla.** The upper head arises from the infratemporal surface of the **great wing of** the **sphenoid.** The fibers of both heads pass backward and laterally and converge to a tendinous insertion into a depression, the pterygoid fossa, on the front of the **neck of** the **mandible.** Some fibers insert into the articular capsule and disk of the temporomandibular joint.

The **buccal nerve** (a branch of the mandibular nerve) usually emerges from between the two heads of the lateral pterygoid. The **deep temporal nerves** usually emerge from under the upper border of the muscle, although the more anterior one may appear between the two heads. Descending from under the inferior border of the lateral pterygoid, two relatively large nerves will be seen. The more anterior one is the **lingual nerve;** it passes downward and forward to reach the inner surface of the mandible in the region of the last molar tooth. Just posterior to the lingual is the **inferior alveolar nerve,** which enters the mandibular foramen on the inner surface of the ramus. Slightly above the mandibular foramen the inferior alveolar gives rise to a small branch, the **mylohyoid nerve,** which descends in the mylohyoid groove on the inner surface of the mandible to reach the digastric triangle. (As shown in Fig. 7.5, the inferior alveolar and lingual nerves pass between the lateral and medial pterygoid muscles, thus helping you to distinguish between the muscles.)

Now clean the **medial pterygoid muscle,** which arises by two heads. The external head, which is the smaller one, arises from the **maxillary tuberosity** and the **pyramidal process of** the **palatine bone.** The large internal head arises from the medial surface of the lateral pterygoid plate; this origin is hidden by the lower head of the lateral pterygoid. The main mass of the medial pterygoid lies below the lateral pterygoid; its fibers run downward, posteriorly, and laterally to insert into the lower half of the internal surface of the **ramus of** the **mandible.**

The **maxillary artery** arises posterior to the neck of the mandible as one of the terminal branches of the external carotid artery. It runs forward, upward, and medially through the **infratemporal fossa** to the **pterygomaxillary fissure,** through which it passes to enter the **pterygopalatine fossa.** It is divided, for descriptive purposes, into **three parts,** the first and second of which lie in the infratemporal fossa. The **first part** extends from the external carotid to the lower border of the lateral pterygoid muscle and lies medial to the neck of the mandible. The **second part** passes from the lower border of the lateral pterygoid muscle to the interval between the two heads of the muscle to enter the pterygomaxillary fissure. The **third part** presently lies hidden in the pterygopalatine fossa. The relationship of the second part of the artery to the lateral pterygoid is variable. In about 50 percent of the cases, the artery crosses the external surface of the muscle; in the other 50 percent, it crosses the deep surface and cannot be exposed until the lateral pterygoid is reflected. Although the structures that receive their blood supply by the maxillary artery are the same in either case, the origin of the branches is somewhat different in the two (see below).

In addition to two small branches, the **anterior tympanic** and the **deep auricular,** the first part of the **maxillary** gives rise to a large branch, the **inferior alveolar artery,** which enters the mandibular foramen in company with the inferior alveolar nerve (Fig. 7.5). When the artery crosses the external surface of the lateral pterygoid, there are additional branches as follows. The first part gives rise to the **middle meningeal artery,** which ascends deep to the lateral pterygoid to enter the **foramen spinosum.** An **accessory meningeal artery** is usually a branch of the middle meningeal, but it can branch directly off the maxillary artery. It courses upward to enter the **foramen ovale.** The second part gives rise to a series of **muscular branches** that supply the temporal, medial and lateral pterygoids and the masseter muscles; and to the **buccal artery,** which accompanies the buccal nerve to the cheek. When the second part of the maxillary crosses the deep surface of the lateral pterygoid, the middle meningeal artery arises from the second part instead of the first and is entirely covered by the lateral pterygoid. The muscular and buccal branches in this case arise from a large common stem off the first part of the maxillary and ascend on the external surface of the lateral pterygoid.

Study the **temporomandibular articulation,** a **synovial** (hinge and gliding) **joint** where the **condyle of** the **mandible** articulates with the **mandibular fossa of** the **temporal bone.** It is enveloped in a loose articular capsule that is strengthened on its lateral aspect by the fibers constituting the **lateral ligament.** This ligament is attached above to the root of the zygomatic process of the temporal bone and narrows inferiorly to its attachment on the lateral aspect of the condyle and neck of the mandible. Define the **sphenomandibular ligament,** an accessory ligament of the joint that is not joined to the capsule but lies medial to it. It is a thin fibrous band running from the spine of the sphenoid to the lingula of the mandible. Cut through the circumference of the capsule and disarticulate the condyle. Observe the **cartilaginous articular disk** that is interposed between the condyle and the mandibular fossa, dividing the articular cavity into distinct superior and inferior parts.

When the condyle is disarticulated, the **lateral pterygoid** may be reflected laterally and forward. If the second part of the maxillary artery lies deep to the lateral pterygoid, it can now be seen, and the **middle meningeal artery** can be traced to the foramen spinosum. At the same time, clean the mandibular nerve and its branches (Fig. 7.6).

The **mandibular nerve** emerges from the cranial cavity through the **foramen ovale** and divides almost immediately into a small anterior and a large posterior part. The anterior division runs forward for a short distance under cover of the lateral pterygoid and then, either by passing between its two heads or, much less frequently, by winding over its upper border, reaches the external surface of that muscle. From this point, it is known as the **buccal nerve,** whose further course has already been seen. While still deep to the lateral pterygoid, the anterior division gives rise to several muscular branches: the **deep temporal nerves** that supply the temporal muscle, and the **nerves** that supply the **masseter** and the **lateral pterygoid** muscles.

The posterior division of the mandibular nerve descends for a short distance and divides into the **lingual,** the **inferior alveolar,** and the **auriculotemporal nerves.** The lingual and inferior alveolar nerves descend deep to the lateral pterygoid, pass between it and the medial pterygoid, and then course along the external surface of the medial pterygoid, where they have already been seen. Observe that the lingual is joined, just below its origin, by a tiny nerve that may be seen running

Figure 7.6 **Deep** dissection of the **infratemporal fossa.**

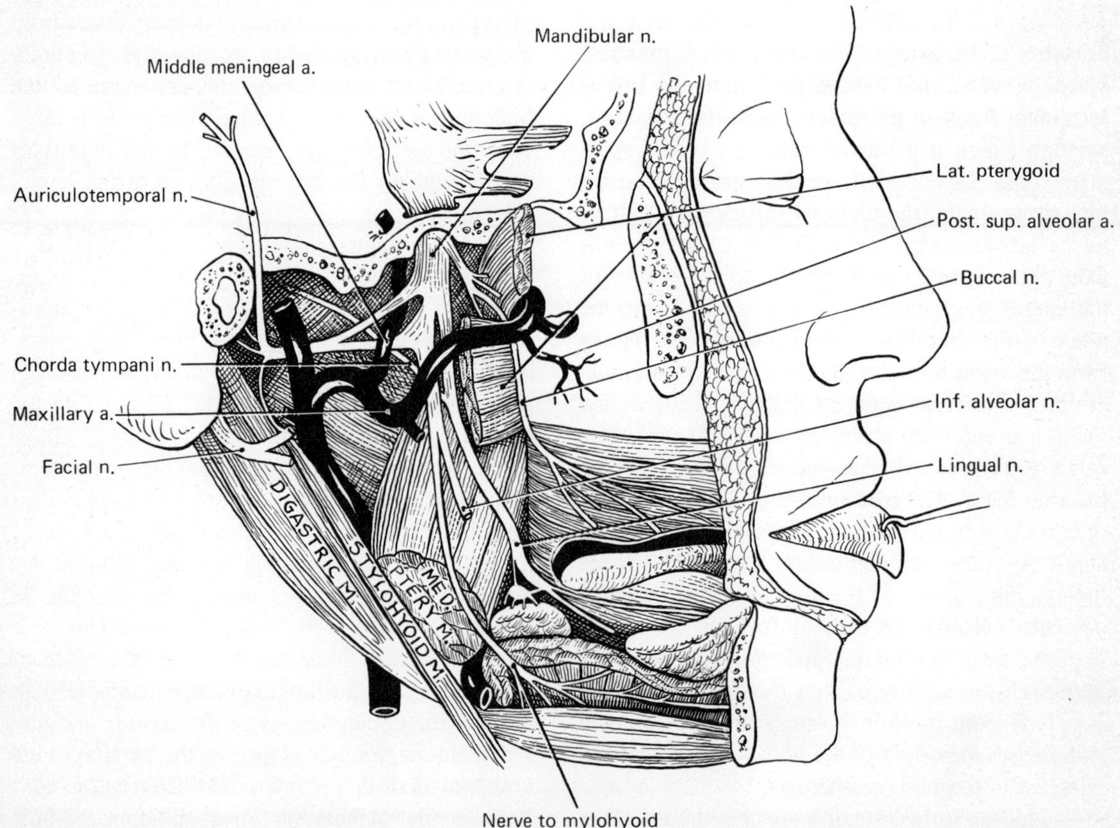

downward and forward medial to the inferior alveolar nerve. This is the **chorda tympani,** a branch of the seventh cranial nerve. It passes through the petrotympanic fissure of the temporal bone to enter the infratemporal fossa, where it joins the lingual nerve.

The **auriculotemporal nerve** usually arises by two roots that embrace the **middle meningeal artery** and join behind it. The nerve then passes posteriorly, winds laterally behind the temporomandibular joint, and turns upward over the root of the zygomatic arch, from which point its further course has been traced.

Attempt to demonstrate the **nerve** supply **to** the **medial pterygoid muscle.** This small nerve usually arises directly from the trunk of the mandibular nerve just below the foramen ovale and enters the upper part of the medial pterygoid muscle.

The **otic ganglion** should be noted on the medial side of the mandibular nerve, just below the foramen ovale. It is one of the parasympathetic ganglia in the head; review the nerves passing to and from this ganglion from one of the standard texts.

CRANIAL CAVITY

To open the cranial cavity, the scalp must be stripped from the bony vault of the skull. Continue the median sagittal incision through the scalp from the **bregma** *(see page 40) to the* **external occipital protuberance.** *At a right angle to this incision make another one at about the midpoint of the* **sagittal suture** *and extend it laterally to each ear. Turn the various layers of the scalp downward and laterally on each side, leaving the external surface of the bones of the cranial vault clean.*

Identify the five layers of the scalp. They are, from superficial to deep, (1) the skin, (2) connective tissue of dense type, (3) the aponeurosis (galea aponeurotica) of the epicranius muscle (frontalis muscle and occipitalis muscle), (4) a loose connective tissue layer, and (5) the periosteum of the skull bones, here called the **pericranium.** Usually, removing the scalp is easy because the fourth layer (i.e., the loose connective tissue layer) acts as a cleavage plane between the pericranium, which is especially adherent to the bone, and the outer three layers, which are nearly inseparable by gross dissection.

The structure of the scalp is the basis for the observations that scalp wounds bleed profusely and that blood and other extravasates may collect and track in the scalp. The rich blood supply of the scalp is distributed through the dense connective tissue layer. Severed blood vessels held open by the connective tissue are unable to collapse, and therefore, bleeding is copious. Blood or infectious substances can track along the loose connective layer unhindered except posteriorly where the occipitalis muscle inserts into the superior nuchal line of the occipital bone. Anteriorly, fluid can collect in the forehead because the frontalis muscle inserts into the skin rather than into bone. Clinically, scalp infections are noteworthy because of the venous interconnections between the scalp and the brain via the **emissary veins.** The loose connective tissue layer is often referred to as the "danger area."

Reflect any remnants of the **temporal muscles** *downward from the upper part of the temporal fossae. Then tie a string around the cranium, and with a wax pencil or piece of chalk, mark a line on the bone along the string. Anteriorly, this line should be about 2.5 cm above the upper margin of the orbits and, posteriorly, about 1 cm above the external occipital protuberance. With a saw, cut through the* **outer table** *of the bones along the line. When the* **diploë** *is reached, the* **inner table** *can be broken through with a chisel. If the cut is made with an oscillating saw, cut through both tables of bone at one time. The* **calvaria** *(skullcap) can then be pulled off, exposing the external surface of the dura mater of the brain.*

CRANIAL MENINGES AND DURAL VENOUS SINUSES

The **cranial dura** consists of two layers: the outer layer, or **endocranium,** is actually the periosteum of the inner surface of the cranial bones; the inner or **meningeal layer** of the cranial dura is analogous to the spinal dura, with which it is continuous at the foramen magnum. In most regions, the two layers of the cranial dura are firmly attached to one another, but in certain places they separate to enclose blood spaces, the **dural venous sinuses.** The dural sinuses are, in fact, veins, but they differ from typical veins in that the actual wall of each vessel consists only of an endothelial layer; the chief support of the wall is provided by the dura mater in which the vessel is enclosed. The endocranium is everywhere closely applied to the inner surface of the cranial bones. The meningeal layer, however, shows reduplications, or double folds, which project into the cranial cavity and partially subdivide it and the brain. The reduplications, which will be seen as the dissection proceeds, are the **falx cerebri,** the **tentorium cerebelli,** the **falx cerebelli,** and the **diaphragma sellae.**

Make a sagittal incision through the dura about 1.5 cm lateral to the midline on each side from the frontal to the occipital region; at each end of these incisions, make transverse incisions. Turn these marked flaps of dura laterally to expose the **subdural space** and the **arachnoid.** The cranial arachnoid is a delicate membrane through which the upper surface of the **cerebral hemispheres** can be readily seen. It, too, is continuous with the arachnoid of the spinal cord.

Observe the numerous **superior cerebral veins** that leave the upper surface of the cerebral hemispheres and pierce the arachnoid to enter the dura close to the median line. These veins carry blood to the **superior sagittal sinus,** which you should now open by making a median sagittal incision in the dura. The superior sagittal sinus, one of the dural venous sinuses, is enclosed within the dura mater. It begins anteriorly at the **crista galli** of the ethmoid bone and extends posteriorly along the cranial vault in the median plane to the **internal occipital protuberance,** where it terminates by joining the right (less frequently the left) **transverse sinus.** Note the lateral extensions, the **lateral lacunae,** from the sinus. In its course, the superior sagittal sinus receives emissary veins from the scalp as well as the superior cerebral veins.

Spread the cerebral hemispheres apart and observe the **falx cerebri.** This double fold of the meningeal layer of the dura mater stretches downward in the median plane **(longitudinal cerebral fissure)** between the two hemispheres. Superiorly, its two layers separate to enclose the superior sagittal sinus and become continuous with the inner layer of cranial dura on each side. Anteriorly, it is attached to the crista galli. Its inferior border is free except posteriorly, where it joins the tentorium cerebelli. The **inferior sagittal sinus** is enclosed within the lower free margin of the falx cerebri.

To study the cranial vault thoroughly and to gain an understanding of the relationships of its structures to the brain, you must now remove the brain. Attempt to remove the entire brain intact, which will facilitate studying the cranial nerves and arteries found on the base of the brain. You will need to refer frequently to a macerated skull for orientation. Cut the falx cerebri from the crista galli and pull its free anterior portion upward and posteriorly, out of the longitudinal cerebral fissure (Fig. 7.7, cut A). Gently separate the posterior poles of the hemispheres **(occipital lobes)** and locate the **tentorium cerebelli,** the double fold of dura that courses in the **transverse cerebral fissure** and roofs the **posterior cranial fossa.** Now carefully make a parasagittal incision in the tentorium extending from its free anterior margin to the occipital bone posteriorly (Fig. 7.7, cut B). Tilt the head well backward and carefully draw the anterior poles **(frontal lobes)** of the cerebrum upward and backward from the floor of the **anterior cranial fossa.** As this is done, you will see the minute filaments of the **olfactory nerves** (CN I) piercing the cribriform plate of the ethmoid bone to reach their respective **olfactory bulbs.** The **optic nerves** (CN II) will next come into view, passing from the optic canals to the optic chiasma at the rostral extent of the brainstem. Cut the optic

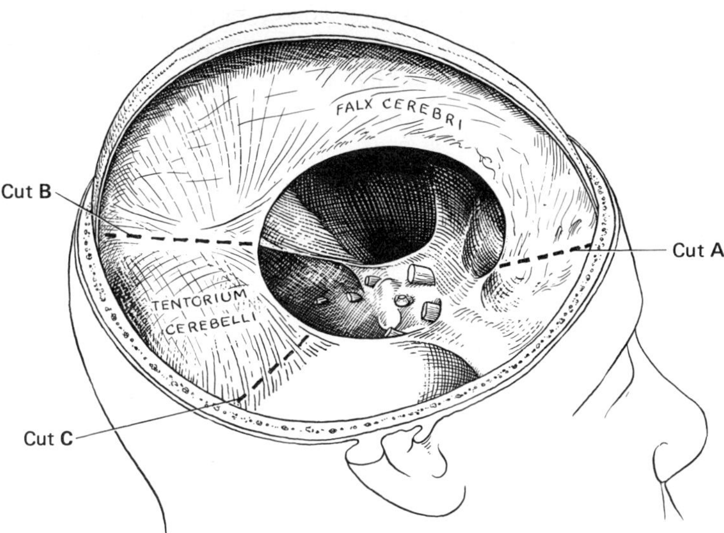

Figure 7.7 Dural reduplications seen with the brain removed to show the positions of the dural incisions needed to remove the brain from the cranium.

nerves just posterior to the optic canals. As you continue to lift the frontal lobes gently, the two **internal carotid arteries** will be seen, one on each side just below the optic canals, running posteriorly to the base of the brain; cut them. In the midline, between the internal carotid arteries, the **infundibulum** will appear. This narrow stalk of nervous tissue connects the base of the brain with the **pituitary gland (hypophysis);** transect it. Now gently dislodge the **temporal lobes** of the cerebral hemispheres from the **middle cranial fossae** and continue to lift the brain slowly farther upward and backward. The anterior part of the tentorium cerebelli will be seen. You should also see a portion of the brainstem, the **midbrain (mesencephalon),** passing upward from the posterior cranial fossa at the free margin of the tentorium. Now carefully make an incision through the tentorium on the right side extending laterally and backward about 1.5 cm medial to the tentorium's line of attachment to the superior border of the petrous part of the temporal bone (Fig. 7.7, cut C). Make a similar incision on the left side. Reflect the tentorium from the transverse fissure posteriorly toward the back of the skull. In so doing, you will expose the **cerebellum** and segments of the brainstem. Attempt to identify the remaining cranial nerves and transect them near their point of attachment to the brainstem.

The **oculomotor nerves** (CN III), which are relatively large, arise from the ventral surface of the midbrain near the median line. The **trochlear nerves** (CN IV) are much smaller; they originate from the dorsal surface of the midbrain and wind ventrally around its lateral border. You will find the filaments that make up the large roots of the **trigeminal nerves** (CN V) arising from the sides of the pons. The **abducens nerves** (CN VI) attach to the caudal border of the **pons,** near the midline. Slightly more laterally at the same level, find the **facial** (CN VII) and **vestibulocochlear** (CN VIII) **nerves.** The **basilar artery** will be found running forward in the midline along the ventral surface of the pons; divide it. Inferior to the pons, the brainstem narrows to become the **medulla oblongata.** The roots of the **glossopharyngeal** (CN IX), **vagus** (CN X), and **accessory** (CN XI) **nerves** arise from the sides of the medulla; the **hypoglossal nerve** (CN XII) arises from its ventral surface. Having severed the roots of the cranial nerves and the basilar artery, transect the medulla just above the **foramen magnum.** Carefully remove the intact brain from the cranial cavity.

Set the brain aside for the time being and resume studying the cranial dural venous sinuses and dural reflections, both of which should still be almost entirely intact.

Examine the **tentorium cerebelli.** It is a transverse reduplication of the meningeal dura interposed in the transverse cerebral fissure between the posterior parts of the cerebral hemispheres and the cerebellum. Its outer border is attached to the anterior and posterior clinoid processes, the superior border of the petrous portion of the temporal bone, the posteroinferior angle of the parietal bone, and the transverse ridges of the occipital bone. Its inner or anterior border is free and forms the margin of an opening, the **tentorial notch,** through which the posterior cranial fossa communicates with the middle cranial fossae. In the midline, the upper surface of the tentorium is joined to the posterior part of the falx cerebri.

Next, in the posterior cranial fossa, find the **falx cerebelli,** a small triangular fold of dura that attaches to the inferior surface of the tentorium and to the median crest of the occipital bone. Its free edge projects between the cerebellar hemispheres.

Using the infundibulum as a central point, make a circular incision through the dura about 1 cm lateral to it. Elevate the circular piece of dura, the **diaphragma sellae,** and observe the pituitary gland sitting in the **hypophyseal fossa of** the **sella turcica.**

Tumors of the pituitary gland often expand superiorly beyond the limits of the fossa. Compression of the optic chiasma, causing visual impairments, usually results.

Open the venous sinuses that are enclosed by the layers of the tentorium. The **straight sinus** is in the median plane, along the junction of the tentorium and the falx cerebri. The sinus begins as a continuation of the inferior sagittal sinus at the tentorial notch, where it also receives the **great cerebral vein,** and passes straight posteriorly to the **internal occipital protuberance.** The straight sinus ends usually by joining the **left transverse sinus.** The **right transverse sinus** most commonly is a continuation of the superior sagittal sinus, as mentioned above. These relationships may, however, be reversed, or all four sinuses may come together as the **confluence of** the **sinuses** at the internal occipital protuberance. The transverse sinus of each side begins at the internal occipital protuberance and passes laterally, enclosed within the attached margin of the tentorium, along the occipital bone. At the lateral end of the superior border of the petrous part of the temporal bone, it turns downward in the dura lining the wall of the posterior cranial fossa. This segment of the sinus is called the **sigmoid sinus.** Observe that it pursues a curved course downward and medially to enter the **jugular foramen.** Inferior to the foramen, the sigmoid sinus is continuous with the **internal jugular vein.**

The **occipital sinus,** which is enclosed in the attached margin of the falx cerebelli, extends from the area of the foramen magnum and drains into one of the transverse sinuses or the confluence of sinuses.

The **cavernous sinuses** lie between the two layers of dura at the sides of the sella turcica. Each receives blood from the **superior** and **inferior ophthalmic veins,** which enter it from the orbit by passing through the **superior orbital fissure,** and from the **sphenoparietal sinus,** which lies within the dura along the free margin of the lesser wing of the sphenoid bone. The cavernous sinuses drain posteriorly through the **superior** and **inferior petrosal sinuses.** The cavernous sinuses of the two sides are united by the **anterior** and **posterior intercavernous sinuses,** which lie in the diaphragma sellae anterior and posterior to the pituitary infundibulum. In close relation to the lateral wall of each cavernous sinus are the trochlear and oculomotor nerves, the trigeminal ganglion, and the ophthalmic and maxillary divisions of the trigeminal nerve. Projecting farther medially into the sinus are the abducens nerve and the internal carotid artery.

The cavernous sinus has numerous connections with the facial vein not only through the ophthalmic veins as mentioned but also through the deep facial vein, the pterygoid venous plexus, and emissary veins that pass from the plexus to the sinus through the foramen ovale, the foramen spinosum, or other foramina in the area. Although the facial area of the lips, nose, and eyes usually drains through the facial vein into the internal jugular vein, it can, under certain conditions, drain into the cavernous sinuses because of the absence of valves in the veins. Infectious materials can then be carried from this "danger area" of the face to the cavernous sinuses, resulting in **cavernous sinus thrombosis,** a very serious condition that often causes neurologic damage by blockage of the venous drainage of the eyes and by pressure on the nerves traversing the sinus.

The **superior petrosal sinus** is enclosed in the outer margin of the tentorium, where it attaches to the superior border of the petrous part of the temporal bone. It begins just lateral to the posterior clinoid process, where it receives blood from the cavernous sinus, and ends by joining the transverse sinus at the point where the latter turns inferiorly as the sigmoid sinus.

The **inferior petrosal sinus** lies in the groove between the basal portion of the occipital bone and the petrous portion of the temporal bone. Running from the lower posterior part of the cavernous sinus, it passes through the jugular foramen to join the internal jugular vein.

BRAIN

This section is designed to acquaint you with some of the larger structures that can be seen grossly on the surface of the brain. When these are studied in conjunction with the dissection that follows, your primary objective should be to correlate the surfaces and surface structures of the brain with the subdivisions, foramina, and dural folds of the cranial vault. A detailed account of brain structure and function should be sought in a neuroscience course.

Use the intact brain that you removed from the cranium. Some of the meningeal coverings should still be present, although most, if not all, of the dura mater has probably already been removed from the surfaces of the brain. The **arachnoid** and **pia mater** should still be present; they are structurally similar to the respective spinal meninges with which they are continuous at the **foramen magnum.** The outer parts of the brain can be seen through them, and you will note that the arachnoid is a thin, weblike covering that extends over the convolutions and processes of the brain. The **subarachnoid space** is continued into the spinal subarachnoid space, and like it, contains cerebrospinal fluid. In certain areas, particularly on each side of the superior sagittal sinus, projections of the arachnoid, **arachnoid granulations,** protrude through the dura into the venous sinuses and lateral lacunae.

Currently, the granulations are thought to serve as part of the turnover mechanism for cerebrospinal fluid eliminating it into the venous system.

Look at the internal surface of the calvaria and note the pits that the granulations create in the bone. Gently remove the arachnoid from the brain and be particularly careful to avoid destroying the blood vessels and cranial nerves.

The **pia mater,** unlike the arachnoid, is closely applied to the outer surface of, and sends trabecular prolongations into, the substance of the brain.

The two **cerebral hemispheres** are the most conspicuous parts of the human brain. As a result of the growth of the hemispheres, their cortex is convoluted and folded in the form of elevations (**gyri**) and furrows (**sulci**). The various gyri and sulci are topographically similar in all brains and all are named. One of the main sulci is the horizontal **lateral sulcus.** It is on the lateral convexity of each hemisphere, beginning anteriorly and extending posteriorly (Figs. 7.8 and 7.9). The **central sulcus** is also on the lateral surface of the cerebrum, running from the middle of the superior margin of the hemisphere downward toward the lateral fissure. Note that superiorly and medially it extends onto the medial surface of the hemisphere. Gently pull the posterior poles of the

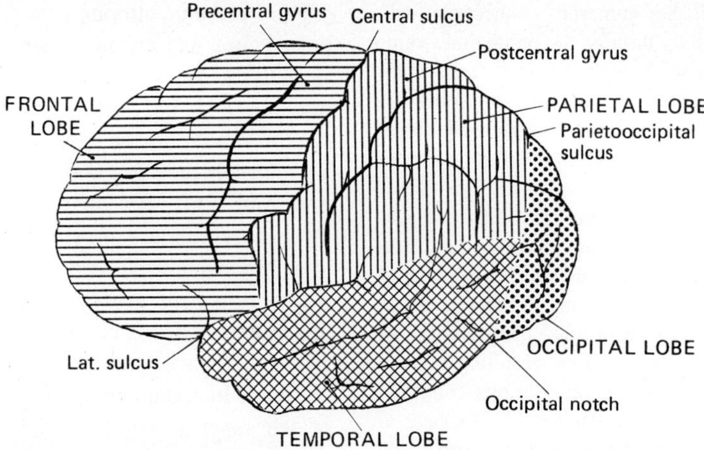

Figure 7.8 Cerebral hemisphere, lateral view.

cerebral hemispheres apart and locate the **parieto-occipital sulcus.** As mentioned below, it helps to distinguish the **parietal** and **occipital lobes** from one another.

Identify the **precentral** and **postcentral gyri;** they are anterior and posterior to the central sulcus, respectively. The precentral gyrus is the primary motor area, and the postcentral gyrus is the primary sensory area.

Each hemisphere is composed of four major lobes: **frontal, parietal, occipital,** and **temporal** (Figs. 7.8 and 7.9). They are named after the bones that cover them. The **frontal lobe** is the largest, extending posteriorly from the anterior aspect of the cerebral hemisphere to the central sulcus and inferiorly to the lateral sulcus. The **temporal lobe** lies inferior to the lateral sulcus. The **parietal lobe** is bounded anteriorly by the central sulcus, inferiorly by a line along the lateral sulcus, and posteriorly by an imaginary vertical line drawn from the parietooccipital sulcus. The **occipital lobe,** which rests on the tentorium, is bounded anteriorly by the same imaginary line.

Note the **cerebellum** lying inferior to the occip-

Figure 7.9 Cerebral hemisphere, medial view.

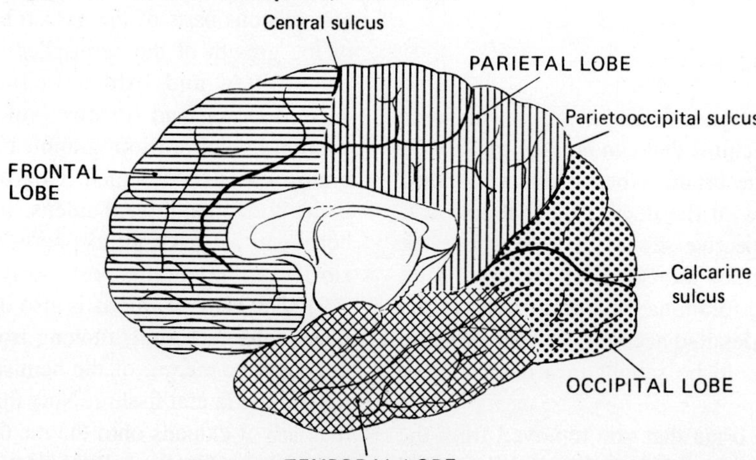

ital lobes of the cerebral hemispheres, from which it is separated in the living by the tentorium cerebelli. The cerebellum is also divided into lobes, processes, and hemispheres, the surfaces of which are noticeably wavy, but a detailed knowledge of them is not necessary here.

Turn the brain over and study its inferior surface (base) (Fig. 7.10). The frontal and temporal lobes of the cerebral hemispheres and the cerebellum are again quite obvious. Direct your attention to the centrally placed **brainstem** and its subdivisions. Starting with the cut end of the spinal cord, observe that it is continuous rostrally with the **medulla oblongata,** which has a well-defined **anterior median sulcus.** The medulla is about 2.5 cm long and ends at the **pons,** which is easily recognized as a prominent ridge of transverse fibers extending laterally into the hemispheres of the cerebellum. The **midbrain** (mesencephalon) is found immediately rostral to the pons. The only parts of the midbrain visible are the paired, cordlike, right and left **crura cerebri.** The space between the crura is the **interpeduncular fossa.** Between the crura and the **optic chiasma,** you will notice a small, cone-shaped piece of tissue, the **tuber cinereum,** with which the infundibulum is continuous. The tuber represents the most inferior aspect of the diencephalon. Finally, most anteriorly, the **olfactory bulbs** and their posterior extensions, the **olfactory tracts,** will be seen running along the medial aspects of the frontal lobes.

Now study the cranial nerves and give particular emphasis to the area of the brain's surface with which each is associated (see page 53; also see Fig. 7.10).

The entire brain receives its blood supply from the two **vertebral** and two **internal carotid arteries.** On the base of the brain near the optic

Figure 7.10 Cranial nerves on the inferior surface of the brain.

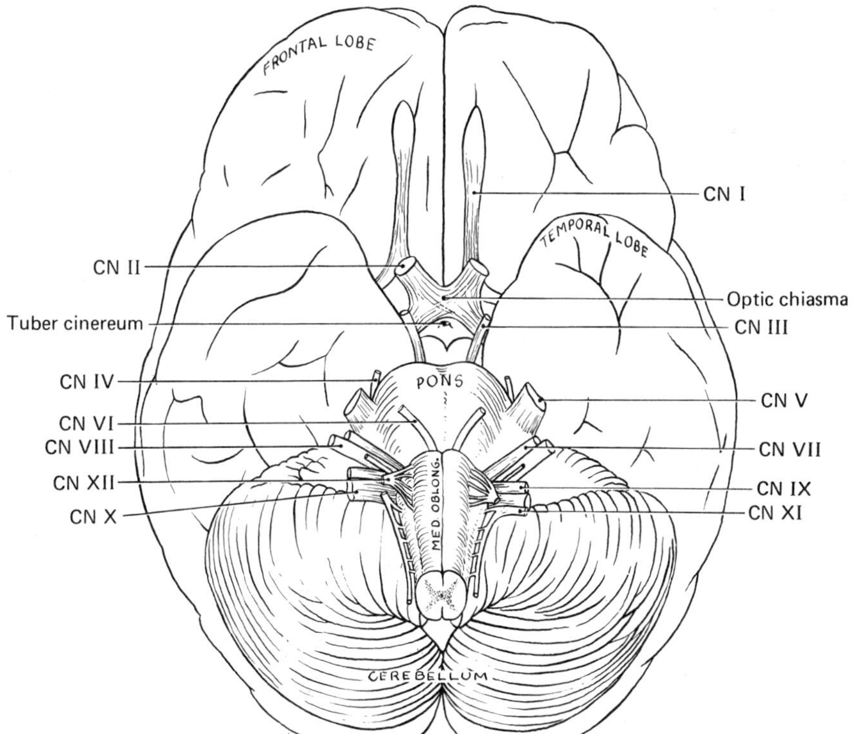

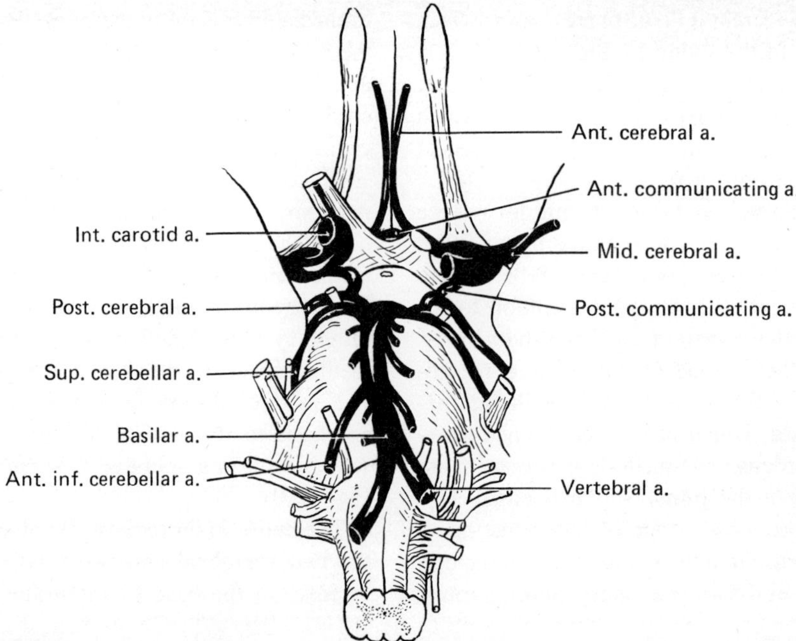

Figure 7.11 The **cerebral arterial circle.**

chiasma, locate the cut ends of the internal carotid arteries (Fig. 7.11). After contributing numerous small branches to the brain, each internal carotid terminates by dividing into **anterior** and **middle cerebral arteries,** which distribute to the medial aspect of the frontal and parietal lobes and to the lateral aspects of the frontal, parietal, and temporal lobes, respectively. Follow the anterior cerebral artery anteriorly into the longitudinal cerebral fissure, and notice the short **anterior communicating artery** that joins the two anterior cerebrals just rostral to the optic chiasma. The middle cerebral artery courses laterally between the temporal and frontal lobes; near its origin, it gives rise to the **posterior communicating artery** that passes posteriorly along the ventral surface of the brain to anastomose with the posterior cerebral artery (see below).

After entering the posterior cranial fossa through the foramen magnum, the two vertebral arteries give rise to the **anterior spinal, posterior spinal,** and **posterior inferior cerebellar arteries**; they then unite to form the unpaired **basilar artery** in the region of the medullary-pontine junction. The basilar artery runs forward along the median plane of the pons and provides numerous **pontine branches** and most of the blood supply to the cerebellum through the **anterior inferior** and **superior cerebellar arteries.** In the interpeduncular region, the basilar artery bifurcates into the **posterior cerebral arteries,** each of which courses rostral to the oculomotor nerve and winds laterally around the midbrain to distribute primarily to each of the occipital lobes and a little to each temporal lobe. As mentioned above, each posterior cerebral artery anastomoses with the posterior communicating artery of the same side.

Having identified the major arteries, you should examine the **cerebral arterial circle** (of Willis), a seven-sided arterial ring situated around the optic chiasma, the tuber cinereum, and the interpeduncular region. It is formed by the anastomosis of the anterior cerebral, the anterior communicating, the posterior communicating, and the posterior cerebral arteries. The numerous branches that arise from the circle course dorsally into the brain tissue.

Although it has not been well proved, the arterial circle is said to help equalize the distribution of blood to various brain regions and to dampen the blood pressure in the small and delicate brain arteries and arterioles.

CRANIAL FOSSAE

Now returning to your cadaver, relate the gross structures of the brain that you have just learned to the bony cranial vault. For example, notice that the frontal lobes of the cerebral hemispheres occupy the anterior cranial fossa, the floor of which forms the roof of the orbits. Notice that the temporal lobes sit snugly in the middle cranial fossae and that the cerebellum, midbrain, pons, and medulla are housed in the posterior cranial fossa.

Compare the floor of the cranial cavity as it now appears with the internal base of a macerated skull. The differences that will appear depend on the fact that the meningeal layer of the cranial dura does not closely follow the contour of the bones in all regions, but is separated to some extent from the endocranium by structures that are interposed between the two layers. This is particularly true in the **middle cranial fossa**, where you should note that nothing can be seen of the superior orbital fissure, the foramen rotundum, the foramen ovale, the carotid canal, or the foramen spinosum as long as the meningeal layer of the dura is intact, bridging the openings. Some cranial nerves pierce the inner layer of the dura at a considerable distance from the foramina through which they leave the skull, passing forward between the two layers to reach these foramina.

Observe the points at which the oculomotor, trochlear, trigeminal, and abducens nerves pierce the meningeal dura. The **oculomotor nerve** is most anterior, entering the dura at the side of the posterior clinoid process. The **trochlear nerve** enters the dura at the most anterior point of attachment of the tentorium cerebelli. The point of entry for the **trigeminal nerve** is slightly posterior and inferior to that of the trochlear; it is covered superiorly by the narrow anterior part of the tentorium. The **abducens nerve** enters the dura well back on the floor of the posterior fossa. To follow the further course of these nerves, the inner layer of the dura must be carefully stripped from the floor of the middle cranial fossa at the side of the sella turcica. As this is done, the cavernous sinus is opened.

Clean the **trigeminal nerve**. Shortly after it enters the dura, its root fibers expand to form the **trigeminal ganglion.** This large ganglion is covered by the inner layer of dura, forming the lower lateral wall of the cavernous sinus. From the ganglion, the **ophthalmic division** of the trigeminal nerve passes forward in the lateral wall of the sinus to reach the **superior orbital fissure.** As it reaches the fissure, the ophthalmic nerve divides into the lacrimal, frontal, and nasociliary nerves, but those nerves probably cannot be identified until the orbit is opened. Below the ophthalmic nerve, in the lower part of the lateral wall of the cavernous sinus, the **maxillary division** of the trigeminal nerve runs forward to the **foramen rotundum**. The **mandibular division** passes directly inferiorly from the posterior part of the ganglion to the **foramen ovale**.

The **oculomotor** and **trochlear nerves** pass forward in the upper part of the lateral wall of the cavernous sinus. The oculomotor is the highest of all the nerves, with the trochlear lying between it and the ophthalmic nerve. These three nerves enter the orbit at the superior orbital fissure. The **abducens nerve** passes farther medially into the cavernous sinus; it runs forward medial to the ophthalmic nerve and lateral to the internal carotid artery to enter the orbit at the superior orbital fissure.

The **internal carotid artery** enters the cranial cavity at the internal opening of the carotid canal, which lies just superior to the **foramen lacerum.** Running forward between the two layers of the dura, the artery enters the cavernous sinus. Below the anterior clinoid process, it turns upward medially and then backward to pierce the meningeal layer of the dura just inferior and posterior to the **optic foramen.** As it emerges from the dura, it gives rise to the **ophthalmic artery,** which passes forward into the orbit through the optic foramen, where it lies immediately inferior to the optic nerve.

Observe that the **facial** and **vestibulocochlear nerves** leave the posterior cranial fossa by entering the **internal auditory meatus** in the petrous part of the temporal bone. The **glossopharyngeal, vagus,** and **accessory nerves** enter the medial end of the **jugular foramen.** Medial to the jugular foramen but in the anterolateral wall of the foramen magnum is the **hypoglossal canal,** through which the **hypoglossal nerve** leaves the cranial cavity. Observe that the **vertebral artery** enters the cranium on each side at the lateral margin of the **foramen magnum.** Passing forward and medially over the floor of the posterior fossa, the two vertebral arteries join to form the basilar artery. Separate the facial from the vestibulocochlear nerve and attempt to identify the smaller, intervening **nervus intermedius.**

Observe the distribution of the **middle meningeal artery.** This vessel, a branch of the **maxillary artery,** enters the cranial cavity at the **foramen spinosum** and divides almost at once into anterior and posterior branches, which are distributed to the dura mater of the floors of the anterior and middle cranial fossae and of the cranial vault. These vessels are embedded in the outer layer of the dura but can usually be clearly seen through the dura without dissection. The dura of the posterior cranial fossa is supplied by one or two small **meningeal branches** of the occipital artery, which reach the dura by passing through the jugular foramen.

Use Table 7.1 as a guide to the structures that traverse the various foramina, canals, and fissures of the cranial fossae.

ORBIT

The orbit is approached by removing the **orbital plate** *of the frontal bone; use a chisel to break through the orbital plate about 2.5 cm lateral to the crista galli. Then chip away the remaining part of the plate, noting the position of the* **frontal sinus** *within the bone. Using the handle of a forceps, depress the orbital periosteum (***periorbita***) and orbital contents downward in the front part of the orbital cavity. Then make two saw cuts down through the squamous portion of the frontal bone to the floor of the* **anterior cranial fossa;** *the first opposite the end of the* **cribriform plate** *of the ethmoid and the second downward and medial, opposite the end of the lesser wing of the sphenoid. Then reflect the cut section of the frontal bone forward. In order to observe the mucous membrane lining of the* **ethmoid air cells** *and the course of the* **anterior** *and* **posterior ethmoid vessels** *and* **nerves,** *gently remove the lateral part of the cribriform plate of the ethmoid bone with the aid of a chisel or bone forceps. The lesser wing of the sphenoid bone may be carefully chipped away with the bone forceps, to open the superior orbital fissure completely from above; it is advisable, however, to leave the bony rim of the optic canal intact.*

If the orbit has been carefully opened, the **periorbita** of its roof, which is very loosely attached to the bone, will remain intact. The periorbita should be slit longitudinally and reflected to each side to expose the orbital contents from above. The structures contained in the orbit are embedded in loose fatty tissue, which must be removed piecemeal as the dissection proceeds.

Three nerves—the **trochlear,** the **frontal,** and the **lacrimal**—are the most superior structures in the orbit and should be cleaned first. All enter the orbit through the upper part of the superior orbital fissure. The trochlear nerve is the most medial; it passes forward and medially to end in the **superior oblique muscle,** which may be seen occupying the angle between the roof and the medial wall of the orbit (Fig. 7.12).

The **frontal nerve** is the largest of the three terminal branches (the lacrimal and the nasociliary being the other two) of the **ophthalmic nerve.** Passing forward in the midline of the orbit, it lies immediately above the **levator palpebrae superioris muscle.** About midway in its course through

Table 7.1 Structures That Traverse the Foramina, Canals, and Fissures of the Cranial Fossae

- **I** Anterior fossa
  - ***A*** Foramen cecum
    - **1** Vein from nose to superior sagittal sinus
  - ***B*** Anterior ethmoidal foramen
    - **1** Anterior ethmoidal vessels and nerve
  - ***C*** Posterior ethmoidal foramen
    - **1** Posterior ethmoidal vessels and nerve
  - ***D*** Foramina in cribriform plate
    - **1** Olfactory nerves (CNI)
- **II** Middle fossa
  - ***A*** Superior orbital fissure
    - **1** Ophthalmic veins
    - **2** Oculomotor nerve (CN III)
    - **3** Trochlear nerve (CN IV)
    - **4** Ophthalmic nerve (V_1)
    - **5** Abducens nerve (CN VI)
    - **6** Orbital branch of middle meningeal artery
    - **7** Recurrent (dural) branch of lacrimal artery
  - ***B*** Optic canal
    - **1** Optic nerve (CN II)
    - **2** Ophthalmic artery
  - ***C*** Foramen rotundum
    - **1** Maxillary nerve (V_2)
  - ***D*** Foramen ovale
    - **1** Mandibular nerve (V_3)
    - **2** Accessory meningeal artery
    - **3** Emissary veins
  - ***E*** Foramen lacerum
    - **1** Meningeal branch of ascending pharyngeal artery
    - **2** Emissary veins
    - **3** Nerve of pterygoid canal (or its components)
  - ***F*** Carotid canal
    - **1** Internal carotid artery
    - **2** Internal carotid venous plexus
    - **3** Internal carotid nervous plexus (sympathetic)
  - ***G*** Foramen spinosum
    - **1** Middle meningeal vessels
    - **2** Recurrent (dural) branch of mandibular nerve
  - ***H*** Hiatus of facial canal
    - **1** Greater petrosal nerve
    - **2** Petrosal branch of middle meningeal artery
- **III** Posterior fossa
  - ***A*** Internal acoustic meatus
    - **1** Internal auditory vessels
    - **2** Facial nerve (CN VII)
    - **3** Vestibulocochlear nerve (CN VIII)
  - ***B*** Jugular foramen
    - **1** Sigmoid sinus
    - **2** Inferior petrosal sinus
    - **3** Glossopharyngeal nerve (CN IX)
    - **4** Vagus nerve (CN X)
    - **5** Accessory nerve (CN XI)
    - **6** Meningeal branches of the occipital and ascending pharyngeal arteries
  - ***C*** Hypoglossal canal
    - **1** Hypoglossal nerve (CN XII)
    - **2** Emissary veins
    - **3** Meningeal branch of ascending pharyngeal artery
  - ***D*** Foramen magnum
    - **1** Vertebral arteries
    - **2** Accessory nerves (spinal contribution to CN XI)
    - **3** Medulla oblongata and meninges
    - **4** Anterior and posterior spinal arteries
    - **5** Membrana tectoria
    - **6** Apical dental ligament
  - ***E*** External aperture of vestibular aqueduct
    - **1** Endolymphatic duct and sac
    - **2** Small vessels
  - ***F*** Mastoid foramen
    - **1** Emissary vein
  - ***G*** Condyloid canal
    - **1** Emissary vein

the orbit, the frontal nerve divides into a small **supratrochlear nerve** and a larger **supraorbital nerve.** The supratrochlear nerve passes forward and medially to emerge on the face at the superior margin of the orbit just above the trochlea for the superior oblique muscle. The supraorbital nerve continues forward to turn upward on the forehead at the **supraorbital notch** or **foramen;** it frequently divides into two or more branches before exiting from the orbit through the supraorbital notch or foramen.

The **lacrimal nerve** is the smallest of the three branches of the ophthalmic nerve. It passes forward along the junction of the roof and the lateral wall of the orbit. It gives a few small twigs to the lacrimal gland and ends in minute twigs to the skin of the lateral part of the upper eyelid.

The **ophthalmic artery,** a branch of the internal carotid artery, enters the orbit through the optic canal inferior to the optic nerve (Fig. 7.12). Winding around the lateral side of the optic nerve and then crossing above it, it runs forward close to the

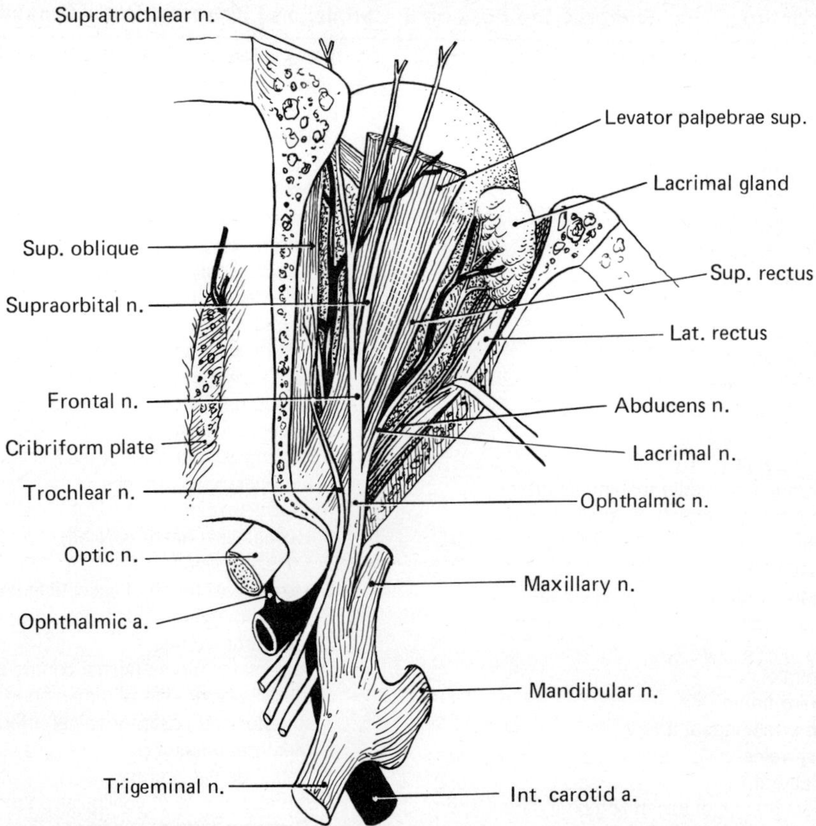

Figure 7.12 The right **orbit** seen from above after removal of its roof.

medial wall of the orbit deep to the superior oblique muscle. In its course, the ophthalmic artery gives rise to **lacrimal, supraorbital, posterior ethmoidal,** and **anterior ethmoidal arteries,** which accompany the nerves of the same name. In addition to these branches, it supplies twigs to the ocular muscles and a group of small **ciliary arteries** that enter the posterior pole of the eyeball. It ends by dividing into two small branches, the **supratrochlear artery** and the **dorsal nasal artery,** which emerge onto the face close to the infratrochlear nerve.

Find the **lacrimal gland,** a small, oval, lobulated structure that lies in the upper anterolateral part of the orbit. Its secretion enters the upper part (superior fornix) of the conjunctival sac through a number of minute lacrimal ducts.

Clean the **levator palpebrae superioris muscle** (Fig. 7.12). This narrow, flat muscle arises from the upper margin of the optic canal immediately above the superior rectus muscle and runs forward, just below the roof of the orbit, to insert into the **superior tarsus.** It also inserts into the skin of the upper eyelid and into the conjunctiva. The superior tarsus is a thin but strong plate of fibrous tissue that lies in the upper eyelid posterior to the orbicularis oculi muscle and in front of the palpebral conjunctiva.

Immediately below the levator palpebrae superioris is the **superior rectus muscle.** This is also a flat, bandlike muscle, somewhat wider than the levator, which arises from the upper margin of the optic canal and inserts into the sclera of the eyeball. Although all the ocular muscles cannot be exposed at present, it is well for you to have a general idea of their arrangement and attachments before proceeding with the dissection of the orbit. The **superior, medial, inferior,** and **lateral rectus muscles** are all flat, bandlike muscles that arise at the apex of the orbit from a common tendon, the **anulus tendineus.** The anulus tendineus attaches to the superior, medial, and inferior aspects of the bony rim of the optic canal, and laterally to the sphenoid bone, where the lateral rectus muscle will be seen to originate. Because the origin of the lateral rectus spans the superior orbital fissure, the muscle is often said to have two heads of origin, one medial and one lateral to the fissure. Spreading forward through the orbit, the ocular muscles are all inserted into the **sclera** at points anterior to a plane that would divide the eyeball into anterior and posterior halves. The **superior oblique muscle,** which should now be cleaned, arises from the margin of the optic canal, between the origins of the superior and medial recti but superior to the anulus tendineus. Its fibers pass forward to the **trochlea** at the upper medial angle of the orbital rim of the frontal bone; from here the muscle turns downward, laterally and posteriorly, passing under the superior rectus, to reach the sclera, where it is inserted on the lateral side of the globe posterior to the plane dividing the eyeball into anterior and posterior halves.

Divide the frontal nerve a short distance anterior to the optic canal and turn it forward. Divide the levator palpebrae superioris and the superior rectus muscles at about the middle of the orbit and turn the anterior segments of the two muscles forward. Then turn the posterior segments backward. As this is done, you will find the **superior division of** the **oculomotor nerve** entering the deep surface of the superior rectus, which it supplies; a small branch of the nerve either pierces the superior rectus or winds around its medial border to supply the levator palpebrae superioris.

As the dissection proceeds, you will notice that some of the structures that enter the orbit (i.e., optic, nasociliary, oculomotor, and abducens nerves and ophthalmic artery) pass through the superior orbital fissure and optic canal **within** the ring created by the anulus. The nerves already displayed near the roof of the orbit (i.e., lacrimal, frontal, and trochlear), however, enter the upper part of the superior orbital fissure **above** the anulus tendineus.

The **nasociliary** is the third branch of the ophthalmic nerve. Passing forward and medially, it crosses above the optic nerve and ends near the upper anterior part of the medial wall of the orbit by dividing into **infratrochlear** and **anterior ethmoidal nerves.** Before its termination, it gives rise to the communicating root to the ciliary ganglion, the long ciliary nerves, and the posterior ethmoidal nerve. The **communicating root** to the **ciliary ganglion** (often called the sensory root) is a small nerve that arises from the nasociliary far back in the orbit and passes forward along the lateral side of the optic nerve to reach the ciliary ganglion (Fig. 7.13). The **long ciliary nerves,** three or four fine filaments, arise from the nasociliary nerve as it crosses above the optic nerve; they pass forward to pierce the posterior part of the sclera. The **posterior ethmoidal nerve** passes medially above the medial rectus and enters the **posterior ethmoidal foramen** to reach the mucosa of the posterior ethmoidal air cells and sphenoid sinus. The **anterior ethmoidal nerve** is the largest branch of the nasociliary. It crosses above the medial rectus and enters the **anterior ethmoidal foramen,** eventually reaching the nasal cavity, where its distribution will be studied later. The **infratrochlear nerve** passes forward above the anterior part of the medial rectus and below the trochlea of the superior oblique to supply the skin on the lateral side of the nose and the medial aspect of the upper eyelid.

The **oculomotor nerve,** as it passes through the two heads of the lateral rectus muscle, divides into a superior and an inferior division. The **superior division** turns upward, lateral to the optic nerve, to supply the superior rectus and the levator palpebrae superioris, as already observed. The **inferior division** runs forward for a short distance and then divides into three branches. Of these, one crosses below the optic nerve to supply the medial rectus; another supplies the inferior rectus muscle; the third runs forward along the floor of the orbit to reach the inferior oblique muscle. The **oculomotor root** of the ciliary ganglion arises from the branch to the inferior oblique.

The **ciliary ganglion** is very small. It lies in the posterior part of the orbit at the lateral side of the optic nerve medial to the lateral rectus muscle. It receives sensory and motor roots from the **nasociliary** and **oculomotor nerves,** respectively. The branches that arise from the ganglion are the **short ciliary nerves.** They are numerous, fine filaments that pass forward in close relation to the optic nerve to pierce the posterior part of the sclera (Fig. 7.13).

The **abducens nerve** enters the orbit through the superior orbital fissure within the anulus and passes forward directly into the lateral rectus muscle, which it supplies.

Separate the lids as widely as possible, or, if the contents of the orbit are dried, remove the lids and locate the insertions of the ocular muscles on the eyeball. By blunt dissection free the orbital contents from the lateral and inferior walls of the orbital cavity and reflect them medialward and upward. Identify the course of the **zygomatic nerve** in the lateral wall of the orbit. The **zygomaticotemporal** and **zygomaticofacial nerves** are branches of this nerve. From the front of the orbit dissect the **inferior oblique muscle.** It arises from the maxilla at the anterior medial angle of the floor of the orbit and passes laterally and backward, below the inferior rectus, to insert into the lateral part of the sclera, posterior to a plane dividing the eyeball into anterior and posterior halves.

Figure 7.13 Deep dissection of the right **orbit.**

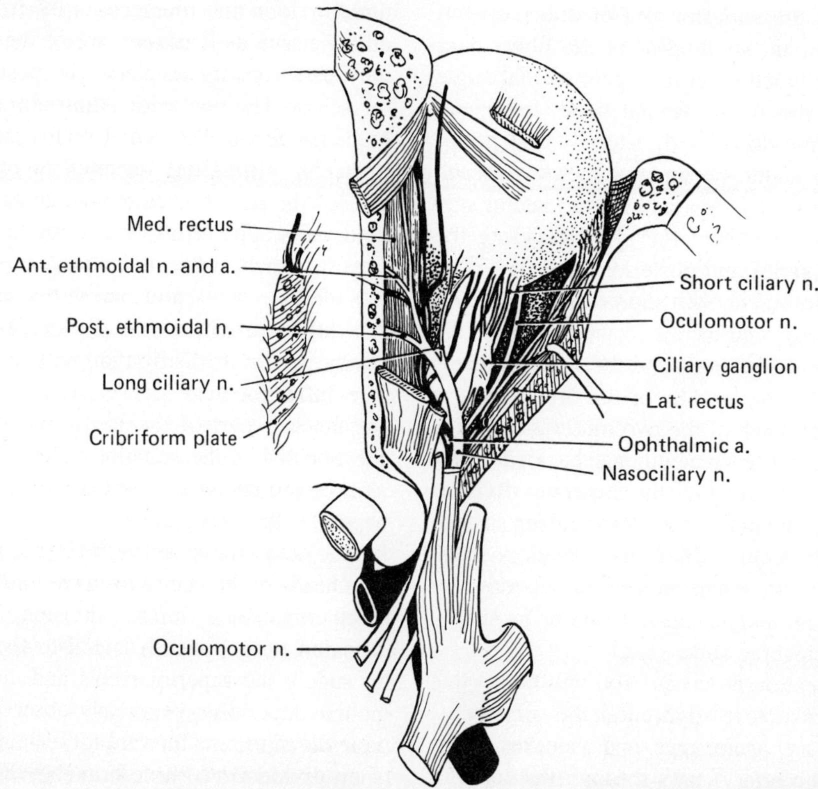

EYEBALL

Normally, the eyeball occupies only the anterior half of the orbital cavity, the posterior half of the cavity being filled by the ocular muscles and the periorbital fat, which you removed during the previous dissection. Remove one eyeball from the orbit by cutting the muscles, vessels, and optic nerve, so that at least 1.5 cm of each of these structures is left attached to the eyeball. Observe the **fascia bulbi,** a thin, enveloping layer of connective tissue that surrounds the eyeball and the distal portion of the ocular muscles. It forms a socket that holds the eyeball in position relative to the orbit and yet allows for free movement in three planes. The connections of the ocular muscles to the eyeball and their relationship to the fascia bulbi should be noted; then reflect the muscles anteriorly towards the **cornea.**

If the eyeballs of the cadaver are not suitable for study or are missing (enucleated), the following dissection should be done using eyes from sheep, pigs, or cattle. The dissection can be facilitated if the animal eyes are previously hardened in alcohol or formalin. Ideally, several eyes should be dissected: in one the various coats can be stripped off the eyeball in succession, in one they can be bisected along the equator, and in a third they can be bisected on the long axis of the eyeball. However, if only one eyeball is available, you are advised to cut it in half transversely at the equator; then bisect the anterior half along the long axis. This approach should help display most of the structures to maximum advantage.

Observe the positions of the attachment of the ocular muscles to the eyeball and identify the optic nerve and the ophthalmic vessels and nerves. Then remove the conjunctiva, the fascia bulbi, and the muscles and vessels from the eyeball, by using a forceps to pick up the conjunctiva and fascia bulbi close to the corneal margin. Then make a cut through the fascia bulbi around the corneal margin and divide the fascia from the underlying tissues. Dissect the structures progressively backward toward the optic nerve. The **vorticose veins** (two superior and two inferior) will be found a little posterior to the equator of the eyeball, and a little farther posteriorly, the **posterior ciliary arteries** and the **ciliary nerves** will be found piercing the sclera around the entrance of the optic nerve.

The dura mater, extending along the course of the optic nerve and surrounding it, should be cleaned and its attachment to the eyeball noted. If a fresh eye is being used, the central artery may be seen within the optic nerve, if that nerve is transected close to its entrance into the eyeball.

The wall of the eyeball is made up of three concentric coats: (1) the outer coat consists of the transparent **cornea,** which constitutes the anterior one-sixth of the outer coat and the **sclera,** which makes up the posterior five-sixths; (2) the middle vascular coat is composed of the **choroid,** the **ciliary muscles** and the **ciliary process,** and the **iris;** (3) an inner **retinal coat** consists of an outer pigmented layer and an inner nervous layer. These three coats enclose three **transparent media:** the **lens,** the **aqueous humor,** and the **vitreous body.** Attempt to demonstrate as many of these structures as possible; a detailed account of the coats, the transparent media, and the apparatus necessary for adjusting the focal length of the eye should be studied in one of the descriptive texts.

Study the contents of the eyeball (Fig. 7.14). The space behind the cornea is the **anterior chamber,** which is continuous through the **pupil of** the **iris** with the **posterior chamber.** The posterior chamber is bordered by the pigmented **iris** anteriorly and the **lens** posteriorly. Both of these chambers contain **aqueous humor.** Behind the lens and within the confines of the retinal surface, note the gelatinous **vitreous humor.**

Observe that the cornea is more convex than the sclera. These two parts of the outer coat become continuous at the **corneoscleral junction,** often called the **limbus.** The **ciliary body,** which is continuous in front with the iris and behind with the choroid, is a whitish zone about 6 mm broad. It contains the **ciliary muscle,** which is firmly attached to the sclera at the corneoscleral junction. Note also the **iridocorneal angle,** the acute angle

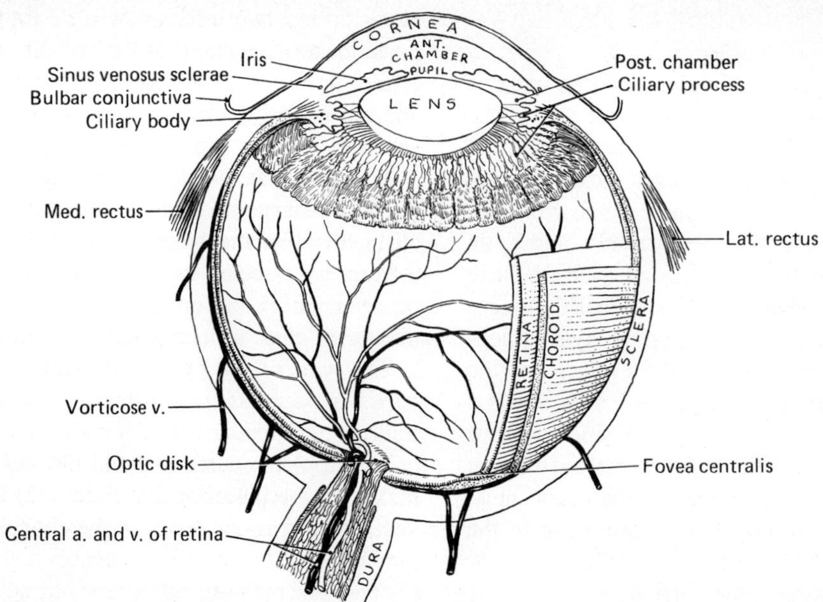

Figure 7.14 Horizontal section of the right **eyeball** with some of the retina and choroid left intact.

between the cornea and the iris. This angle is crossed by strands of connective tissue that pass from the back of the cornea to the iris and sclera. Here you may find spaces enclosed by this connective tissue that communicate with the **sinus venosus sclerae.** The sinus in turn communicates with the scleral veins.

Produced by the epithelium lining the posterior chamber, aqueous humor circulates through the pupil into the anterior chamber, the spaces, and the sinus venosus sclerae, and then out through the scleral veins. If for some reason aqueous humor is not eliminated at the same rate as it is produced, pressure builds up in the eyeball; blindness may result. The condition is known as glaucoma.

The **ciliary processes,** about 70, are fingerlike infoldings of the ciliary body. Anteriorly, they are continuous with the periphery of the iris. Their free margins project toward the lens to which they are attached by suspensory ligaments. Since the pigmented layer of the retina attaches to them, the processes are black.

The **lens** is a biconvex, elastic, transparent structure. It is posterior to the iris and anterior to the vitreous body. The lens is suspended in place by the **suspensory ligament,** which extends from the capsule of the lens to the free margins of the ciliary processes.

One in whom the lens or its capsule loses its transparency is said to have cataracts. Alteration of lens shape for focus adjustment is one aspect of the accommodating process, i.e., change of view from a distant object to a close object. With advancing age, the lens often hardens, making accommodation for vision increasingly difficult (presbyopia).

Locate the optic nerve. The meningeal layer of the dura mater, arachnoid, and pia mater extends along the optic nerve to attach to the posterior aspect of the eyeball. Can you demonstrate the subarachnoid space? Observe that the nerve pierces the sclera as a bundle, about 3 mm to the nasal side of the posterior pole of the eyeball. At this point the sclera is thin. The optic nerve fibers next pierce the choroid and the outer layer of the retina, which is adherent to the choroid. These nerve fibers form a circle, the **optic disk** or papilla, which is called the **blind spot,** since this area is devoid of light-sensitive elements (rods or cones). The nerves then spread out as the inner **nervous layer** of the retina. The central artery and vein pass through the disk and subdivide to supply the inner surface of the retina.

Occlusion of the central artery results in blindness, since it is the sole blood supply to the nervous retina.

About 3 mm lateral to the optic disk, note a yellowish, oval area, the **macula,** in the center of which is a depression, the **fovea centralis.** This area is in the direct axis of vision, and is the most sensitive part of the retina.

As you approach the ciliary body, note that a short distance behind it, the retina becomes thin at a wavy line, the **ora serrata.** The retina posterior to the ora serrata is the true nervous (optic) retina, whereas the retina anterior to the ora serrata is reduced to a single layer of epithelial cells attached to the pigmented layer of retina. The nonnervous layer covers the ciliary body and iris to the margin of the pupil.

PREVERTEBRAL REGION

Preparation for this dissection involves disarticulating the skull and attached soft tissues of the neck from the vertebral column at the atlanto-occipital joint. The structures passing through the jugular foramen are of primary importance, so be sure to avoid severing them during the dissection.

With the cadaver on its back, make a vertical saw cut on each side of the skull, starting on the external surface about 1 cm posterior to the **mastoid process** *and passing anteriorly and medially into the* **foramen magnum,** *just posterior to the* **jugular foramen.** *In the midline, cut through the dura and ligaments connecting the atlas to the occipital bone by a horizontal incision through the foramen magnum. Insert a chisel through the foramen magnum between the anterior arch of the atlas and the occipital bone and/or between the* **occipital condyle** *and the* **superior articular process of** *the* **atlas** *on each side, or chisel through the occipital condyles if necessary. Pry the anterior part of the cranium forward, cutting the anterior parts of the sternocleidomastoid, trapezius, and splenius muscles that hinder retraction. Identify the insertions of the* **longus capitis** *and the* **rectus capitis anterior** *and* **lateralis muscles** *on the base of the skull; cut the muscles near their insertions to facilitate the dissection.*

As you retract the anterior part of the cranium, the pharynx, larger nerves, and vessels forward and downward, try to leave the **cervical sympathetic trunks** *on the surface of the deep prevertebral muscles that are attached to the cervical vertebrae. Remove the posterior part of the* **jugular foramen** *and* **hypoglossal canal** *with a chisel or bone forceps.*

Now study the course of the **glossopharyngeal** (CN IX), **vagus** (CN X), **accessory** (CN XI), and **hypoglossal** (CN XII) **nerves** and their relationships to the pharynx and large vessels of the neck (Fig. 7.15).

Study the **cervical portion** of the **sympathetic trunk.** It lies posterior to the carotid sheath in the prevertebral fascia covering the anterior surfaces of the prevertebral muscles. It begins anterior to the second cervical vertebra and courses inferiorly to the neck of the first rib, in front of which it passes, to become continuous with the thoracic portion of the trunk. The cervical portion usually exhibits three ganglionic enlargements. The largest is the **superior cervical ganglion,** which lies anterior to the second and third vertebrae and represents the superior extent of the trunk. The **middle cervical ganglion** is small, sometimes lacking, and lies anterior to the sixth vertebra. The **inferior cervical ganglion** lies just below the seventh vertebra; it is frequently fused with the first thoracic ganglion to form a large ganglionic mass, the **stellate ganglion,** anterior to the neck of the first rib. Note the **ansa subclavia,** a loop of nerve fibers around the subclavian artery that connects the middle and inferior cervical ganglia (Fig. 7.17). A number of the fine nerve fibers that you will notice arise from each of the cervical sympathetic ganglia; they are **cardiac branches** that descend into the thorax to join the cardiac plexus. In addition to these, communicating branches (gray rami) pass laterally to join the cervical spinal nerves. The superior ganglion usually communi-

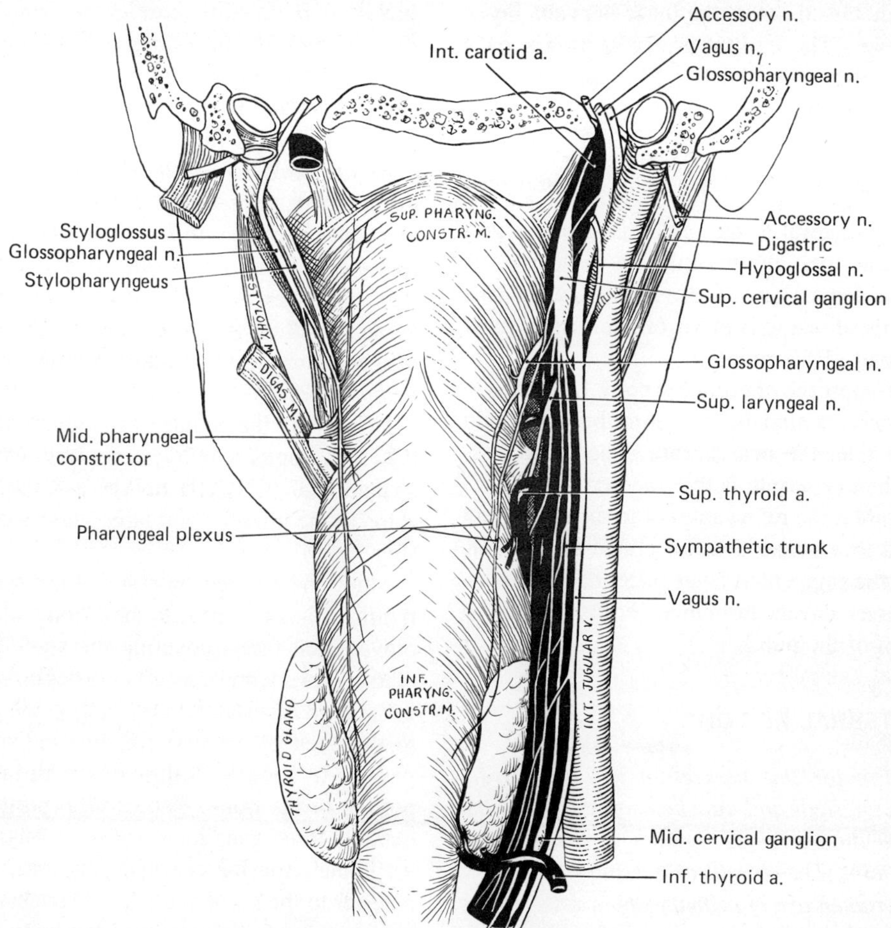

Figure 7.15 Posterior view of the **pharynx** and related structures.

cates with the first four cervical nerves, the middle ganglion with the fifth and sixth, and the inferior ganglion with the seventh and eighth. The superior cervical ganglion contributes large **internal** and **external carotid nerves** that accompany the internal and external carotid arteries, respectively. The sympathetics ramify with all the arterial branches and in this way provide the structures of the head with sympathetic innervation.

Review the position of the jugular foramen, the hypoglossal canal, and the external orifice of the carotid canal. As the structures that traverse these foramina descend in the neck, they all pass deep to the posterior belly of the digastric muscle. In order to expose the upper portions of the structures, the posterior belly of the digastric should be elevated as far as possible from its attachment to the internal aspect of the mastoid process; review the course of the occipital artery.

Note the **stylohyoid muscle** and its origin on the styloid process. Observe that the **stylopharyngeus** and **styloglossus muscles** (Fig. 7.24) as they run downward to reach the pharynx and the tongue, respectively, pass between the internal and the external carotid arteries. Identify the origin of the **stylohyoid ligament** from the styloid process (the **stylomandibular ligament,** which extends from the styloid process to the angle of the mandible, may also be seen). Then identify the glossopharyngeal, vagus, accessory, and hypoglossal nerves as they emerge from their respective foramina at the base of the skull (Fig. 7.15).

Observe that the glossopharyngeal, vagus, and accessory emerge from the medial end of the **jugular foramen,** medial and slightly anterior to the beginning of the internal jugular vein. The **glossopharyngeal nerve** descends vertically for a short distance and then turns forward across the lateral aspect of the internal carotid artery to wind laterally around the stylopharyngeus muscle. In the upper part of its course, the glossopharyngeal gives **pharyngeal branches** to the wall of the pharynx. As it winds around the **stylopharyngeus,** it supplies the muscle and continues forward to the posterior part of the tongue.

The vagus and accessory nerves are bound by a fibrous sheath in the jugular foramen. The **vagus** descends almost vertically within the carotid sheath, where you have already seen the greater part of its cervical course. Just below the jugular foramen, it receives a communicating branch from the accessory. The vagus exhibits a swelling, the **superior ganglion,** as it lies in the foramen. Slightly lower, it exhibits another ovoid swelling, the **inferior ganglion.** Just below the ganglion, the vagus gives off its **pharyngeal branch,** which runs forward, lateral to the internal carotid artery, to reach the wall of the pharynx, where it joins with the pharyngeal branches of the glossopharyngeal and the sympathetic fibers to form the **pharyngeal plexus** (Fig. 7.15). Somewhat below the origin of the pharyngeal branch, the vagus gives rise to a larger branch, the **superior laryngeal nerve.** Running downward and forward, and passing deep to the internal carotid artery, the superior laryngeal nerve divides into the **internal** and **external laryngeal nerves,** which you have already exposed in the dissection of the carotid triangle.

The **accessory nerve** (spinal root), inferior to its communication with the vagus, bends laterally to cross either anterior or posterior to the internal jugular vein. Turning posteriorly and downward to pass deep to the posterior belly of the digastric and the occipital artery, it reaches the deep surface of the sternocleidomastoid, from which point it has already been studied.

Emerging from the **hypoglossal foramen,** the **hypoglossal nerve** lies medial to the vagus and accessory nerves. As it descends, it spirals first posterior to and then lateral to the vagus nerve.

The **internal carotid artery** begins at the level of the upper border of the thyroid cartilage as one of the terminal branches of the common carotid and ascends anterior to the upper three cervical vertebrae to the base of the skull, where it enters the external orifice of the **carotid canal.** The internal carotid is adjacent to the lateral pharyngeal wall and has no branches in the neck. Note that the nerves described above have the following relationships to the external and internal carotid arteries: *the hypoglossal is lateral to both, the glossopharyngeal and pharyngeal branches of the vagus pass between the two, and the superior laryngeal branch of the vagus is medial to both* (Fig. 7.16).

Attempt to display the three small arteries that supply the upper part of the pharyngeal wall. They are the **ascending pharyngeal,** the **ascending palatine,** and the **tonsillar arteries.** All three vessels are not usually present in a single person; however, the one that is lacking is frequently replaced by branches from the other two. The **ascending pharyngeal** is usually the first branch of the external carotid, arising from its medial aspect. It ascends on the wall of the pharynx, where it lies medial to the internal carotid artery. The **ascending palatine** and the **tonsillar arteries** are small branches that arise from the **facial artery** as it lies deep to the digastric muscle. They ascend on the upper lateral part of the pharyngeal wall, the ascending palatine lying slightly posterior to the tonsillar. You can differentiate them by the fact that the ascending palatine passes deep to the styloglossus muscle, whereas the tonsillar artery crosses it superficially (Fig. 7.24).

Review the attachments of the **scalenus ante-**

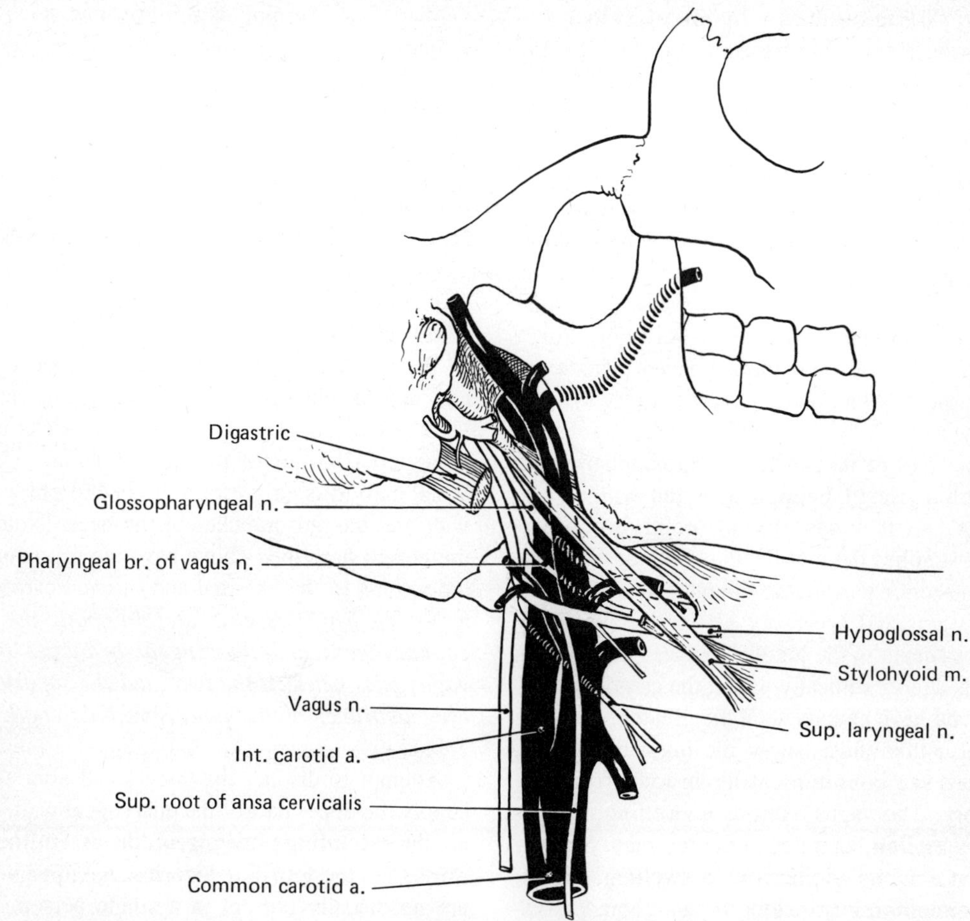

Figure 7.16 Right lateral view of the **carotid arteries** and the **nerves** associated with them.

rior muscle and then study the **scalenus medius** and **scalenus posterior.** All three muscles originate from the transverse processes of the **cervical vertebrae** (the scalenus anterior from the anterior tubercles, and the scalenus medius and scalenus posterior from the posterior tubercles). The scalenus anterior and medius insert on the **first rib.** The scalenus posterior inserts on the **second rib.** The **longus capitis,** which was cut when you retracted the head, arises from the anterior tubercles of the transverse processes of the third through the sixth **cervical vertebrae** and inserts on the basilar part of the **occipital bone** (Fig. 7.17).

The **longus colli** is a complex muscle that is usually regarded as consisting of three parts: vertical, superior oblique, and inferior oblique. Note, however, that the three parts are continuous and cannot be entirely separated from one another.

Because they were severed when you retracted the head, the **rectus capitis anterior** and the **rectus capitis lateralis,** two small, flat muscles that pass from the upper border of the atlas to the basilar portion of the occipital bone, must be studied from one of the standard texts. The ventral ramus of the first cervical nerve emerges between these two muscles and turns downward in front of the transverse process of the atlas (Fig. 7.17).

The anterior aspects of the transverse processes

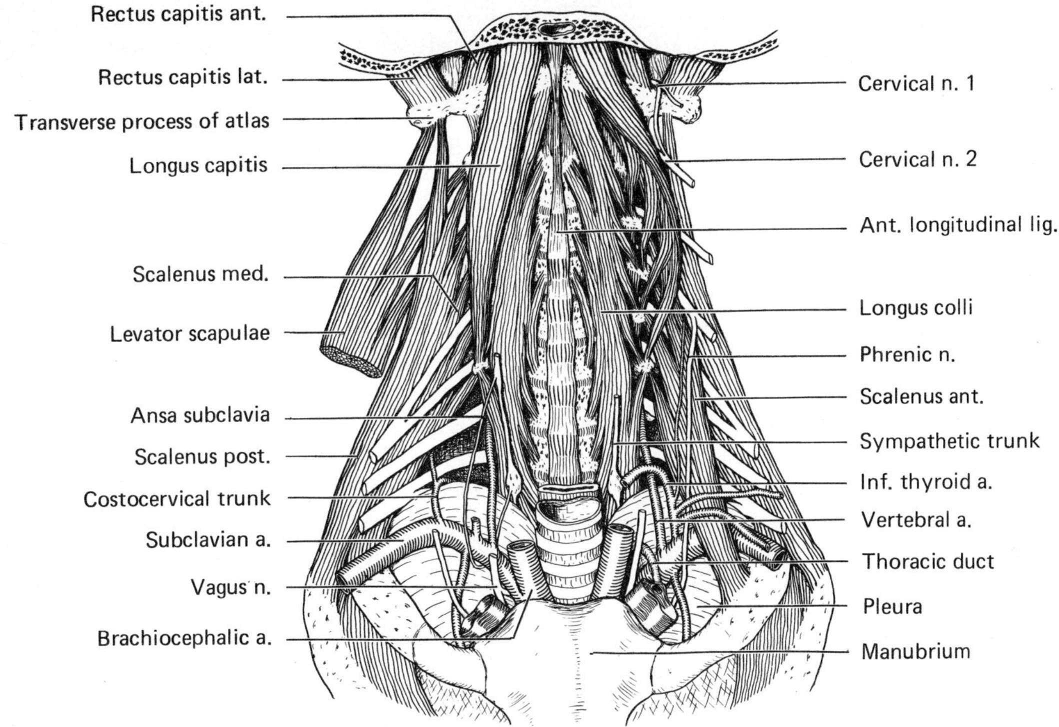

Figure 7.17 The **prevertebral region.** The left longus capitis muscle has been pulled laterally to display its slips of origin.

of the successive cervical vertebrae are connected by a series of small anterior intertransverse muscles. Remove them to expose the course of the cervical portion of the **vertebral artery.** This has already been seen to arise from the **subclavian** and to run upward anterior to the transverse process of the seventh cervical vertebra to enter the transverse foramen of the sixth cervical vertebra. Coursing upward through the **transverse foramina** of the upper six vertebrae, it turns posteriorly and medially in the groove on the upper surface of the posterior arch of the atlas to enter the cranial cavity through the **foramen magnum.** It is surrounded by a plexus of small veins, which unite inferiorly to form the **vertebral vein.** In its upward passage through the neck, the vertebral artery gives rise to a series of small spinal branches that enter the vertebral canal at the intervertebral foramina.

Observe that the cervical nerves, as they emerge from the intervertebral foramina, pass posterior to the vertebral artery.

FASCIAL SPACES OF THE HEAD AND NECK

There have been many diverse descriptions of the fascia and fascial spaces of the head and neck. Their importance as factors that limit or aid the spread of infection in the head and neck is as applicable today, even with the widespread use of antibiotics, as it was in the past. Of the numerous fasciae and spaces that could be listed, only a few of the more significant ones are described below as they relate to disease processes. Keep in mind that, in the strict sense of the term, only those spaces that are filled with loose connective tissue bounded by dissectable, dense connective tissue sheets should be described as fascial spaces.

The concentric arrangement of the connective tissue around the structures in the neck forms four definite fascial cylinders or compartments. The outermost one, defined by the superficial fascia, contains the external and anterior jugular veins, fat, and the platysma; it can be instrumental in the spread of superficial infections from the face to the neck. The superficial muscles of the neck region, the sternocleidomastoid and the trapezius, are enclosed in a collar (the enclosing cylinder) of deep fascia, the **investing fascia,** which attaches to the bony structures at the superior and inferior margins of the neck. The attachment of the investing fascia to the manubrium is split, forming a pocketlike area just above the jugular notch called the **suprasternal space** (of Burns).

The infrahyoid muscles are enclosed in the **middle cervical fascia,** which is most often considered a subdivision of the investing fascia.

Deep to the investing layer, the cervical vertebrae and their associated muscles are enclosed in the **prevertebral fascia;** it forms the musculoskeletal compartment. Another compartment (visceral), more anteriorly located around the lower part of the pharynx, larynx, trachea, thyroid gland, and esophagus, is limited by the **visceral fascia.** Posteriorly, between the prevertebral and visceral fasciae, there is a loose connective space called the **retropharyngeal space.**

It allows for independent movement of the cervical viscera over the cervical vertebrae, and through it infections can travel from the region of the nasal or oral pharynx into the posterior mediastinum.

This space can be studied by inserting your fingers or an instrument into it and tracing it downward into the posterior mediastinum. Potential spaces also exist within the visceral compartment around the esophagus **(paraesophageal)** and around the trachea **(paratracheal),** which also extend down into the thorax.

When studying the spaces around the facial portion of the skull, you must remember that the investing layer of cervical fascia extends superiorly above its attachment to the inferior border of the mandible, and in so doing helps to define various compartments structurally. For example, the investing fascia blends with the masseteric and pterygoid fasciae; encapsulates the submandibular, sublingual, and parotid glands; contributes to the stylomandibular ligament; and attaches to the zygomatic arch, above which it is continuous with the temporal fascia.

The **masseteric space** encloses the mandible, the masseter and pterygoid muscles, and the associated nerves and vessels. This space is subdivided into the **buccal space** (containing the buccal fat pad) anteriorly and the **pretemporal space** superiorly. The latter extends deep to the zygomatic arch upward along the temporalis muscle. It is limited superficially by the attachment of the temporal fascia to the zygomatic arch and superiorly by the attachment of the fascia to the superior temporal line.

Infections can extend from the mandibular area—for example, from abscesses of the lower molar teeth—to the anterior part of the temporal region or anteriorly into the buccal fat-pad region.

Another subdivision of the masseteric space has been described, the **pterygomandibular space.** It is bounded laterally by the inner surface of the mandible, medially by the medial pterygoid muscle, and superiorly by the lateral pterygoid muscle. The contents of the infratemporal fossa are in this space.

The **parotid gland** is generally considered to occupy its own space, although some describe the space enclosing it and the masseter muscle as the **parotideomasseteric fascial space.** Either way, this space is important in limiting the spread of infections from the parotid gland.

Now place a probe in the mouth and pass it through the lateral wall of the pharynx in the vicinity of the palatine tonsils. Note that as the pharyngeal constrictor is perforated, the tip of the probe enters the **lateral pharyngeal** (parapharyngeal) **space,** lateral to the constrictors, through which course the carotid artery, the internal jugular vein, and the vagus, hypoglossal, glossopharyngeal, and spinal accessory nerves (Fig. 7.15). Some investigators subdivide this space into a prestyloid and a retrostyloid area, using the styloid process as the dividing line.

Susceptible to infection from numerous sources, the lateral pharyngeal space is clinically quite important because it communicates posteriorly with the retropharyngeal space.

The **submandibular space** is the potential space bounded inferiorly by the mylohyoid muscle, the mucous membrane on the inferior lateral side of the tongue superiorly, and the geniohyoid and genioglossus muscles medially.

An infection in the anterior part of this space, anterior to the second molars, will usually be confined to the floor of the mouth, but posterior to the last molars, the infection will spread to the connective tissues of the neck.

MOUTH

The interior of the mouth can be studied more effectively in a living person than in the cadaver. The mouth is divided into two parts, the vestibule and the oral cavity proper. The **vestibule** is the narrow, cleftlike space that is bounded by the cheeks and lips externally and the teeth and gums internally. The **oral cavity proper** is bounded anteriorly and laterally by the teeth and gums; posteriorly, it is continuous with the oral portion of the pharynx (oropharynx). The vestibule and the oral cavity proper are lined with **mucous membrane,** which is interrupted only at the points where the teeth erupt through the gums. The mucous membrane is continuous anteriorly with the lips and the skin of the face, and posteriorly, with the mucous membrane lining the pharynx. The **parotid duct** passes through the cheek and opens into the vestibule at the **parotid papilla,** which is at the level of the second upper molar tooth.

The arched roof of the mouth is formed by the **hard** and **soft palates.** The actual boundary between the mouth and the oropharynx is formed by the **palatoglossal arches** (Fig. 7.18). To see them, open the mouth wide and depress the tongue; the arches extend upward, one on each side, from the side of the base of the tongue to the undersurface

Figure 7.18 The **oral cavity.**

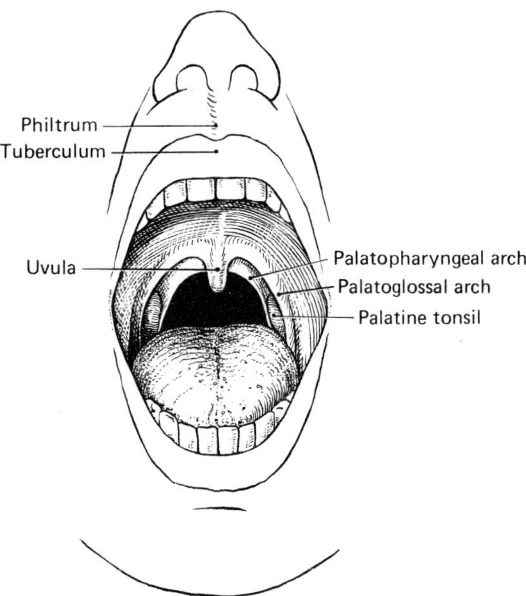

of the soft palate. Farther posteriorly, extending upward from the lateral wall of the pharynx to the free edge of the soft palate, you will see the **palatopharyngeal arches.** The space enclosed between the palatoglossal and the palatopharyngeal arches on the right and left sides creates a passageway through which the oral cavity communicates with the oropharynx; the opening is called the **isthmus of** the **fauces.** It is itself, however, actually a part of the oropharynx. The **palatine tonsil** is lodged within the wall of the isthmus, i.e., between the palatoglossal and the palatopharyngeal arches (Fig. 7.18).

The **tongue** projects from the floor of the mouth and is covered by oral mucous membrane. Observe the vertical fold of mucous membrane running from the undersurface of the anterior free portion of the tongue to the floor of the mouth; it is the **lingual frenulum** (Fig. 7.19). At each side of the base of the frenulum, the opening of the **submandibular duct** can be seen at the summit of a small papilla, the **sublingual caruncle.** Extending posterolaterally along the floor of the mouth from the caruncle is a low ridge, the **sublingual fold (plica).** It is caused by the **sublingual gland,** which lies immediately below the mucous membrane. At the summit of the fold, the minute **orifices of** the **sublingual ducts** can sometimes be recognized.

ORAL CAVITY (DETAIL)

This material is presented for the student who requires a more detailed knowledge of the oral cavity than that given in the preceding section. You will find it easier to learn most of this material if you either use a mirror to study your own oral cavity or study that of one of your fellow students.

Locate the **nasolabial groove,** which separates the cheek from the upper lip on each side. It extends downward and laterally from the wing of the nose toward the corner of the mouth. Also observe the transverse **labiomental groove,** which separates the chin from the lower lip (Fig. 7.19).

In addition to the facial muscles around the mouth described previously (see page 41), the upper and lower lips **(labia)** are composed of skin and subcutaneous tissue on the outer surface, and **labial glands** covered by mucous membrane on the inside. The glands vary in size and form an almost continuous layer in both the upper and lower lips. The larger ones can be felt through the mucous membrane by moving the tip of the tongue against the inner surface of the lips.

Open your mouth and note that the angles where the lips are connected, the **labial commissures,** are very thin and may be torn by forcibly stretching the lips apart. The red zone of the lips is due to blood vessels showing through the thin epithelium. In the upper lip, the red zone protrudes downward in the midline as the **tuberculum;** a shallow depression in the skin of the upper lip, the **philtrum,** extends from just above the tuberculum to the nose (Fig. 7.18).

The oral cavity or mouth is divided into the **oral vestibule** and the **oral cavity proper.** The **vestibule** is the space between the teeth and alveolar processes internally and the lips and cheeks externally. Its anterior opening is the **oral fissure (rima oris).** Pull the lips outward and find the fold of mucous membrane in the midline, the **frenulum,** that extends from the gum to the lip. The frenulum is usually better developed in the upper than in the lower lip.

The **oral cavity proper** is bounded anteriorly and laterally by the alveolar processes and the teeth. The hard and soft palates form the roof. The floor is formed by the tongue and the **sublingual groove,** the mucous membrane-lined area around the front and sides of the tongue. Posteriorly, the oral cavity proper communicates with the oropharynx through the **isthmus of** the **fauces** (see above).

Next study the mucous membrane lining the inner surface of the cheeks. The point of reflection of the membrane from the cheek onto the alveolar process is referred to as the **fornix of** the **vestibule** or the **mucobuccal fold.** A tendinous slip, the **pterygomandibular raphe,** which extends between the pterygoid hamulus and the posterior ex-

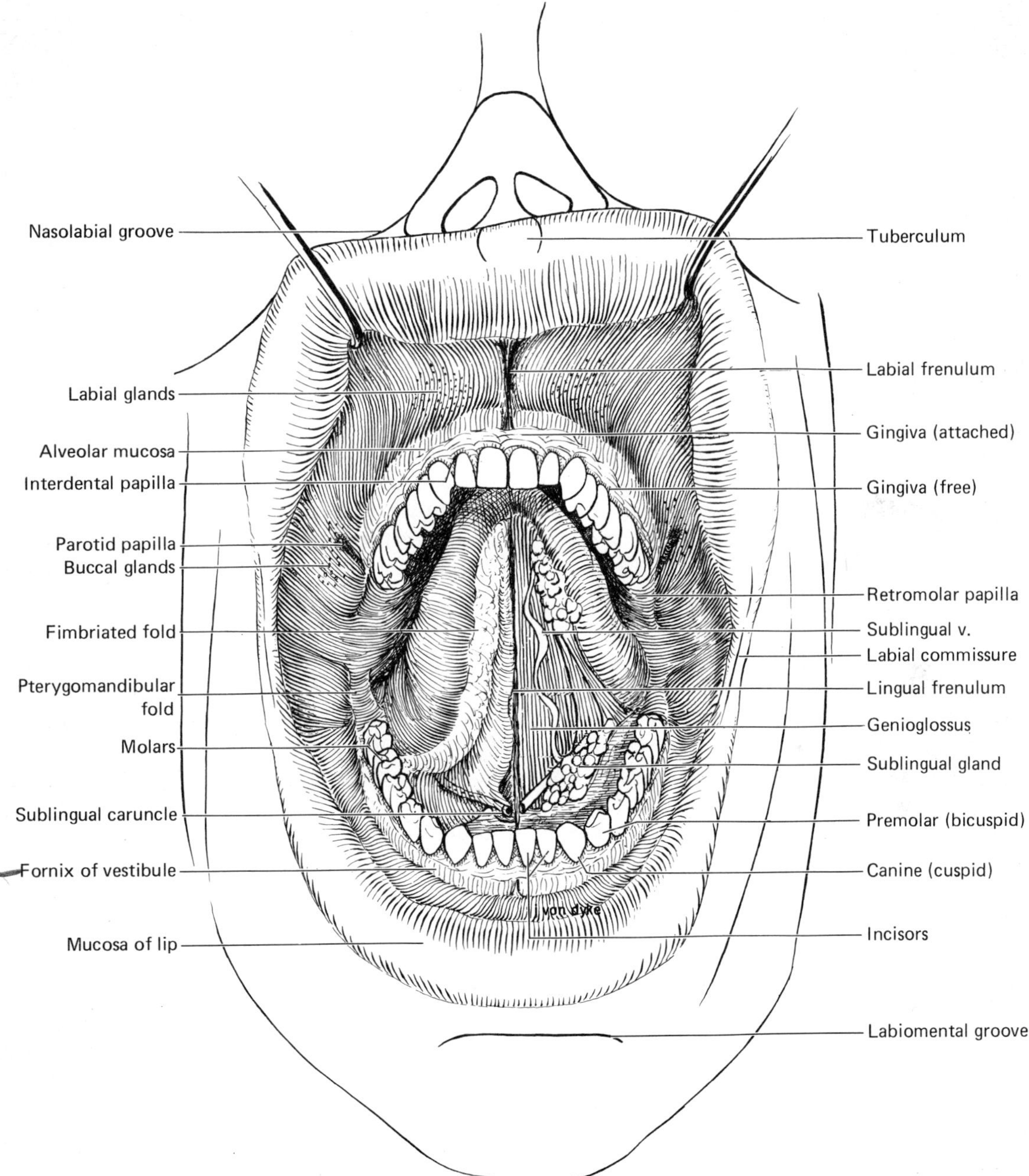

Figure 7.19 The **oral cavity** with the tongue elevated and the mucous membrane removed from one-half of its inferior surface.

tent of the mylohyoid line of the mandible, produces a fold, the **pterygomandibular fold,** in the mucous membrane. **Buccal glands** are present in the submucous tissue of the cheek; in the molar region they may be so numerous as to form a solid-appearing glandular body. Isolated sebaceous glands, which can become enlarged with age and may be visible (as yellowish bodies) through the mucous membrane, are found in the buccal mucosa just lateral to the angles of the mouth.

Locate the **parotid papilla,** an elevation in the mucous membrane opposite the second upper molar, where the parotid duct opens into the oral vestibule. Carefully strip the mucous membrane from the inner surface of the cheek and lips to see the buccal and labial glands and the muscles that form the peripheral borders of the oral cavity. While doing this, note that the mucous membrane is tightly attached to the labial and buccal muscles. The part of the mucous membrane in the fornix of the vestibule, however, is loosely attached to the submucous tissue, which allows one to pull the lips and cheeks away from the alveolar processes and teeth. Posteriorly, however, in the region of the molars, the mucous membrane in the fornix is more firmly attached.

Now direct your attention to the mucous membrane covering the alveolar processes and the base of the teeth. If the cadaver specimen is edentulous or has only a few teeth, study the **alveolar mucosa** and the **gingiva** (gums) in a living subject. The **alveolar mucosa** is characterized by its thin texture, its dark red color, and its mobility. The **gingiva** is harder, very slightly movable, lighter in color, and stippled with prominent sulci, giving it an orange-peel appearance. The **marginal portion** of the gingiva is a collar extending around the cervical region of the tooth. It tapers to a sharp edge, the **gingival margin** or **free margin,** which is separated from the tooth surface by a shallow crevice. A shallow depression, the **gingival groove,** separates the marginal gingiva from the stippled, **attached gingiva.** Another line, the **mucogingival junction,** separates the attached gingiva from the alveolar mucosa. Also note that the mucous membrane may extend between the teeth as **interdental papilla.** If some teeth are present in the cadaver, these subdivisions of the mucous membrane should be defined by probing around the teeth and by stripping the mucous membrane from the teeth and jaws. As you strip the mucous membrane, note that the **alveolar tubercle,** covered by gingiva, forms a round, large prominence on the posterior end of each upper alveolar process.

Also observe that behind the last molars, the gingiva may be elevated, forming the **retromolar papilla.** The **retroalveolar notch** is a groove varying in depth and extending from the junction of the maxilla and the palatine bones to the lower end of the pterygoid process. The **retromolar pad** may also be present where the retromolar papilla of the lower jaw and the buccal glands (retromolar glands) are adjacent to one another, forming an almost continuous pad.

Review the bony structure of the hard palate, muscular soft palate, and the mucous membrane that covers them (Fig. 7.20). The posterior lateral part of the membrane was removed when you traced the course of the descending palatine nerves and vessels, but enough of it should be present for you to see that the peripheral part of the mucous membrane is continuous with that of the vestibular gingiva. Note the **incisive** or **palatine papilla** immediately behind the upper central incisors; this papilla covers the opening of the **incisive canal.** A low ridge, the **palatine raphe,** extends posteriorly from the papilla along almost the entire length of the hard palate. **Transverse palatine folds (plicae)** extend across the anterior part of the hard palate. Strip the palatine mucous membrane and note that the submucosa contains fat anteriorly and **palatine glands** mainly in the posterior part. These glands empty into the **palatine foveola,** which may be bilateral or present only on one side of the midline (Fig. 7.20). In the molar region, the connective tissue embedding the palatine vessels and nerves is usually thicker than in other areas of the palate. The connective tissue strands that extend from the periosteum of the hard palate to the mucous membrane should also be exam-

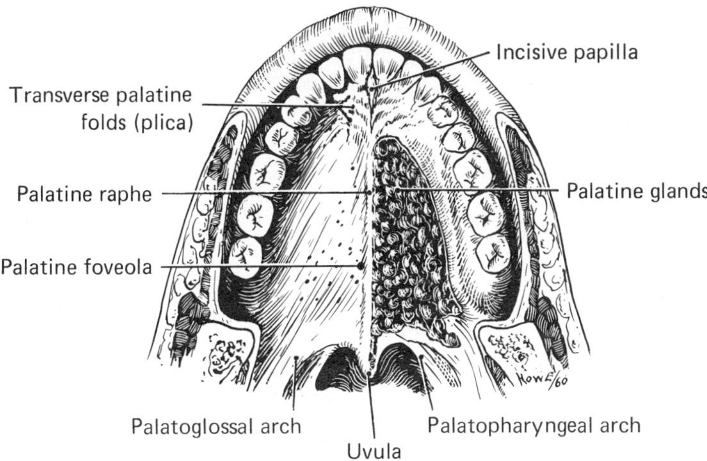

Figure 7.20 The inferior surface of the **palate** with the mucous membrane removed from its left side.

ined, since they greatly limit the movement of the membrane over the hard palate. The muscles of the soft palate will be studied in a forthcoming dissection (see page 81).

The mucous membrane on the lingual surface of the alveolar process is subdivided into mandibular and alveolar mucosa. The submucosa, near the sublingual groove, is loose to allow for greater motility of the tongue. Elevate the tongue and observe the sickle-shaped fold of mucous membrane, the **lingual frenulum,** on its underside (Fig. 7.19), which extends from the mandibular process to the tongue. The frenulum varies in length in different persons.

When there is a congenital abnormally short frenulum (ankyloglossia), the person is said to be tongue-tied.

Fimbriated folds extend from the end of the frenulum laterally and posteriorly along the underside of the tongue. Large, tortuous sublingual veins can be seen on each side of the ventral surface of the tongue. Other veins (deep and dorsal lingual veins) accompany branches of the lingual artery.

Note the **sublingual fold** that contains the sublingual gland and the duct of the submandibular gland (see page 86). This fold ends in a small papilla, the **sublingual caruncle,** near the mandibular attachment of the lingual frenulum, upon which the submandibular duct and the larger duct of the sublingual gland open (Fig. 7.19). There are 15 or more smaller ducts from the sublingual gland that open along the crest of the **sublingual fold.** Strip the mucous membrane from the floor of the oral cavity to identify the sublingual gland, to locate the duct of the submandibular gland, and to observe the relationship of this duct to the lingual nerve. Note the course of this duct in relationship to the mylohyoid muscle.

TONGUE

Next, while studying the surface of the **tongue,** observe that the oral surface of the anterior two-thirds, the **body** and **tip,** is turned up toward the hard palate, whereas the posterior one-third, the **base,** faces backward toward the pharynx. On the oral surface of the tongue, the V-shaped **sulcus terminalis** separates the body from the base. A small depression, the **foramen cecum,** is located where the two limbs of the sulcus terminalis come together. This depression marks the point of embryological origin of the thyroid gland.

Just as the **transverse palatine folds** are well developed and are instrumental in mastication in some animals, the roughened tongue also serves a similar purpose, but in humans the rough mucosa merely takes the form of several types of papillae. The remains of food, mucus, etc., should be washed from, or gently scraped off, the lingual mucosa to identify the various types of papillae. The larger **vallate (circumvallate) papillae,** 8 to 12 in number, are located just anterior to the sulcus terminalis, and they decrease in size from the midline laterally. These papillae have circular furrows around elevated prominences; serous glands empty into the deepest part of the furrows. The line of circumvallate papillae demarcates fairly well the area of the tongue supplied by the lingual nerve (taste, via the chorda tympani) anteriorly and the glossopharyngeal nerve posteriorly. In front of the vallate papillae, numerous, hairlike **conical** and **filiform papillae** give the rest of the oral surface of the tongue a velvety, grayish pink color in the living individual. Between the filiform papillae notice the isolated, irregularly distributed **fungiform papillae.** They too are small, mushroomlike elevations on the sides of which taste buds are located.

Posterior to the sulcus terminalis, the pharyngeal surface of the tongue is irregularly folded due to the presence of prominent accumulations of lymphoid tissue, the **lingual follicles.** The **lingual tonsil** is the term applied to the aggregate of the lingual follicles. The **lingual crypt,** a narrow depression, can be seen in the center of most of the follicles, where the ducts of small mixed glands, the **posterior lingual glands,** open. The muscles of the tongue will be studied in a later dissection.

Since the microanatomy of the teeth forms a specialized part of dental training, it will have to suffice here merely to name the teeth. In the adult there are 32 permanent teeth; there are **two incisors** located on each side in the anterior medial part of the maxilla and in the mandible. Lateral to these, on each side is a strong, pointed tooth, the **canine.** More lateral and posterior to the canines are **two premolars** on each side in each jaw, and **three molars** (Fig. 7.19).

When the permanent teeth are lost, the alveolar bone is resorbed, and the contours of the jaws become more rounded. If the central incisors are missing in your cadaver, palpate the inner surface of the mandible for the **mental spines,** which may appear prominent under these conditions.

If any of the maxillary molar teeth are present, study the relationship of their roots to the maxillary sinus and the distribution of the superior alveolar nerves to these teeth.

PHARYNX

The wall of the pharynx is composed of four layers. From external to deep, they are the **buccopharyngeal (visceral) fascia,** the **muscular layer,** the **pharyngobasilar fascia,** and the **mucous membrane.** The buccopharyngeal fascia and the plexus of veins that it contains should be removed, when you clean the muscles. The principal muscles of the pharyngeal wall are the **superior, middle,** and **inferior pharyngeal constrictors** (Fig. 7.21). Because the muscular layer is not complete superiorly, the pharyngobasilar fascia, a strong submucosal layer, defines the pharyngeal wall. The constrictors arise anterolaterally and spread posteromedially around the wall of the pharynx to insert into a fibrous **median raphe** that represents a thickening of the pharyngobasilar fascia; it runs from the pharyngeal tubercle on the base of the occipital bone down the posterior wall of the pharynx in the median line. Posteriorly, as they spread to their insertions, the constrictors overlap one another from below upward. You are, therefore, advised to clean the inferior constrictor first.

The **inferior pharyngeal constrictor** is covered at its origin by the upper part of the sternothyroid muscle. It arises from the **thyroid cartilage** just posterior to the oblique line, from a **fibrous arch** bridging the cricothyroid muscle between the thyroid and cricoid cartilages, and from the lateral surface of the **cricoid cartilage.** As it approaches its insertion into the median raphe, it spreads superiorly, so that its upper fibers overlap the insertion of the middle constrictor.

The most caudal fibers of the inferior pharyngeal constrictor can function as a separate muscle,

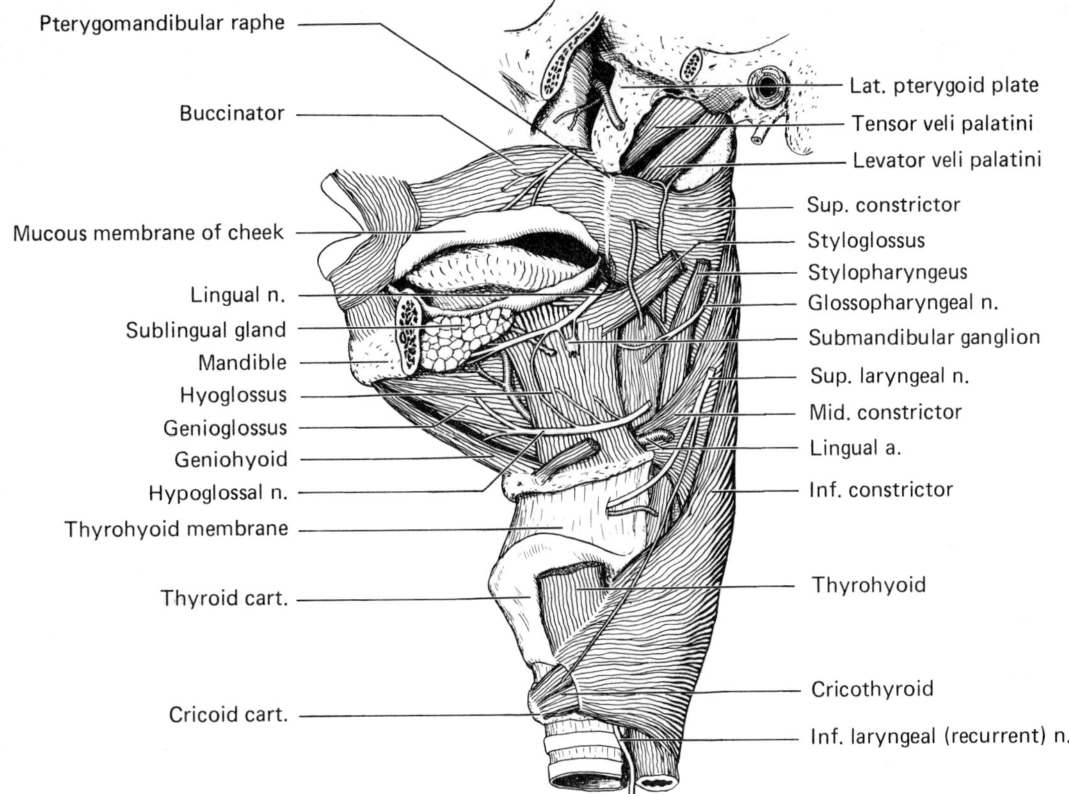

Figure 7.21 The left lateral **pharyngeal wall.**

the **cricopharyngeus.** It helps to occlude the esophageal opening so that one does not continuously swallow air.

The **middle constrictor** arises from the upper border of the **greater horn** and from the posterior border of the **lesser horn** of the **hyoid bone;** it is overlapped at its origin by the hyoglossus muscle. Its fibers radiate toward their insertion into the median raphe, almost entirely covered by the inferior constrictor.

The **superior constrictor** arises from the lower part of the posterior border of the **medial pterygoid plate,** from the **pterygomandibular raphe,** and from the highest part of the **mylohyoid line** on the inner surface of the mandible. The **pterygomandibular raphe** separates the fibers of the buccinator from those of the superior constrictor. The uppermost fibers of the superior constrictor insert as high as the **pharyngeal tubercle** of the occipital bone; the remainder insert into the median raphe under cover of the insertion of the middle constrictor.

The **stylopharyngeus muscle,** already seen arising from the **styloid process,** reaches the wall of the pharynx at the upper border of the middle constrictor. Passing downward deep to that muscle, most of its fibers blend with the **constrictors,** although a few insert on the **thyroid cartilage.**

Open the pharynx by making a transverse incision in its posterior wall just below the base of the skull and a longitudinal incision along the median raphe. Study the interior of the pharynx (Fig. 7.22).

Observe that the **wall of** the **pharynx** is com-

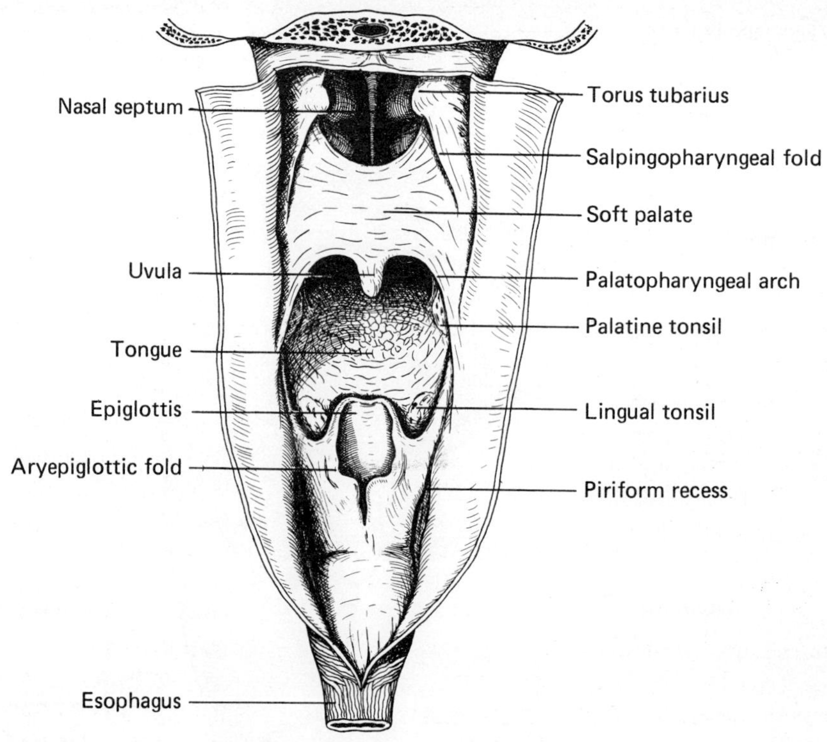

Figure 7.22 A posterior view of the **interior** of the **pharynx.**

plete laterally and posteriorly, but that anteriorly it is incomplete, since the pharynx communicates freely with the nasal cavities, the oral cavity, and the larynx. The pharynx is lined by a **mucous membrane** that is continuous with the mucous membranes lining the nasal cavities, the oral cavity, and the larynx. The pharynx is divisible from above downward into three parts: the **nasopharynx,** the **oropharynx,** and the **laryngopharynx.**

The **nasopharynx** lies below the body of the sphenoid and the basal portion of the occipital bone and posterior to the nasal cavities, with which it communicates at the two **choanae.** At the upper anterior part of the lateral wall of the nasopharynx on each side you may be able to see the opening of the **auditory tube** (it is more easily seen after the head is bisected). It is bounded superiorly and posteriorly by a prominent ridge, the **torus tubarius.** A flexible probe introduced into the opening will pass laterally and backward into the **cavity of** the **middle ear.** Observe the **salpingopharyngeal fold,** a slight fold of mucous membrane descending on the side wall of the pharynx from the torus tubarius; it gradually disappears inferiorly. Just posterior to the torus tubarius and the salpingopharyngeal fold is a pocketlike depression in the lateral wall, the **pharyngeal recess.** In the posterior wall of the nasopharynx, between the two pharyngeal recesses, there is a collection of lymphoid tissue known as the **pharyngeal tonsil.**

When enlarged owing to chronic inflammation, this tonsil is commonly referred to as the "adenoids."

The **soft palate** projects backward and downward into the pharynx, separating the nasal from the oral portion. Below the soft palate, the palatoglossal arches and the posterior surface of the base of the tongue separate the oral cavity from the oropharynx. The palatopharyngeal arches appear as prominent folds on the lateral wall of the oropharynx. Note the **palatine tonsil** between the palatoglossal and palatopharyngeal folds on each side.

When swollen, they are called the "tonsils."

The **lingual tonsil** is a similar but more diffuse aggregation of lymphoid tissue at the base of the tongue.

The **laryngeal portion of** the **pharynx** is an inferior continuation of the oral portion, below the level of the hyoid bone. The **epiglottis** is in the upper part of its anterior wall. The **superior aperture of** the **larynx** is below the epiglottis and is bounded by the **aryepiglottic folds.** They are folds of the mucous membrane passing upward and forward from the arytenoid cartilages (which may be felt but not seen through the mucous membrane) to the lateral borders of the epiglottis. Below the laryngeal aperture, the anterior wall of the pharynx is formed by the mucous membrane covering the posterior aspect of the cricoid cartilage. The pharynx ends inferiorly at the level of the lower border of the cricoid cartilage, where it becomes continuous with the esophagus. Lateral to the lower part of the aryepiglottic fold on each side is a deep pocket in the pharyngeal wall, the **piriform recess.**

Now direct your attention to the **soft palate.** It is covered on its superior and inferior surfaces by mucous membrane. Anteriorly, it is attached to the posterior border of the hard palate; posteriorly, it presents a free margin at the center of which is a conical projection, the **uvula;** laterally, the soft palate joins the wall of the pharynx. The soft palate consists primarily of muscle fibers, most of which are inserted into the **palatal aponeurosis**—a sheet of fibrous tissue that extends posteriorly into the soft palate from the bony margin of the hard palate.

The muscles of the soft palate can be studied more easily after the facial portion of the skull is divided into two parts. Therefore, cut through the soft palate with a scalpel in a parasagittal plane slightly to the left of the median line. Starting at the left nostril, divide the fleshy and cartilaginous portions of the left side of the nose in the same plane. Then complete the division by sawing (in the same plane) through the roof of the left nasal cavity, the hard palate, and the mental symphysis. Then bisect the tongue with a scalpel in the midsagittal plane. In order to expose the muscles of the soft palate, carefully remove the mucous membrane from the superior surface of the soft palate and from the lateral wall of the nasal and oral portions of the pharynx.

The principal muscles of the soft palate are the **tensor veli palatini** and the **levator veli palatini,** which tense and raise the palate, and the **palatoglossus** and **palatopharyngeus muscles,** which depress it. The palatopharyngeus and the levator are nearest to the superior surface of the palate; clean them first (Fig. 7.23).

The **palatopharyngeus muscle** is lodged in the **palatopharyngeal fold.** It arises on each side from the posterior border of the **thyroid cartilage** and from the **pharyngeal aponeurosis** in close relation to the inner surface of the inferior constrictor. Running upward into the soft palate, its fibers insert into the **palatal aponeurosis** in two strata, of which the superior one crosses above the levator and the inferior (and more anterior) one below it.

The **levator veli palatini** originates from the petrous part of the **temporal bone.** Sweeping downward and medially into the soft palate, most of its fibers insert into the **palatal aponeurosis** near the median line; a few are continuous across the median line with fibers of the corresponding muscle on the opposite side.

The **tensor veli palatini** arises from the scaphoid fossa of the **sphenoid bone** and the inferior surface of the **auditory tube.** To expose its insertion, the palatal portions of the levator and the palatopharyngeus must be removed. Passing downward from its origin, the belly of the tensor muscle lies just lateral to the medial pterygoid plate. At the hamulus it becomes tendinous; the tendon turns medially inferior to the **hamulus,**

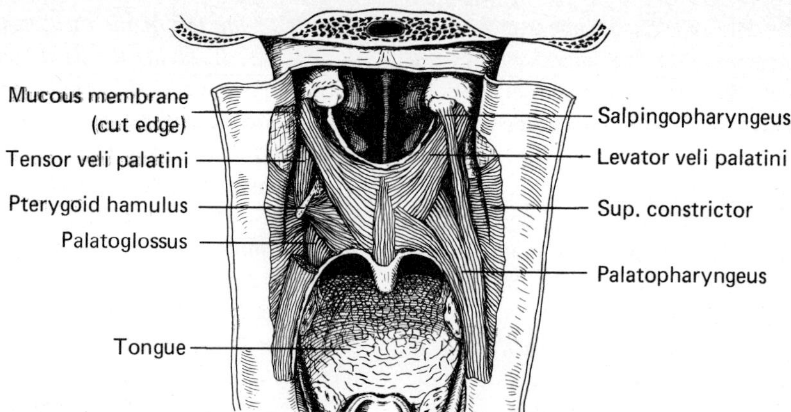

Figure 7.23 A posterior view of the **muscles of** the **soft palate.**

enters the soft palate, and spreads out to insert directly into the **palatal aponeurosis** and the posterior border of the hard palate.

The **palatoglossus muscle,** which is lodged in the palatoglossal fold, arises from the side of the posterior part of the **tongue.** Its fibers ascend to the undersurface of the **palatal aponeurosis,** into which they insert. It is the most inferior muscle of the soft palate.

NASAL CAVITIES

There are two nasal cavities; each has a medial wall, the **nasal septum,** and a complex lateral wall, which is described below. The mucous membrane of the nasal cavities, in general, is thick and spongy, due to the presence of numerous small mucous glands. The upper third of the nasal mucosa is called the **olfactory area,** since it contains the minute filaments of the **olfactory nerves,** which enter the cavity through the small openings in the cribriform plate of the ethmoid bone. The lower two-thirds of the mucosa, which is thicker and more glandular, is called the **respiratory area.** Anteriorly, the nasal cavity communicates with the exterior at the **nostril.** Just internal to the nostril, the hair-containing area that is circumscribed by the ala is called the **nasal vestibule.** Posteriorly, the nasal cavity opens into the nasopharynx at the **choana.**

Study the **nasal septum.** It is a bony and cartilaginous plate covered on each side by mucous membrane. It usually deviates somewhat to one side, most frequently to the right. Strip the mucous membrane from the left side of the septum and observe its bony and cartilaginous framework. The bony portion is formed principally by the **vomer** and the **perpendicular plate of** the **ethmoid bone.** Anteriorly the septum is completed by the **septal cartilage.** Anterosuperiorly, the septal cartilage joins the suture between the two **nasal bones.** Posterosuperiorly, it joins the anterior border of the perpendicular plate of the ethmoid, and posteroinferiorly, it joins the anterior border of the vomer.

With forceps, carefully remove, a bit at a time, the bony portion of the septum to expose the deep surface of the mucous membrane of the right side of the septum and the vessels and nerves that course through it. In addition to the **olfactory nerve,** the septal mucosa receives nerves, derived from the **ophthalmic** and **maxillary nerves,** that convey the general sensory modalities of temperature, pain, and touch. The anterior third of the septum is supplied by the **medial nasal branch** of the **anterior ethmoidal nerve,** which may be found descending on the deep surface of the anterior part of the septal mucosa, accompanied by a small branch of the **anterior ethmoidal artery.** The posterior two-thirds of the septum is supplied mostly by the **nasopalatine nerve.** It is a branch of the **pterygopalatine ganglion** (see page 85) but is principally composed of afferent nerve fibers derived from the maxillary nerve. It reaches the upper posterior part of the septum by crossing the posterior portion of the roof of the nasal cavity. From there it runs downward and forward between the mucosa and the bone of the septum to reach the **incisive canal,** through which it passes to terminate in the mucosa of the anterior portion of the hard palate. It is accompanied by the **sphenopalatine artery,** a branch of the third part of the maxillary artery.

Study the left lateral wall of the nasal cavity. (If it was destroyed when you bisected the head, cut the septal mucosa to expose the right lateral wall.) The **superior, middle,** and **inferior nasal conchae** project from the lateral wall; they partially subdivide the nasal cavity into several regions. The portion of the cavity lying anterior to the conchae and communicating with the vestibule and the nostril is known as the **atrium.** The small portion of the cavity that lies above and behind the superior concha is known as the **sphenoethmoidal recess.** The portion of the cavity lying below the superior concha and above the middle concha is the **superior meatus.** The **middle meatus** lies below the middle concha, and the **inferior meatus** below the inferior concha. The uninterrupted medial portion of the nasal cavity (between the conchae and the septum), with which the atrium, the three meatuses, and the sphenoethmoidal recess are all in free communication, is known as the **common meatus.**

After you have examined the conchae, turn them upward or break them from the lateral wall with forceps to expose the various openings in the lateral wall that lie under them. The **posterior ethmoidal air cells** communicate with the nasal cavity through one or more openings in the lateral wall of the superior meatus. Through the openings, the nasal mucosa is continuous with the mucous membrane of the ethmoidal cells. The **middle meatus** is considerably wider than the superior meatus. The portion of the middle meatus lying just inferior to the anterior end of the middle concha leads upward into a closed passage known as the **infundibulum;** through it the **frontal sinus** communicates with the middle meatus. Running downward and posteriorly from the infundibulum is a curved groove, the **hiatus semilunaris.** In the hiatus, observe the openings of the **anterior ethmoidal air cells** anteriorly and the **maxillary sinus** more posteriorly. Posterior to the infundibulum and superior to the hiatus is a bulging prominence in the lateral wall known as the **ethmoidal bulla;** the orifice of the **middle ethmoidal air cells** is on it. The opening of the **nasolacrimal duct** is in the wall of the **inferior meatus;** through it tears are conveyed from the **lacrimal sac** into the nasal cavity. The **sphenoidal sinus** opens into the nasal cavity in the wall of the **sphenoethmoidal recess.**

Observe the **sphenopalatine foramen** in a macerated skull; through it the nasal cavity communicates with the **pterygopalatine fossa.** It is not visible in the cadaver as long as the nasal mucosa is in place. Therefore, carefully strip the mucous membrane from the lateral wall of the nasal cavity to expose the **sphenopalatine foramen** and the vessels and nerves that pass through it.

The nasopalatine nerve and the posterior superior nasal nerves enter the nasal cavity through the sphenopalatine foramen. All are branches of the **pterygopalatine ganglion.** The **nasopalatine nerve** has been observed (see page 82). The **posterior superior nasal nerves** are small twigs, usually very difficult to demonstrate, that are distributed to the posterior parts of the lateral nasal walls. The **sphenopalatine artery** also enters the nasal cavity at the sphenopalatine foramen. Its branches accompany the nerves in their distribution to the lateral wall and the septum.

The anterior part of the lateral wall of the nasal cavity is supplied by the **lateral nasal branches of** the **anterior ethmoidal nerve,** which has already been seen in the orbit as one of the terminal branches of the **nasociliary nerve.** Leaving the orbit through the anterior ethmoidal foramen, it enters the cranial cavity. Here, lying external to the dura, the anterior ethmoidal nerve crosses the cribriform plate of the ethmoid bone and enters the nasal cavity through a foramen at the side of the crista galli. Descending in a groove on the inner surface of the nasal bone, it divides into medial nasal, lateral nasal, and external nasal nerves. The **medial nasal branch** is distributed to the anterior part of the nasal septum, as already noted. The **lateral nasal branch** supplies the anterior part of the lateral wall of the nasal cavity. The **external nasal branch** emerges between the nasal bone and the nasal cartilage to supply the skin of the nose. The anterior ethmoidal nerve is accompanied in its distribution by the anterior ethmoidal branch of the ophthalmic artery.

MAXILLARY NERVE AND PTERYGOPALATINE FOSSA

Before you attempt to display the **pterygopalatine fossa** and its contents, locate and define the boundaries of the fossa in a macerated skull.

The **pterygopalatine ganglion** *can be located in either of two ways. First locate the palatine nerves and vessels by stripping the mucous membrane from the posterior lateral part of the hard palate. Then trace them cranially to the area of the pterygopalatine ganglion by removing, with a chisel or bone forceps, the perpendicular part of the palatine bone.*

In the other method, the approach is from the top downward. Open the superior orbital fissure more widely by removing, with a saw, a wedge-shaped piece of bone that includes the great wing of the sphenoid and the anterior portion of the squamous part of the temporal bone. The apex of the wedge should reach the superior orbital fissure just above and anterior to the **foramen rotundum;** *preserve the bony rim of the foramen rotundum. Then remove the periorbita and any structures that remain within the orbit. Trace the course and distribution of the maxillary nerve.*

Arising from the **trigeminal ganglion,** the **maxillary nerve** passes forward in the lower part of the lateral wall of the cavernous sinus to the foramen rotundum. Here it leaves the middle cranial fossa and enters the upper part of the **pterygopalatine fossa.** Running forward through the highest part of the pterygopalatine fossa, the maxillary nerve bends laterally through the **pterygomaxillary fissure** to enter the infratemporal fossa, which it leaves almost at once by entering the posterior end of the **infraorbital canal.** From this point on, it is known as the **infraorbital nerve.** Remove the roof of the infraorbital canal with a chisel. Passing straight forward through the canal, which lies in the portion of the maxilla forming the floor of the orbit and the roof of the maxillary sinus, the infraorbital nerve emerges at the **infraorbital foramen** and breaks up, under cover of the zygomaticus minor and the levator labii superioris muscles, into a number of cutaneous branches (see page 46).

In the pterygopalatine fossa, the maxillary nerve gives rise to two short, thick **pterygopalatine branches** (sensory roots) that descend to join the **pterygopalatine ganglion.**

In the short portion of its course through the infratemporal fossa, the maxillary nerve gives rise to two branches, the zygomatic nerve and the posterior superior alveolar nerve. The **zygomatic nerve** passes upward through the inferior orbital fissure to reach the lateral wall of the orbit, external to the periorbita. Here it divides into **zygomaticofacial** and **zygomaticotemporal branches,** both of which enter canals in the zygomatic bone, through which they reach the face, where their distribution has been seen (see page 46). The zygomaticotemporal nerve gives a communicating branch to the lacrimal nerve, which conveys postganglionic parasympathetic fibers to the lacrimal gland. The **posterior superior alveolar nerve** usually divides into two branches, which descend on the infratemporal surface of the maxilla, where they enter small canals in the bone; they are conveyed, in the lateral wall of the maxillary sinus, to the roots of the upper molar teeth.

In the infraorbital canal, the infraorbital nerve gives rise to **anterior** and **middle superior alveolar nerves,** which pass through canals in the bony wall of the maxillary sinus to the upper incisor, canine, and premolar teeth. The superior alveolar nerves also supply the mucous membrane of the upper gums.

In addition to the maxillary nerve, the **pterygopalatine fossa** contains the pterygopalatine ganglion and the terminal part of the maxillary artery. The **pterygopalatine ganglion** lies inferior to the maxillary nerve and lateral to the sphenopalatine foramen. From the maxillary nerve it receives the two **pterygopalatine nerves,** which are described as the **sensory roots** of the ganglion. Posteriorly, it receives the **nerve of** the **pterygoid canal,** its **motor root.** This nerve enters the fossa at the anterior end of the pterygoid canal. The principal branches that arise from the ganglion can be grouped as medial and descending branches.

The medial branches pass through the sphenopalatine foramen to enter the nasal cavity. They include the **posterior superior nasal nerves** and the **nasopalatine nerve.** The descending branches are the **greater** and **lesser palatine nerves.** They descend in the palatine canal to reach the palate. Carefully strip the mucous membrane from the hard palate to expose the distribution of these nerves. The **greater palatine nerve** emerges at the greater palatine foramen and is distributed to the mucous membrane and glands of the hard palate. The **lesser palatine nerves,** which are much smaller, emerge at the lesser palatine foramen and turn posteriorly into the soft palate.

Another branch of the ganglion, one that is very small and difficult to find, is the **pharyngeal nerve.** It courses posteriorly from the ganglion and is inferior and medial to the nerve of the pterygoid canal. It distributes to the superior wall of the nasopharynx.

The **third part of** the **maxillary artery** is very short. As it enters the pterygopalatine fossa, it breaks up almost immediately into its four terminal branches. The **posterior superior alveolar artery** can arise from the second part of the maxillary. It accompanies the posterior superior alveolar nerve. The **sphenopalatine artery** enters the nasal cavity through the sphenopalatine foramen and divides into branches whose distribution has already been observed (see page 83). the **infraorbital artery** enters the infraorbital canal in company with the infraorbital nerve and gives rise to small branches corresponding to the branches of the nerve. The **descending palatine artery** descends in the palatine canal, gives rise to two small palatine arteries, which are distributed to the soft palate with the lesser palatine nerves, and then accompanies the greater palatine nerve into the hard palate.

With bone forceps, attempt to open the pterygoid canal to expose the nerve that traverses it. The **nerve of** the **pterygoid canal** is formed at the posterior end of the canal (which is at the anterior wall of the foramen lacerum) by the union of the **greater** and the **deep petrosal nerves.** The former is a branch (nervus intermedius) of the facial nerve, which conveys preganglionic parasympathetic nerve fibers to the pterygopalatine ganglion. The deep petrosal nerve is composed of postganglionic sympathetic fibers derived from the superior cervical ganglion and delivered through the internal carotid plexus. Note that the branches of the **pterygopalatine ganglion** consist of **sensory fibers** derived from the **maxillary nerve** through its pterygopalatine branches, but that they also contain the **sympathetic postganglionic neurons of** the **deep petrosal nerve** and **parasympathetic postganglionic neurons** derived from the postganglionic neurons whose cell bodies lie in the pterygopalatine ganglion.

SUBMANDIBULAR REGION

Review the boundaries and contents of the submandibular triangle and the attachments of the mylohyoid muscle (see page 29). Cut the membrane at the lateral inferior sides of the tongue and by retracting it medially, separate it and the adjacent structures from the mylohyoid muscle. By doing this, you will expose the sublingual gland, the deep portion and duct of the submandibular gland, the terminal parts of the lingual and hypoglossal nerves, the submandibular ganglion, and the extrinsic muscles of the tongue.

Clean the **sublingual gland,** a lobulated structure that is flattened from side to side. Its superior surface is related to the mucous membrane on the floor of the mouth. The sublingual gland does not possess a single excretory duct but a series of small, short ducts that pass upward from its superior surface to open along the sublingual fold into the floor of the mouth. Observe that the **duct of** the **submandibular gland** runs forward and upward across the muscles of the tongue, passing deep to the lingual nerve and the sublingual gland, to open into the floor of the mouth at the sublingual caruncle near the anterior end of the sublingual gland.

The **lingual nerve** has already been traced from its origin to the point where it lies between the internal surface of the mandible and the mucous membrane lining the mouth in the region of the last molar. Now follow it downward and forward across the muscles of the tongue to the deep surface of the sublingual gland, where it breaks up into its terminal branches, which are distributed to the mucous membrane of the tongue. The lingual nerve is the **sensory nerve** of the anterior two-thirds of the tongue. It mediates impulses of general sensibility (pain, temperature, and touch) and of the special sense of taste from this area. The former are carried through the **lingual branch of** the **mandibular nerve;** the latter, through the **chorda tympani nerve of** the **facial nerve,** which joins the lingual high in the infratemporal fossa.

Identify the **submandibular ganglion.** It is connected to the **lingual nerve,** in the region of the submandibular gland, by short communicating branches (usually two). It contains the cell bodies of **postganglionic parasympathetic neurons** that are secretomotor to the submandibular and sublingual salivary glands. **Preganglionic nerve fibers,** which are derived from the facial nerve (CN VII), are conveyed to the ganglion first through the chorda tympani, and then through the lingual nerve. Of the postganglionic fibers that leave the ganglion, some pass directly into the submandibular gland for its supply, while others pass back into the lingual nerve to be distributed to the sublingual gland (Fig. 7.24).

The **hypoglossal nerve** passes forward lateral to the hyoglossus, giving branches to it and to the

Figure 7.24 Deep dissection of the **submandibular** and **infratemporal regions.**

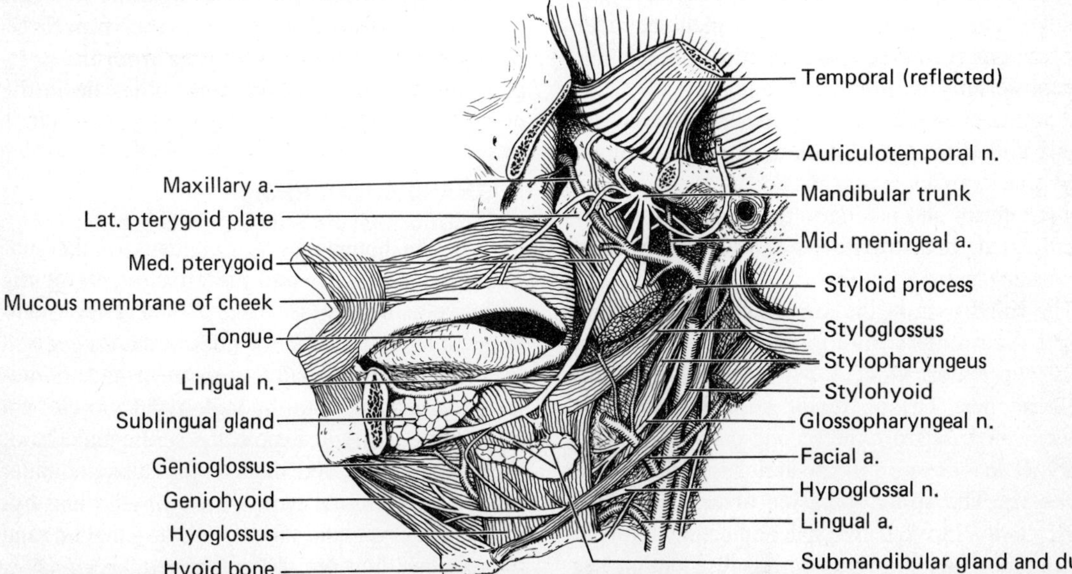

styloglossus. After giving a branch (actually derived from the first cervical spinal nerve) to the geniohyoid, it breaks up into terminal branches that supply the **genioglossus** and the **intrinsic musculature** of the tongue. It is usually connected, near the anterior border of the hyoglossus, to the lingual nerve by a communicating loop. The hypoglossal is the **motor nerve of** the **tongue,** supplying all of its extrinsic and intrinsic muscles.

Injury to the hypoglossal nerve will cause paralysis of the tongue musculature on the same side as the injury. When protruded, the tongue will deviate to the side of the injury.

Now clean the **extrinsic muscles of** the **tongue.** They all have bony origins and insert into the fleshy mass of the tongue, where their fibers mingle with one another and with the **intrinsic muscles.**

The **hyoglossus** is a thin, quadrilateral muscular sheet that arises from the lateral part of the **body** and the upper border of the **greater horn of** the **hyoid bone.** Its fibers pass vertically upward into the **tongue** and interlace with the intrinsic muscle fibers and with the styloglossus (Fig. 7.24).

The **geniohyoid,** which is not actually a muscle of the tongue but is best considered with them, is a flat, triangular muscle that arises from the inferior **mental spine** on the internal aspect of the mental symphysis. It is inserted on the upper border of the **body of** the **hyoid bone.** Immediately above it, find the **genioglossus,** which takes origin from the superior mental spine. Its fibers radiate upward and posteriorly into the tongue, the lower ones passing deep to the hyoglossus; a few of its lowest fibers insert on the hyoid bone.

The **styloglossus** is a slender muscle that arises from the tip of the **styloid process** and runs downward and forward to the side of the tongue, where its fibers interlace with those of the hyoglossus.

The **stylohyoid muscle** has already been cleaned. Observe now that it arises from the base of the **styloid process** and winds downward and forward, lateral to the external carotid artery. The **stylopharyngeus,** another slender muscle, arises from the styloid process between the origins of the stylohyoid and the styloglossus. It passes downward, forward, and medially to enter the wall of the **pharynx.** Observe the terminal part of the **glossopharyngeal nerve** running downward and forward across the external surface of the stylopharyngeus. Near the posterior border of the hyoglossus, it breaks up into terminal branches that supply the mucous membrane of the posterior third of the tongue with impulses of general sensation and taste.

The origin of the **lingual artery** from the external carotid has already been seen. The first part of the lingual artery extends from the external carotid to the posterior border of the hyoglossus. The second part extends forward deep to the hyoglossus a short distance above the hyoid bone. Spread the fibers of the hyoglossus muscle in the area between the tendons of the digastric muscle, just inferior to the hypoglossal nerve, to expose the vessel. Two or three **dorsal lingual branches** arise from the second part of the lingual artery; they ascend into the posterior part of the tongue. Near the anterior border of the hyoglossus, the lingual artery terminates by dividing into the sublingual and deep lingual arteries. The **sublingual artery** runs forward and upward, across the genioglossus, to supply the sublingual gland and neighboring structures. The **deep lingual artery** runs upward on the genioglossus and bends forward into the free portion of the tongue, where it reaches as far as the tip.

INTERNAL EAR AND FACIAL NERVE

This section is not meant to be an exhaustive study of the human auditory system; such an objective cannot be achieved in the gross anatomy laboratory. The gross dissection of the internal and middle ears, however, can be quite rewarding, if you proceed carefully and patiently. With the help of a good atlas, model, or text, you should orient yourself and be somewhat familiar with the topographical location of the structures embedded in the petrous portion of the temporal bone (Fig.

7.25), before you begin to locate them in the cadaver. As you chip away at the bone, the semicircular canals, cochlea, facial nerve, geniculate ganglion, and ear ossicles will be revealed a bit at a time. It is unlikely that all of the structures will be visible at the same time, so approach your dissection with a "chip a little and look" technique.

Identify the **facial** (CN VII) and **vestibulocochlear** (CN VIII) **nerves** entering the **internal auditory meatus** (Fig. 7.25). With a sharp chisel, chip away, a little at a time, the upper wall of the meatus, following the course of the nerves laterally and anteriorly. Note the location of the **geniculate ganglion** of the facial nerve. Examine the anterolateral surface of the temporal bone and identify the **greater petrosal nerve** leaving the ganglion to exit the **hiatus of** the **facial canal.** The **lesser petrosal nerve** exits the temporal bone lateral and inferior to the greater petrosal nerve. Just inferior to the facial nerve dissect the bone from the vestibulocochlear nerve and note its division into the cochlear and vestibular nerves.

Follow the **cochlear nerve** forward and chip away part of the bone to identify the location of the **cochlea.** It lies anteriorly along a line that joins the internal auditory meatus and the hiatus of the facial canal. Similarly, carefully chip away the bone to identify the **vestibular nerve** and one or more of the **semicircular canals,** deep to the arcuate eminence.

MIDDLE EAR

Remove the **tegmen tympani** to expose the cavity of the middle ear, the **tympanic cavity.** Without the aid of magnification, only the more gross structures will be seen. Identify the **malleus, incus,** and **tympanic membrane** through the opening made in the tegmen tympani. Insert the handle of a probe into the external auditory meatus and, while gently pushing the probe inward, note the movement of the tympanic membrane and the ear ossicles.

Chip away the posterior wall of the middle ear and the posterior part of the **mastoid process,** and

Figure 7.25 The **internal** and **middle ears** superimposed on the temporal bone.

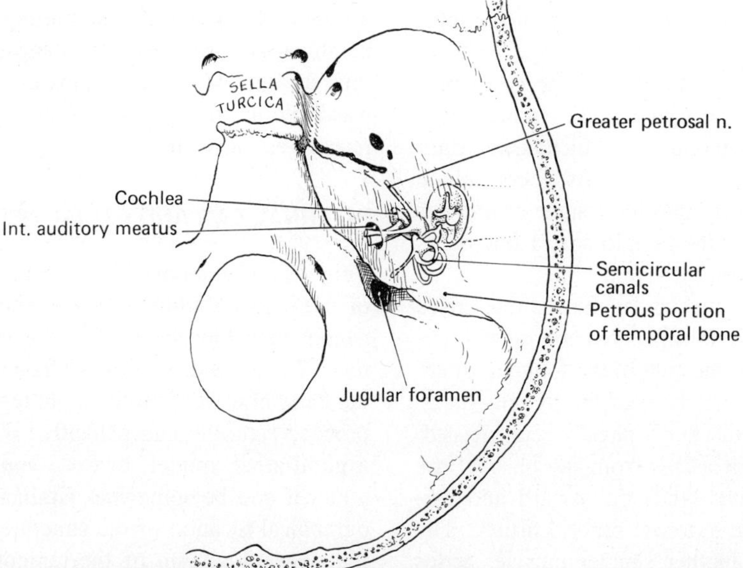

follow the course of the facial nerve inferiorly. Note the course of the **chorda tympani** in relation to the tympanic membrane, malleus, and incus. The chorda tympani is a component of the nervus intermedius of the facial nerve, transmitting preganglionic parasympathetic impulses to the submandibular ganglion and taste sensation from the tongue (see page 86). Attempt to locate the **stapes** and the **tensor tympani muscle.**

The **tympanic cavity** is irregularly shaped and compressed from the sides, resulting in the vertical dimension being two to three times longer than the transverse dimension. Using the superior and inferior limits of the tympanic membrane as a guide, the cavity is divided into the **tympanic cavity proper,** on the same plane as the membrane, and the **attic** or **epitympanic recess,** above the level of the membrane. The very small **hypotympanic cavity** lies below the plane of the membrane. The tegmen tympani, the roof of the cavity, was removed in the preceding dissection.

The tympanic cavity is described as consisting of six walls. The **anterior** or **carotid wall** tapers, being wider above than below. It is separated from the carotid canal by a thin plate of bone. Identify the **auditory tube,** which connects the pharynx with the tympanic cavity. The **tensor tympani muscle,** located in a semicanal above the auditory tube, should also be identified. It may have been damaged in opening the cavity of the middle ear, but attempt to ascertain its insertion into the malleus.

The **medial wall** contains a rounded prominence, the **promontory,** formed over the first turn of the cochlea. Using the promontory as a guide, locate the oval window **(fenestra vestibuli)** on its superoposterior edge; it usually contains the base of the stapes. A little below and posterior to the oval window, locate the **round window (fenestra cochleae),** which is closed by a membrane.

The **posterior** or **mastoid wall** contains a variable number of **mastoid air cells,** particularly in the caudal part of the mastoid process. Above the cells is a cavity, the **mastoid antrum,** which communicates with the epitympanic recess through the **aditus.** Also on the posterior wall find the **pyramidal eminence,** which is immediately posterior to the oval window and in front of the vertical portion of the facial canal. It contains the **stapedius muscle.**

The **lateral** or **membranous wall** consists mainly of the **tympanic membrane** and the ring of bone into which it inserts. The malleus and the incus may be still attached to the tympanic membrane. If they are, review their attachments and the course of the chorda tympani nerve.

The **floor** or **jugular wall** is narrow and is separated from the jugular vein by a thin plate of bone.

The **roof** has been described.

The mucous membrane that lines the auditory tube is continuous with the lining of the cavity of the middle ear and the structures that traverse it. Note also that the mastoid air cells are lined by small outpouchings of this mucous membrane.

The relationship of these walls to the middle cranial fossa, the jugular vein, and the carotid artery is particularly important clinically; a severe and unattended infection within the middle ear cavity may erode any of the walls, endangering the structures adjacent to them.

EXTERNAL EAR

The external ear should be studied next. Identify the **auricle** (pinna) and its subdivisions: the helix, anthelix, tragus, antitragus, lobule, concha, and auricular tubercle. Remove the skin from the auricle and attempt to identify some of the intrinsic and extrinsic muscles and ligaments of the auricle and the **auricular cartilage.** Review the cartilaginous and osseous portions of the **external auditory meatus** and its nerve and blood supplies from one of the standard descriptive texts.

Chapter 8

Larynx

Before you start to dissect the larynx, you should have a clear idea of its cartilaginous and membranous structure (Fig. 8.1). A good model showing the laryngeal cartilages and their articulations is helpful. The cartilages that form the main skeleton of the larynx are the thyroid cartilage, the cricoid cartilage, and the paired arytenoid cartilages. The **thyroid cartilage** consists of **two laminae** that are joined in the midline anteriorly at the laryngeal prominence, which is often called "Adam's apple." It is opened posteriorly; the free posterior margin of each lamina is prolonged superiorly and inferiorly as the **superior** and **inferior horns,** respectively. The **cricoid cartilage,** which lies below the thyroid cartilage at the level of the sixth cervical vertebra and above the first ring of the trachea, forms a complete ring. The ring, like a signet ring, is relatively narrow anteriorly and laterally but is expanded posteriorly to form a broad plate or **lamina.** The medial surface of the tip of the inferior horn of the thyroid cartilage articulates with the posterolateral aspect of the cricoid. The **arytenoid cartilages** are small, pyramid-shaped cartilages resting, one on each side, upon the upper border of the cricoid lamina, with which they articulate by true diarthrodial joints. Each arytenoid cartilage exhibits a superior prolongation, the **apical process,** a lateral prolongation, the **muscular process,** and an anterior prolongation, the **vocal process.** At its pointed apex, the arytenoid cartilage articulates with a small cartilaginous nodule, the **corniculate cartilage,** which lies within the aryepiglottic fold. A very small **cuneiform cartilage** is also usually embedded within the aryepiglottic fold, anterior and superior to the corniculate cartilage.

The cartilages of the larynx are connected to one another by ligaments and muscles. The most important ligament, the **conus elasticus,** is a membranous ligament whose inferior margin is attached to the upper border of the anterior and lateral parts of the cricoid cartilage; its superior

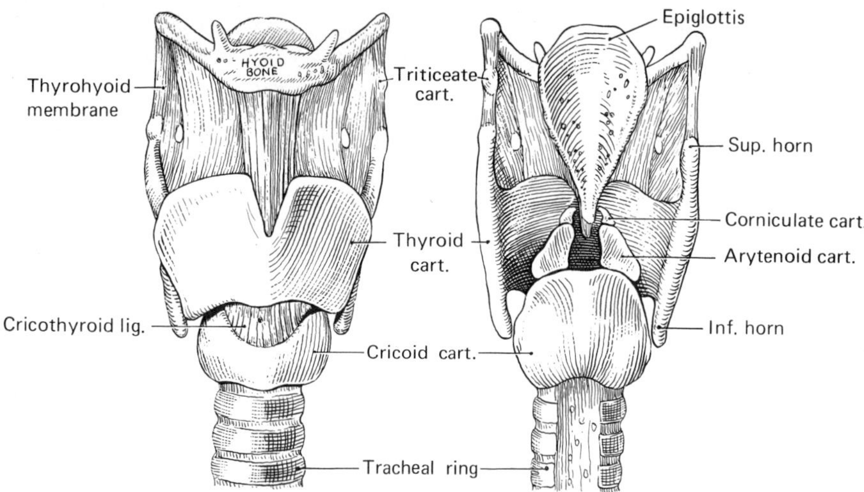

Figure 8.1 The **laryngeal cartilages.**

margin is attached anteriorly to the inner surface of the thyroid lamina and posteriorly to the vocal process of the arytenoid cartilage. Between these two superior attachments, the conus elasticus presents a free superior border, known as the **vocal ligament.** The vocal ligament is covered medially by laryngeal mucous membrane and laterally by muscle and mucous membrane to become the **true vocal fold** or **cord.**

Clean the **thyrohyoid membrane,** which extends from the upper border of the thyroid cartilage to the lower border of the body and greater horn of the hyoid bone. The thyrohyoid membrane is pierced on each side by the **internal laryngeal nerve** and the **superior laryngeal artery.** Its free posterolateral border, which runs from the superior horn of the thyroid cartilage to the greater horn of the hyoid, is rather strong and is often referred to as the **lateral thyrohyoid ligament.** A small cartilaginous nodule, the **triticeate cartilage,** is sometimes found in the ligament.

Study the interior of the larynx as seen through the **superior laryngeal aperture.** The larynx is clothed internally by a layer of mucous membrane that is continuous superiorly with the mucous membrane of the pharynx and inferiorly with that of the trachea. Beginning superiorly at the superior laryngeal aperture, which is bounded by the epiglottis and the aryepiglottic folds, the larynx is partially subdivided into three compartments by two pairs of transverse folds in its lateral walls. The upper pair of folds is the vestibular folds, or **false vocal cords.** Below these are the vocal folds, or **true vocal cords,** which are easily seen from above, since they project farther medially than do the ventricular folds. The highest compartment of the laryngeal cavity is the **vestibule of** the **larynx;** it lies posterior to the epiglottis and superior to the vestibular folds. The portion of the laryngeal cavity between the vestibular folds and the vocal folds is the **ventricle of** the **larynx.** The area below the vocal folds is the **infraglottic compartment,** which widens inferiorly to become continuous with the trachea. The ventricle communicates with the infraglottic compartment through the **rima glottidis,** the narrow interval between the two vocal folds. The term "glottis," often used interchangeably but erroneously with "rima glottidis," actually refers to the vocal folds inclusive of the rima glottidis.

Next direct your attention to the muscles of the larynx. By moving the arytenoid cartilages upon the cricoid cartilage or by changing the relative positions of the cricoid and thyroid cartilages, the muscles act to tense or relax, to approximate (adduct) or separate (abduct), the vocal cords.

First clean the **cricothyroid muscle.** It arises from the anterolateral part of the arch of the **cricoid.** Running upward and backward, its fibers radiate slightly to insert on the lower border and inferior horn of the **thyroid cartilage.** It is supplied by the external branch of the superior laryngeal nerve (Fig. 7.21).

Turn to the posterior aspect of the larynx and remove the mucous membrane that forms the anterior wall of the pharynx below the superior laryngeal aperture. Then clean the posterior cricoarytenoid and the arytenoid muscles (Fig. 8.2). As you remove the mucous membrane, identify and retain in position the **inferior laryngeal nerve** (the terminal portion of the recurrent laryngeal nerve above the cricoid cartilage), which ascends on the posterior aspect of the larynx and is closely related to the external surface of the pharyngeal mucosa.

The paired **posterior cricoarytenoid muscle** arises on each side from the posterior aspect of the **cricoid lamina.** Its fibers converge upward and laterally to insert into the muscular process of the **arytenoid cartilage.** The **arytenoid muscle** is an unpaired median muscle, whose fibers take origin from the posterior surface of one **arytenoid cartilage** and insert into the posterior surface of the other. It is roughly divisible into **transverse** and **oblique portions.** The transverse fibers run horizontally across the interarytenoid space from one arytenoid cartilage to the other. The oblique fibers arise from the posterior aspect of the muscular process of one arytenoid cartilage and run upward and medially across the median line to reach the apex of the arytenoid cartilage of the opposite side. A few of them are prolonged laterally and anteriorly within the aryepiglottic fold to the epiglottis as the **aryepiglotticus muscle** (Fig. 8.2).

Turn to the lateral aspect of the larynx. Remove one lamina of the thyroid cartilage according to the following procedure. Sever the attachment of the thyrohyoid membrane to the thyroid cartilage on one side and disarticulate the inferior horn of the thyroid cartilage from the cricoid. Detach the cricothyroid muscle from its origin on the cricoid cartilage. Then, on the same side, cut vertically through the lamina of the thyroid cartilage about 1 cm posterolateral to the median line and remove it.

Clean the lateral cricoarytenoid and the thyroarytenoid muscles (Fig. 8.3). The **lateral cricoarytenoid muscle** arises from the upper border of the lateral part of the **cricoid arch.** Its fibers run upward and posteriorly, and converge to insert into the muscular process of the **arytenoid cartilage.** The **thyroarytenoid muscle** is variable in

Figure 8.2 **Posterior** aspect of the **larynx** after removal of the pharyngeal mucosa.

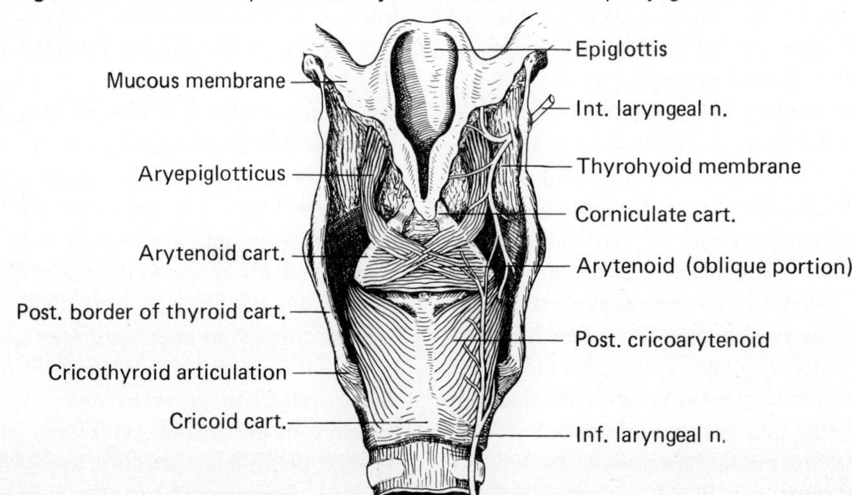

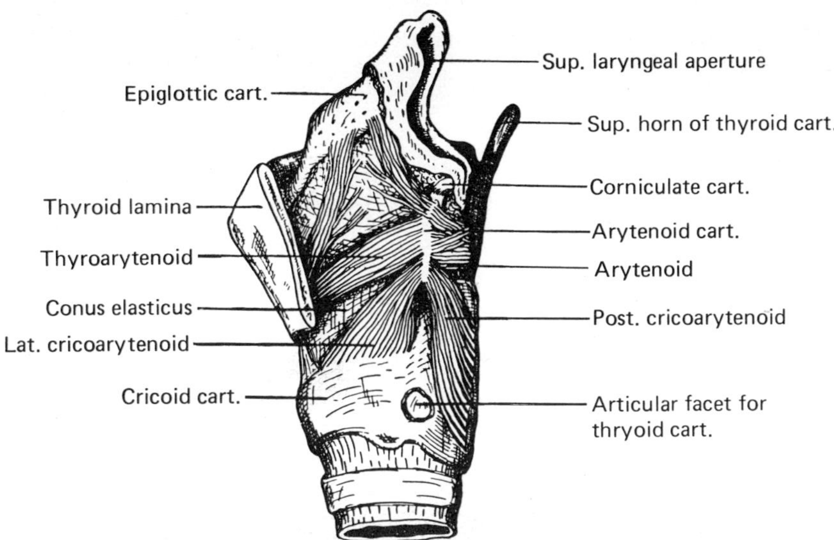

Figure 8.3 Left **lateral** view of the **larynx** after the lamina of the thyroid cartilage has been removed.

size and frequently appears to be continuous with the upper border of the lateral cricoarytenoid. It extends from the inner surface of the angle of the **thyroid laminae,** anteriorly, to the lateral border of the **arytenoid cartilage** posteriorly. Although it is indistinguishable in the gross dissection, the **vocalis muscle,** which is a medial subdivision of the thyroarytenoid muscle, inserts into the vocal ligament. Both lie within the vocal fold, just lateral to the vocal ligament.

The muscles of the larynx, with the exception of the cricothyroid, are supplied by the **inferior laryngeal nerve.** Ascending in the groove between the trachea and the esophagus, it generally divides at the lower border of the cricoid cartilage into an anterior and a posterior branch. The **posterior branch** ascends on the posterior cricoarytenoid to supply that muscle and the oblique and transverse arytenoid muscles. The **anterior branch** runs forward and upward to supply the lateral cricoarytenoid, the thyroarytenoid, and the vocalis muscles. The inferior laryngeal nerve provides some of the sensory supply to the mucosa below the vocal folds.

The **internal laryngeal nerve** is the sensory nerve of the larynx, primarily above the vocal folds, but there is some overlap with the inferior laryngeal nerve. After piercing the thyrohyoid membrane, it ramifies on the deep surface of the laryngeal mucosa (Fig. 8.2).

Carefully remove the lateral cricoarytenoid and the thyroarytenoid muscles and attempt to display the **conus elasticus.** As mentioned (see page 90), it runs upward and medially, deep to these two muscles, from the upper border of the arch of the cricoid. Observe that its free upper border, the **vocal ligament,** lies within the vocal fold, where it is lateral to the mucous membrane but medial to the vocalis muscle.

Briefly examine the **aryepiglottic folds.** They are formed principally by the **quadrangular membrane,** which runs from the lateral aspect of the arytenoid cartilages posteriorly, to the superior lateral borders of the epiglottis anteriorly. The aryepiglotticus and thyroepiglotticus muscles pass upward into the folds to insert into the quadrangular membrane and the epiglottis. Covered laterally and medially by mucous membrane, the superior free margin of the folds forms the superior laryngeal aperture. The free inferior margin of the mucous membrane-covered quadrangular membrane is the vestibular fold or the false vocal cord.

Chapter 9

Thorax

THORACIC WALL

For the dissection of the thoracic wall and the thoracic cavity, the body lies supine. Review the **anterior** and the **lateral cutaneous branches of** the **intercostal nerves.** The latter emerge through the external intercostal muscles near the costal attachment of the serratus anterior muscle and run forward and slightly downward to be distributed to the skin on the lateral and anterolateral aspect of the trunk.

The bony wall of the thorax is made up of the 12 **thoracic vertebrae,** the **sternum,** and the 12 pairs of **ribs** and their **costal cartilages.** The spaces between the ribs, known as the **intercostal spaces,** are filled by the **external** and **internal intercostal muscles,** the **intercostal nerves,** and the **intercostal blood vessels.** The upper spaces are most favorable for a detailed study of the intercostal structures.

Study the **external intercostal muscles.** These are 11 pairs of thin muscular sheets whose fibers run downward and forward around the thoracic wall. Each takes origin from the **inferior border of** a **rib** and is inserted on the **superior border of** the next **rib below.** Posteriorly, the external intercostals begin at the **tubercles** of the ribs and extend anteriorly only as far as the junctions of the ribs with their costal cartilages. Between the cartilages, the muscle is replaced by a membranous layer, the **external intercostal membrane,** through which the fibers of the internal intercostal muscle are usually visible. Divide the external intercostal muscle and the external intercostal membrane along the upper border of the rib in several spaces and turn them upward to expose the internal intercostal muscle.

The **internal intercostal muscles,** also 11 pairs, run downward and posteriorly. Each takes origin from the **inner surface of** a **rib,** at the upper border of the **costal groove** when the groove is present, and inserts at the **upper border of** the next **rib below,** close to the insertion of the corresponding external intercostal muscle. The costal groove is thus enclosed by the two layers of intercostal muscle. Anteriorly, the internal intercostal muscles reach the lateral border of the sternum; posteriorly, they extend only to the **angles of** the **ribs,** from which point they continue to the tubercles of the ribs as the **internal intercostal membrane.**

The **intercostal nerves** and **vessels** are situated for the greater part of their course in the costal grooves, under cover of the lower borders of the ribs. To display them, you must chip away the lower part of the rib, but this must be done carefully to avoid damaging the nerves and vessels. In the lateral and anterior portions of the thoracic wall, the nerves and vessels are small and are usually impossible to demonstate satisfactorily. You will be more successful in finding them if you dissect posterior to the midaxillary line, where they are larger.

The **intercostal nerves** are the ventral rami of the first 11 pairs of thoracic nerves. In the present dissection, several of them should be exposed in the costal grooves as far posteriorly as convenient and traced anteriorly. In the costal groove, the nerve lies between the internal intercostal and the innermost intercostal,[1] to each of which it gives twigs of supply. Each intercostal nerve gives rise to a relatively large **lateral cutaneous branch,** which pierces the external intercostal muscle along the midaxillary line. Continuing anteriorly, the intercostal nerve enters the substance of the internal intercostal muscle a little anterior to the midaxillary line. Near the junction of the rib and costal cartilage, it reaches the deep surface of the muscle. From this point, it runs forward between the internal intercostal muscle and the pleural membrane or the transversus thoracis muscle, which it also supplies; near the lateral border of the sternum, it bends anteriorly and pierces the internal intercostal muscle, the external intercostal membrane, and the pectoralis major muscle to end superficially as an **anterior cutaneous nerve of** the **chest.** This description pertains to the terminal parts of only the upper five nerves. The lower six intercostal nerves, after reaching the anterior ends of the intercostal spaces, run downward and forward into the anterior abdominal wall; their distribution will be investigated when the abdominal wall is dissected.

[1]The intercostal vein, artery, and nerve, in their course in the costal groove, cause the deeper portions of the internal intercostal muscles to split off as separate layers known as the **innermost intercostal muscles** (musculi intercostales intimi).

The **intercostal arteries** occur in two paired groups, the anterior and the posterior intercostal arteries. The **posterior intercostal arteries** of the first two spaces are derived from the **supreme intercostal artery,** a branch of the costocervical trunk of the subclavian artery. The remaining nine pairs of posterior intercostals are direct branches of the **thoracic aorta.** Running forward in the costal groove, they give off numerous small twigs that supply the intercostal muscles. The **anterior intercostal arteries** are small vessels, usually two to each space, that run posteriorly in the anterior parts of the intercostal spaces and end by anastomosing with the terminal twigs of the posterior intercostals. Notice that in the costal groove the artery lies inferior to the vein but superior to the corresponding nerve. The anterior intercostals of the upper five spaces are branches of the **internal thoracic artery;** those of the lower six spaces are branches of the **musculophrenic artery.**

When a needle is inserted into the thoracic cavity to remove excess fluid (thoracentesis), it should be guided through the intercostal space along the superior border of the rib, thus ensuring the safety of the nerves and vessels that are lodged in the costal groove.

Expose the **internal thoracic artery** by removing the internal intercostal muscles in the upper five spaces for about 2.5 cm lateral to the sternum. This artery arises in the neck as a branch of the first part of the **subclavian artery** and enters the thorax by passing downward behind the sternoclavicular joint. It will be seen running on the inside of the anterior thoracic wall behind the first five costal cartilages, usually accompanied by two veins. In the upper two spaces, it lies between the internal muscles and the pleura; more inferiorly, it is separated from the pleura by slips of the transversus thoracic muscle. The internal thoracic artery terminates behind the sixth costal cartilage by dividing into the **superior epigastric** and the **musculophrenic arteries.**

The **transversus thoracis** is a small muscle of the anterior thoracic wall, of which only an imperfect view can be obtained at present. It arises from the posterior surface of the lower half of the **body** and the **xiphoid process of** the **sternum.** From this origin, flat, fibrous bands run upward and laterally to insert on the posterior surfaces of the **third** to the **sixth costal cartilages.** It will be seen when the sternum and costal cartilages are removed in opening the thoracic cavity.

THORACIC CAVITY

Before opening the **thoracic cavity,** you should have an idea of the general plan of its contents. Refer to a skeleton at this point. The **thoracic wall,** which has already been studied, is made up of the 12 thoracic vertebrae, 12 pairs of ribs and their costal cartilages, the sternum, the external and internal intercostal muscles, and the transversus thoracis muscle. The intercostal vessels and nerves are found in the wall, and the internal thoracic vessels are in close relation to the inner surface of the anterior part of the wall.

The thoracic cavity communicates freely with the root of the neck through the **superior thoracic aperture** (thoracic inlet), which is bounded by the upper border of the manubrium sterni, the first pair of ribs and their cartilages, and the upper border of the first thoracic vertebra.

The **inferior thoracic aperture** (thoracic outlet) has a more irregular outline and a greater diameter than the superior aperture. It can be shown on the skeleton by a line beginning at the lower border of the twelfth thoracic vertebra and passing around on each side along the lower border of the twelfth rib, thence to the tip of the eleventh rib, the lowest part of the tenth costal cartilage, and along the continuous lower margins of the ninth, eighth, and seventh costal cartilages to the xiphoid process. This line will also indicate the approximate line of origin of the peripheral portion of the **diaphragm,** a sheet of muscular and fibrous tissue that separates the thoracic cavity from the **abdominal cavity.** The diaphragm does not, however, bridge this aperture in a transverse plane but is dome-shaped; its central portion reaches considerably higher than its peripheral attachment. Thus the abdominal cavity is enclosed within the lower part of the thoracic skeleton.

The contents of the thoracic cavity consist of two pleural sacs, each enclosing a lung, and the mediastinum. The **pleural sacs** are **laterally** placed, lying internal to the ribs and intercostal muscles; the **mediastinum** is **centrally** placed, lying between the two pleural sacs, in relation to the sternum anteriorly and the bodies of the vertebrae posteriorly (Fig. 9.1).

Each pleural sac is formed by one continuous serous membrane called the **pleura.** The entire lung indents the membrane-bound sac and, in so doing, comes into intimate and inseparable contact with part of the serous membrane. The portion that forms the external covering of the lung is the **visceral pleura,** and the portion more closely related to the thoracic wall is the **parietal pleura.** The visceral and parietal pleurae are continuous only around the **root of** the **lung.** The space that they enclose is the **pleural cavity,** which contains only a thin film of serous fluid. Nowhere are the two pleural cavities in communication with each other.

The parietal pleura is designated as **costal, mediastinal, diaphragmatic,** or **cervical,** depending upon the surface or area with which it is most closely related.

It should be understood that the mediastinum is not a single anatomical entity. The term "mediastinum" is applied to the entire complex of **structures** that lie **between** the **right** and **left mediastinal pleurae.** It extends from the superior thoracic aperture above to the diaphragm below, and from the posterior surface of the sternum anteriorly to

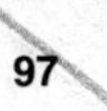

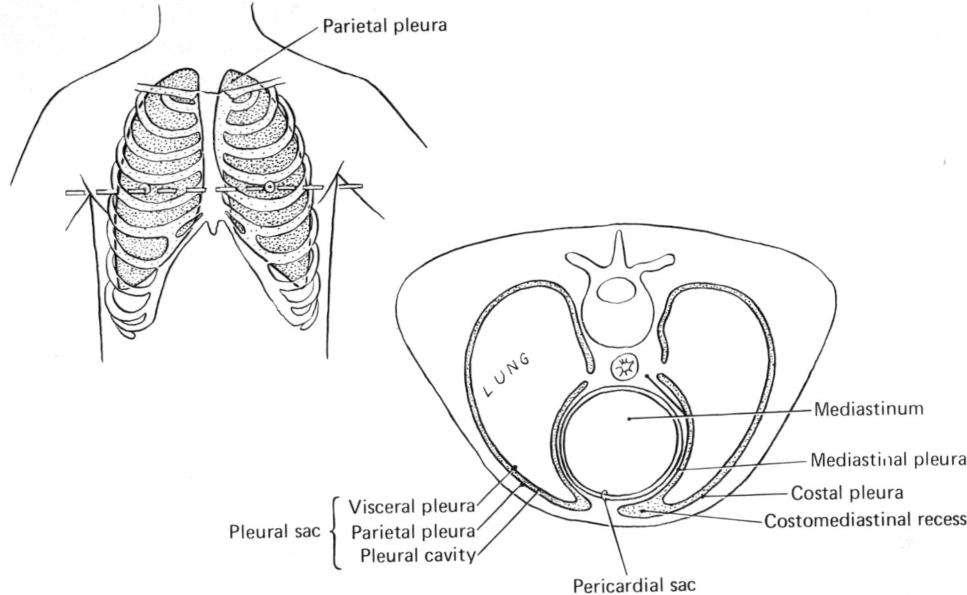

Figure 9.1 A cross section of the thorax to show the **pleural sacs** and the **mediastinum** with the pericardial sac.

the anterior surfaces of the thoracic vertebral bodies posteriorly.

If the musculature of the ventral abdominal wall is not dissected before the thoracic cavity is opened, it is advisable to dissect free and reflect caudally the portions of the rectus abdominis and external oblique muscles that attach to the lower ventral part of the thoracic cage above the level of the eighth rib and costal cartilages. Separate the origin of the serratus anterior muscle from the external intercostal muscles and elevate it from the subjacent ribs as far posteriorly as the midaxillary line, from the first to the eighth rib. In removing the intercostal muscles, as described below, leave the parts of the origins of the pectoralis major and minor and serratus anterior muscles attached to the portion of the thoracic cage that will be removed. This will facilitate review of these muscles and their relationship to the thoracic cage.

Open the **thoracic cavity** *from the front by removing the anterior and lateral portions of its wall, without damaging the underlying* **parietal pleura.** *The* **intercostal muscles** *should be removed from the upper seven spaces on each side as far laterally as the midaxillary line. Do this with care, as the pleura is separated from the internal surface of the internal intercostal muscles by only a very thin fibrous layer, the* **endothoracic fascia.** *Insert your fingers between the ribs and by gently pressing, separate the parietal pleura from the internal surfaces of the ribs as far inferiorly as the eighth rib. Leave the first rib intact for the present, but section the second through the sixth ribs in the midaxillary line on each side. Pass your fingers medially behind the costal cartilages and the sternum, first on one side and then on the other, and separate the pleura as completely as possible from this portion of the thoracic wall. The* **internal thoracic artery** *should be freed from the thoracic wall and left on the surface of the thoracic viscera.*

Now cut the **manubrium sterni** *with a saw transversely, just below its junction with the* **first costal cartilage.** *Make another transverse cut through the lower part of the sternum, between its junction on each side with the sixth and seventh* *costal cartilages. Remove the portion of the sternum between the two cuts, together with the attached portions of the second through the sixth ribs. The xiphoid process and the seventh costal cartilage must be left in place in order not to injure the diaphragm. If the lower part of the neck has not been dissected, the upper part of the manubrium and the first costal cartilage must be left in place throughout the thoracic dissection. If, however, this dissection has been done, the first ribs may be cut at their junctions with their costal cartilages. The manubrium and the attached portion of the second through the sixth ribs can now be removed.*

PLEURA

The anterior lines of reflection of the right and left pleurae should be observed next (Fig. 9.2). These are the lines along which the **costal pleura** of each side turns posteriorly to become the **mediastinal pleura.** In a lean subject, these lines may be readily apparent, but in an obese subject they will be hidden by a considerable amount of adipose tissue, which must be removed. In such a case, it is helpful to make a small opening in the costal pleura 2.5 or 5.0 cm lateral to the midline. The handle of the scalpel may then be introduced through the opening into the pleural cavity and passed medially along the internal surface of the pleura. Its medial excursion will be stopped when it reaches the line of reflection of the pleura. In the region of the **superior mediastinum,** which lies behind the manubrium sterni, the **two pleural margins** diverge from each other. At the lower border of the manubrium, they approach each other and frequently overlap to a slight extent in the midline. The **right pleural margin** passes vertically downward from this point, behind the middle of the sternum, to about the level of the sixth intercostal space, where it turns laterally and inferiorly across the **diaphragm.** Now it can be followed only as far as the junction of the eighth rib with its costal cartilage. Along this inferior part of the margin,

Figure 9.2 The **surface projection of** the parietal **pleurae** and of the fissures and lobes of the **lungs.** Clear area = visceral pleura (lung); clear + shaded areas = parietal pleura.

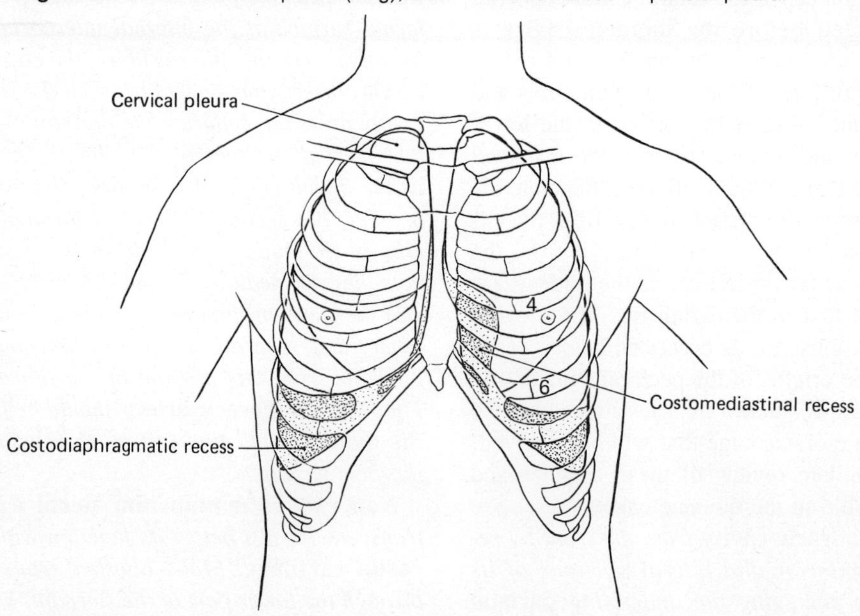

the **costal pleura** is continuous with the **diaphragmatic pleura.**

From the lower border of the manubrium, the **left pleural margin** passes vertically downward close to the right margin to about the level of the fourth costal cartilage; from this point it deviates to the left for a varying distance. Inferiorly, it crosses the diaphragm in a manner similar to the right side. Between the two pleural margins in the region where the left reflection diverges to the left, the anterior surface of the pericardium is exposed. This is known as the **bare area of** the **pericardium** and varies in its extent between individuals. Between the inferior divergent margins of the pleurae and the lower border of the pericardium, a considerable portion of the **diaphragm** is exposed, covered by neither pleura nor pericardium. The muscle of this part of the diaphragm that originates from the xiphoid process and the seventh and eighth costal cartilages may now be seen.

Before proceeding to a study of the mediastinum, the **pleural cavities** should be opened (Fig. 9.4). Make a longitudinal incision through the costal pleura from the level of the first to the seventh rib on each side. From each end of the longitudinal incisions, make transverse incisions laterally and medially, and reflect the folds of pleura thus mapped out to expose the pleural cavities, the very small intervals between the visceral pleura (external surface of the lung) and the internal surface of the parietal pleura. In the cadaver the lungs may be shrunken, thereby increasing the relative size of the pleural cavities. During life, however, each lung is entirely inflated, and the size of the pleural cavity is reduced to merely a potential space. Note that the lungs are not within the pleural cavities, and that the right and left cavities are nowhere in communication with each other.

The embalmed **lungs** now seen within the sacs are usually bluish gray in color with dark patches (carbon debris) scattered over their surface. The external relationships of the lungs may be understood by exploring the walls of the pleural cavities with your fingers. In a perfectly normal and healthy pleural cavity, the **visceral pleura,** which is closely adherent to the outer surface of the lung and may be regarded as a part of the lung, is continuous with the **parietal pleura** only across the **root of** the **lung** and the **pulmonary ligament.** Perfectly healthy lungs are, however, relatively rare in the dissecting room, and numerous secondary adhesions between the visceral and parietal pleurae will usually be found. In many cases, the adhesions can be readily broken down with your fingers.

The **costal portion of** the **pleura** is intimately related throughout with the inner surfaces of the **ribs** and **intercostal muscles.** Its most posterior extent is along the angles of the successive ribs, from which it is continued medially and forward across the lateral aspect of the bodies of the thoracic vertebrae, which may be readily felt through the pleura. Here the costal pleura becomes continuous anteriorly with the **mediastinal pleura.** The uppermost portion of the pleura is dome-shaped and reaches up into the root of the neck above the level of the first rib (Figs. 9.1 and 9.2). This **cervical,** or **apical, portion of** the **pleura,** often called the cupola, is crossed anteriorly, a short distance below its summit, by the subclavian artery, which can usually be felt through the pleura. Along its inferior margin, the costal pleura is reflected upward onto the superior surface of the diaphragm as the **diaphragmatic pleura,** which closely follows the contour of the diaphragm. At the junction of the eighth rib with its costal cartilage, this inferior pleural margin crosses the thoracic wall along a line slightly convex downward, reaching approximately the level of the tenth rib in the midaxillary line and the twelfth in the scapular line. The lateral and posterior portions of the periphery of the diaphragm extend almost vertically upward from this line, so that the lowest portion of each pleural cavity is a pocketlike cleft, the **costodiaphragmatic recess,** between the lowest part of the costal pleura and the peripheral part of the diaphragmatic pleura (Fig. 9.2). The narrow anteromedial prolongation of each pleural cavity to the midline, at the edge of which the costal pleura is reflected posteriorly to become the mediastinal pleura, is known as the **costomediastinal recess.** Even when the lungs are expanded, they do not extend into the recesses.

Some forms of pleurisy (inflammation of the pleura) are accompanied by fluid accumulation in the pleural cavity. The fluid settles in the lowest part of the cavity, the costodiaphragmatic recess, from which it can be safely removed with a needle or cannula.

The contour and relations of the **mediastinal pleura** are not entirely alike on the two sides. On each side, however, the **root of** the **lung** will be seen connecting the lung to the posterior part of the mediastinum at about the level of the fifth to the seventh thoracic vertebrae. The **visceral pleura** covering the lung is reflected across the root to become continuous with the **mediastinal pleura.** Anteriorly, superiorly, and posteriorly, the pleura is closely applied to the root of the lung, but inferiorly, the **pulmonary ligament,** a double fold of pleura, helps to hold the lung in place against the mediastinum. It consists of two layers of parietal pleura fused together with a small amount of fatty areolar tissue. These layers of pleura are continuous laterally with the visceral pleura on the inferior part of the mediastinal surface of the lung, superiorly with the pleura on the lung root, and medially with the mediastinal part of the parietal pleura. Inferiorly, the layers are continuous with each other and present a free margin stretching transversely across the pleural cavity a short distance above the diaphragm.

On the **right side,** in front of the root of the lung and the pulmonary ligament, the right lateral surface of the **heart** may be felt through the mediastinal pleura. This surface of the heart is composed almost entirely of the **right atrium,** which is separated from the mediastinal pleura only by the **pericardium.** Immediately above the diaphragm and anterior to the lowest part of the pulmonary ligament, the **inferior vena cava** can be felt where it traverses the diaphragm to enter the right atrium of the heart. Running upward from the atrium anterior to the upper part of the root, the **superior vena cava** can be felt. Directly continuous with it and running up to the superior thoracic aperture is the **right brachiocephalic vein.** The **arch of** the **azygos vein,** which opens into the posterior aspect of the upper part of the superior vena cava, can be felt immediately superior to the root of the lung. Above the azygos arch and behind the **right brachiocephalic vein,** the right mediastinal pleura is in contact with the **trachea.** Behind the trachea, the pleura is in relation to the **esophagus,** which here lies immediately in front of the vertebral column. A ridge caused by the **right phrenic nerve,** which traverses the mediastinum more or less embedded in the mediastinal pleura, can usually be seen. Superiorly, the nerve is in relation to the brachiocephalic vein and superior vena cava and inferiorly, to the right atrium and the pericardium.

On the **left side,** the mediastinal pleura is also in relation below and anteriorly to the **pericardium,** but it will be seen that the heart projects much farther toward the left than it does to the right, with the result that the capacity of the left lung is less than that of the right. The left surface of the heart is formed principally by the **left ventricle,** but its most superior and anterior part is formed by the **conus arteriosus** of the right ventricle, with a slight contribution from the left atrium. Superior to the root of the left lung in a position similar to that of the **azygos arch** on the right side, the **arch of** the **aorta** can be easily felt through the pleura. Continuous with the posterior part of the arch and coursing vertically downward posterior to the root of the lung and the pulmonary ligament, you will feel the thoracic part of the **descending aorta.** Running upward from the arch, the left **subclavian artery** is in relation to the pleura. The **esophagus** comes into relation with the **left mediastinal pleura** near the trachea and again just before it passes through the diaphragm. The **left phrenic nerve** usually makes a low ridge in the left mediastinal pleura as it crosses, from above downward, the left brachiocephalic vein, the arch of the aorta, and the pericardium.

When the pleural cavities have been thoroughly investigated, the **mediastinum** and its contents should be approached from the front. The subdivisions of the mediastinum are purely arbitrary and depend for their boundaries upon the extent of the **serous pericardium.** The serous pericardium, like each of the pleurae, is a single, uninterrupted membrane that consists of visceral and parietal portions separated from each other by a narrow, enclosed space, the **pericardial cavity.** The **visceral portion of** the **serous pericardium** is closely applied to the external surface of the heart and is to be regarded as a part of that organ. From the surface of the heart, the visceral pericardium is prolonged for a short distance along the external surfaces of the vessels that join the heart and is then reflected from them to become the parietal pericardium. The **parietal pericardium,** which forms the external wall of the pericardial cavity, will appear as a considerably thicker and tougher membrane than the parietal pleura, due to its intimate association with the fibrous pericardium. The **fibrous pericardium** is a layer of relatively dense fibrous tissue intimately blended with the external surface of the parietal serous pericardium, from which it cannot be separated as a definite membrane. It is continuous, through the fibrous sheaths of the vessels in the superior mediastinum, with the **deep fascia of** the **neck.**

The fibrous pericardium is firmly attached inferiorly to the central portion of the diaphragm. On each side, it is in relation to the right and left mediastinal pleurae, from which it is separated only by a small amount of areolar tissue and the phrenic nerves. Anteriorly it is overlapped by the right and left pleurae, except for the small bare area that has already been seen. Posteriorly, it is loosely attached to the esophagus and the descending aorta. The superior extent of the serous pericardium is at the line of its reflection from the ascending aorta, the pulmonary trunk, and the superior vena cava. This is approximately at the level of a plane passing through the **sternal angle** (the junction of the manubrium sterni with the body of the sternum) posteriorly to the disk between the fourth and fifth thoracic vertebrae. Consequently, that plane has been chosen as the separation of the **superior** from the **inferior mediastinum** (Fig. 9.3).

MEDIASTINUM

The **anterior mediastinum** is the portion of the **inferior mediastinum** that lies anterior to the **pericardium.** Superiorly, where the right and left pleurae are in contact with each other, it has virtually no existence. More inferiorly, it is as wide

Figure 9.3 The subdivisions of the **mediastinum.**

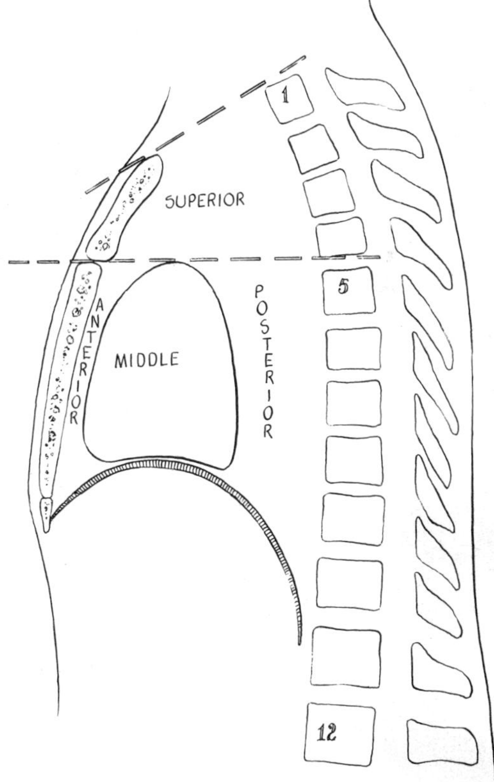

as the bare area of the pericardium, but its antero-posterior extent is very slight and it contains no structures of importance. Occasionally, the remains of the thymus gland reach down into the upper part of the anterior mediastinum between the two pleurae.

The **middle mediastinum** is the portion of the inferior mediastinum that contains the **pericardium.** The only important structures of the middle mediastinum not enclosed within the pericardium are the **two phrenic nerves** and the blood vessels that accompany them. These descend on each side immediately anterior to the roots of the lungs between the mediastinal pleurae and the fibrous pericardium. The middle mediastinum cannot be fully investigated until the pericardial cavity is opened. Now direct your attention to the superior mediastinum.

The **superior mediastinum** lies superior to the pericardium and between the upper portions of the two mediastinal pleurae, extending from the manubrium sterni to the anterior surfaces of the upper four thoracic vertebrae. It communicates with the root of the neck through the superior thoracic aperture, and the structures that connect the thoracic cavity with the neck will be found in the superior mediastinum. To expose the anterior surface of the pericardium and to render the superior mediastinum accessible for study, the mediastinal pleura should be turned laterally as far posteriorly as the roots of the lungs.

The **thymus gland** is the most anterior structure in the superior mediastinum. It is an elongated, bilobed structure that lies behind the middle of the manubrium in relation posteriorly to the left brachiocephalic vein and the arch of the aorta. The size of the thymus varies considerably between individuals and is usually represented in the adult by a mass of adipose tissue. After the position and extent of the thymus have been noted, remove it.

Define the upper limit of the anterior aspect of the pericardium. This is the line along which the parietal pericardium is reflected downward onto the pulmonary trunk, aorta, and superior vena cava as the visceral pericardium of these vessels. In an obese subject, the reflection is obscured by adipose tissue. Make a short transverse incision through the exposed anterior part of the pericardium. The handle of the scalpel can then be introduced through this opening and passed upward within the pericardial cavity between the anterior surface of the heart, which is covered by the visceral pericardium, and the inner surface of the parietal pericardium. The upward passage of the knife will be stopped at the line of reflection between the visceral and the parietal pericardium.

Now clean and study the large vessels of the superior mediastinum. The first rib and the upper part of the manubrium, if still in place for studying their relationship to the subjacent structures, may obscure the structures in the superior mediastinum. Hold the first rib on each side down by pressing against the costochondral junction, and pull up on the lower part of the manubrium until the ribs are fractured. You may have to saw carefully through the first rib on each side. The manubrium can now be retracted and elevated to facilitate study of the structures in the superior mediastinum. Most anteriorly, you will find the brachiocephalic veins and the upper part of the superior vena cava. The **right brachiocephalic vein,** which begins behind the right sternoclavicular joint, is formed by the union of the **right internal jugular** and **right subclavian veins** (Fig. 9.4). From here, it courses downward behind the right border of the manubrium and joins the left brachiocephalic vein at the level of the lower border of the first costal cartilage. The **left brachiocephalic vein** begins at the union of the **left internal jugular** and **left subclavian veins** behind the left sternoclavicular joint. From here it runs downward and to the right to join the right brachiocephalic vein. In addition to the two large tributaries that form them, each brachiocephalic vein receives the **internal thoracic vein** of its respective side. The **inferior thyroid veins,** which descend in the neck anterior to the trachea, usually join the left brachiocephalic vein, either singly or by a common trunk. The **left superior intercostal vein** should also be identified. This vessel drains

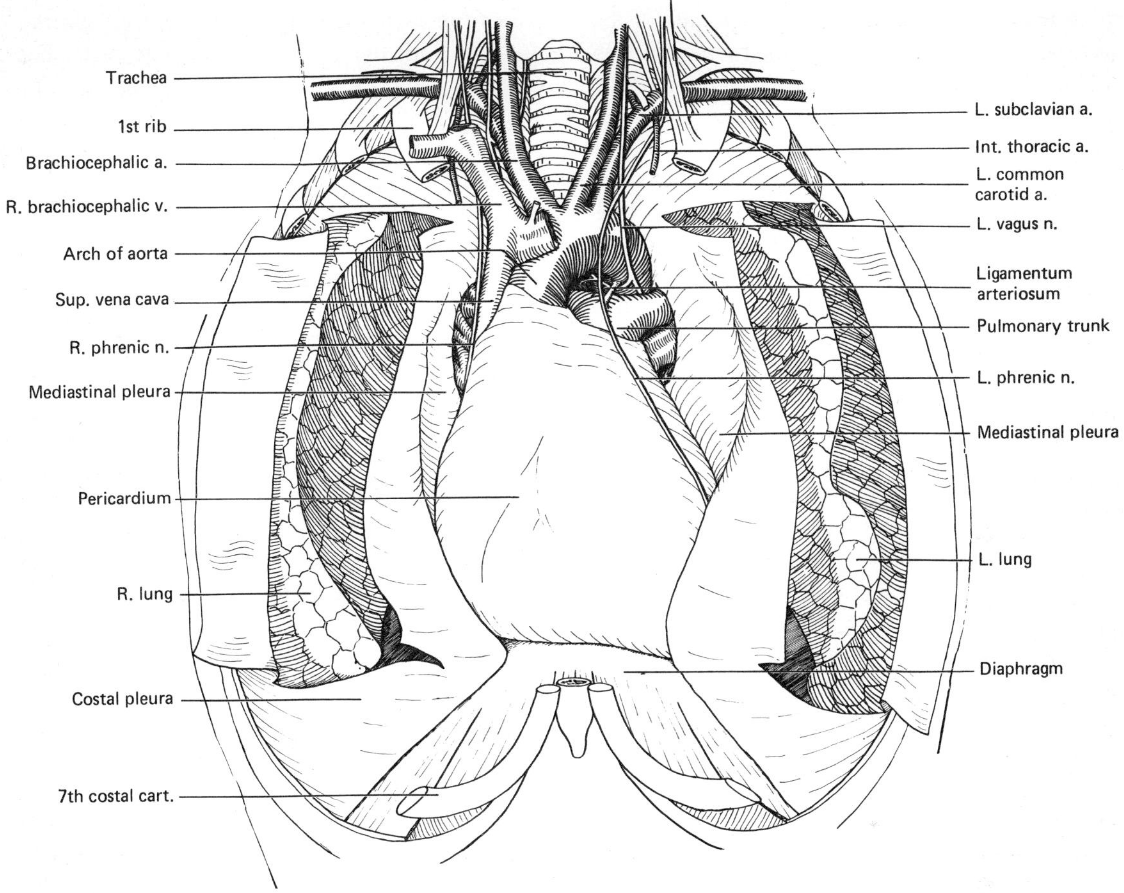

Figure 9.4 The relationships of the **contents of** the **thoracic cavity** after removal of the ventral part of the thoracic cage.

the upper two or three left intercostal spaces. Its terminal portion crosses the left side of the arch of the aorta to enter the inferior aspect of the left brachiocephalic vein.

The **superior vena cava** is formed by the union of the two brachiocephalic veins behind the lower border of the first right costal cartilage. It runs vertically downward to enter the **right atrium of** the **heart.** Its upper portion is in the superior mediastinum, and its terminal portion is in the middle mediastinum, enclosed by the pericardium. In addition to the brachiocephalic veins, the superior vena cava receives the **azygos vein.** Find the terminal portion of this vessel arching above the root of the right lung to enter the posterior aspect of the superior vena cava. The **right superior intercostal vein** drains the upper two or three intercostal spaces and empties into the azygos vein.

For descriptive purposes the **thoracic portion of** the **aorta** is divided into three parts, each of which is in a different subdivision of the mediastinum. The first part, or **ascending aorta,** is in the middle mediastinum, enclosed by the pericardium. The second part, the **arch of** the **aorta,** is in the superior mediastinum and should now be studied. Beginning posterior to the sternal angle, slightly to the right of the midline, it takes an arched course upward, backward, to the left, and downward to become continuous at the left side of the fibrocartilaginous disk between the fourth and fifth thoracic vertebrae with the thoracic portion of the **descending aorta,** which then passes downward through the **posterior mediastinum.**

In order to facilitate studying the **aortic arch** and its branches, you must section the left brachiocephalic vein near its origin and reflect it to the right. The left superior intercostal vein should also be cut where it enters the brachiocephalic and retained in position.

To the left, above the root of the left lung, the arch of the aorta is in contact with the mediastinal pleura. The **left phrenic nerve** and, more posteriorly, the **left vagus nerve** cross the left side of the arch from above downward and separate it from the pleura. If the dissection is carefully done, two much smaller nerves will be found running downward across the arch between the phrenic and the vagus. They are the **superior cervical cardiac branch of** the **left sympathetic trunk** and the **inferior cervical cardiac branch of** the **left vagus;** both join the cardiac plexus, which is described next.

In the ordinary dissection, which must be done in considerable haste by an inexperienced dissector, a complete display of the autonomic nervous system plexuses and their branches of origin and distribution is not practical. They are, however, of the greatest physiological importance, and it is wise to have a general knowledge of their locations so they can be identified as the dissection proceeds.

The nerve supply of the heart and lungs is derived from the **cardiac** and **pulmonary plexuses,** which belong to the **autonomic nervous system.** The **cardiac plexus** is formed by branches from both sympathetic trunks and from both vagus nerves. The **cervical portion of** each **sympathetic trunk** usually contributes three small branches to the plexus, which arise in the neck and enter the superior mediastinum through the superior thoracic aperture. Numerous small twigs are also given to the plexus from the **thoracic portions of** the **sympathetic trunks.** In addition, two branches arise from each **vagus nerve** in the neck and run down to join the plexus, while other branches leave the vagi in the upper part of the thorax. The cardiac plexus consists of superficial and deep parts, which are intimately connected. (Although it has become popular to consider the cardiac plexus as one functional entity, it is discussed here in the more classical form for the benefit of those who teach it that way.) The **superficial cardiac plexus** lies just under the arch of the aorta. It receives the superior cervical cardiac branch of the left sympathetic trunk and the inferior cervical cardiac and thoracic cardiac branches of the left vagus. The remaining cardiac branches of the left vagus and left sympathetic trunk and all the cardiac branches of the right side go to the **deep cardiac plexus,** which lies posterior to the arch, anterior to and at the sides of the terminal part of the trachea. From the cardiac plexuses, small autonomic nerve filaments pass along the vessels to form the pulmonary and coronary plexuses. The **pulmonary plexuses** constitute the nerve supply of the lungs. There is an anterior and a posterior pulmonary plexus on each side; they lie anterior and posterior, respectively, to the pulmonary artery at the root of the lung. From the pulmonary plexuses, autonomic nerves pass into the substance of the lung. The **coronary plexuses** supply the heart; their branches of distribution accompany the coronary arteries.

Beneath and slightly to the left of the arch of the aorta, find the large **pulmonary trunk** emerging from the pericardium. Its extrapericardial course is very short; the pulmonary trunk terminates under the left side of the arch by dividing into right and left branches. The **short left branch** goes horizontally to the left to enter the root of the left lung. The **longer right branch** passes horizontally to the right under the arch of the aorta, posterior to the superior vena cava and under the arch of the azygos vein to reach the root of the right lung. A thick, cordlike structure, the **ligamentum arteriosum,** connects the undersurface of the arch of the aorta to the upper and anterior aspect of the pulmonary trunk (Fig. 9.4). It is the remnant in the adult of the **ductus arteriosus** of the fetus. In the adult it is solid, but during fetal life the ductus arteriosus is an open channel that pemits blood to pass from the pulmonary trunk directly into the aorta, thereby bypassing the nonfunctional lungs. Find the **recurrent laryngeal branch of** the **left vagus** crossing the undersurface of the arch behind the ligamentum arteriosum. As the vagus crosses the left side of the arch, the recurrent branch turns medially and posteriorly beneath the arch to run upward through the superior mediastinum into the neck in close relation to the trachea and esophagus. Under the arch of the aorta, it usually gives a few small twigs to the **superficial cardiac plexus.** Behind the pulmonary artery, the **left bronchus** runs to the left and downward to enter the root of the left lung.

Superiorly, the principal structures in relation to the **arch** are its own three large branches, which should now be cleaned and examined.

The first is the **brachiocephalic artery.** It arises behind the middle of the manubrium and passes upward, backward, and to the right to divide at the level of the right sternoclavicular articulation into the **right subclavian** and the **right common carotid arteries.** The **right vagus nerve** will be found running downward and posteriorly between the artery and the right brachiocephalic vein (Fig. 9.4).

The second branch of the aortic arch is the **left common carotid artery.** It arises just to the left of the brachiocephalic artery and runs upward, to the left, and posteriorly to enter the neck from behind the left sternoclavicular articulation.

The **left subclavian artery** arises from the posterior part of the arch, runs upward to the level of the left sternoclavicular articulation, and arches to the left across the front of the dome of the left pleura. The **left vagus nerve** descends between the left subclavian and left common carotid arteries to reach the left side of the arch of the aorta.

A fourth, much smaller, branch is occasionally found arising from the arch of the aorta between the brachiocephalic and the left common carotid. It is the arteria thyroidea ima, or **lowest thyroid artery,** which runs up into the neck in front of the trachea. Rarely, it may arise from the lowest part of the brachiocephalic artery instead of the aortic arch. In about 90 percent of cases, it is entirely lacking.

The entire thoracic course of the two phrenic nerves can now be studied (Fig. 9.4). Each **phrenic nerve** enters the thorax through the superior thoracic aperture by crossing the medial border of the **anterior scalene muscle.** As it leaves the anterior scalene, it lies anterior to the subclavian artery and immediately comes into relation with the internal thoracic artery. The **right phrenic nerve** runs down along the lateral side of the right brachiocephalic vein and then along the lateral side of the superior vena cava. Continuing inferiorly, it crosses anterior to the root of the right lung and finally, courses along the right lateral surface of the pericardium to reach the diaphragm. The **left phrenic nerve** descends between the left subclavian and left common carotid arteries, crossing in front of the left vagus nerve, then across the left side of the arch of the aorta in front of the root of the left lung, and finally, along the left lateral surface of the pericardium to reach the diaphragm. Small **pericardiacophrenic blood vessels** will be found accompanying the nerves. The arteries are branches of the internal thoracic arteries; the veins drain either into the internal thoracic veins or into the brachiocephalics.

PERICARDIUM

Attention should now be directed to the **middle mediastinum.** Make a transverse incision across the middle of the exposed anterior surface of the fibrous pericardium. From each end of this transverse incision, make longitudinal incisions downward to the diaphragm and upward almost to the upper limit of the pericardium. The two flaps marked out may be turned downward and upward, thus opening the **pericardial cavity** and exposing the anterior surface of the **heart** (Fig. 9.5).

The **pericardial cavity** appears as a narrow interval between thc **external surface of** the **heart**

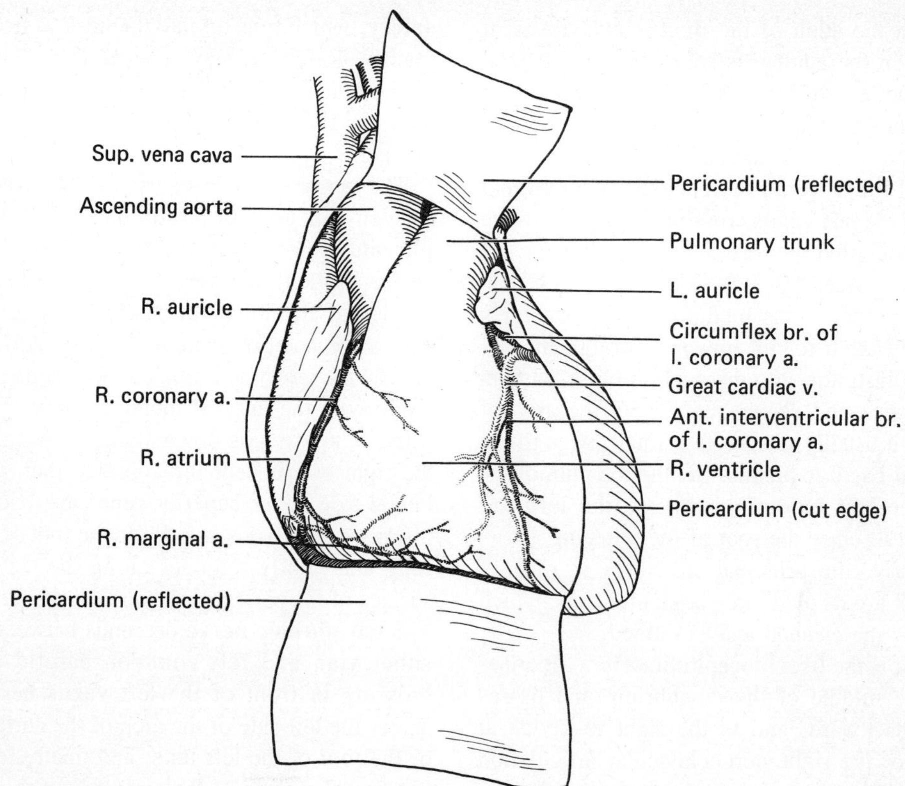

Figure 9.5 The **sternocostal surface of** the **heart,** exposed by reflection of the ventral pericardium.

(enveloped by visceral pericardium) and the internal surface of the **parietal pericardium.** In the cadaver, this cavity is sometimes partially obliterated by pathological adhesions between the heart and the parietal pericardium, or it may be filled with coagulated serous fluid or with an effusion of the embalming fluid. Remove any such material. Anteriorly, inferiorly, and at each side, the heart normally lies quite free in the pericardial cavity, and there is no connection between the **parietal pericardium** and the **visceral pericardium,** which forms the thin, outermost layer of the heart wall. Now identify the vessels that join the base of the heart.

Most anterior is the **pulmonary trunk,** which joins the upper left portion of the anterior surface of the heart. To the right of the pulmonary trunk, and somewhat overlapped by it, is the **aorta.** Still farther to the right and more posterior is the intrapericardial portion of the **superior vena cava.** The **inferior vena cava** pierces the diaphragm to enter the lower posterior part of the heart at the right side. On each side, two **pulmonary veins** enter the upper posterior part of the heart. As seen through the pericardial cavity, all these vessels are covered by prolongations of the visceral serous pericardium.

Two small subdivisions of the pericardial cavity that are formed by the pericardial reflections should be noted. One is the transverse sinus and the other is the oblique sinus. The **transverse sinus** of the pericardium is a tunnellike passageway located posterior to the ascending aorta and the pulmonary artery. It is continuous at each side with the general pericardial cavity. Place your finger or a blunt instrument behind the pulmonary artery from the left side and push transversely to the right. You will traverse the transverse sinus and emerge behind the right side of the ascending aorta in front of the superior vena cava.

The **oblique sinus** is a pocketlike subdivision of the pericardial cavity that lies posterior to the base of the heart. It can be reached by pulling the lower free portion of the heart forward, upward, and to the right. Inferiorly and to the left, the oblique sinus communicates freely with the general pericardial cavity. Its posterior wall is formed by the parietal pericardium, which lies in front of the esophagus and the descending aorta. Its anterior wall is formed by the visceral pericardium on the posterior surface of the left atrium. The right border is formed by the reflection of the parietal to the visceral pericardium across the left side of the right pulmonary veins and the inferior vena cava; the left border is formed by a line of pericardial reflection across the right side of the left pulmonary veins. The superior border is the line of junction of the visceral and parietal pericardium along the upper posterior border of the left atrium. Thus, the **oblique sinus** is bounded entirely by the **venous reflection** of the pericardium.

Although eight large vessels traverse the pericardial cavity to reach the heart, there are only **two lines of pericardial reflection.** This results from the embryonic development of the heart as a simple tube connected to the wall of the pericardial cavity at the two ends—the venous end, through which blood enters the tube, and the arterial end, through which blood leaves it. The **venous portion of** the tubular **embryonic heart** is represented in the adult by the **two atria** and the **veins** that join them; the **arterial portion** is represented by the **two ventricles** and the **arteries** that leave them. Each of the lines of pericardial reflection of the adult heart marks the position of one of the two ends of the embryonic heart tube. These lines of pericardial reflection should now be studied (Fig. 9.6).

The **arterial reflection** can easily be seen at the upper anterior part of the pericardial cavity, where the **aorta** and the **pulmonary trunk** are ensheathed in a common visceral pericardial covering that is reflected from their external surfaces to become the parietal pericardium along a line encircling the vessels. The other line of reflection, the **venous reflection,** is more complex and encircles all six veins that enter the heart. Starting at the right side where the **superior vena cava**

Figure 9.6 Posterior aspect of the **heart.**

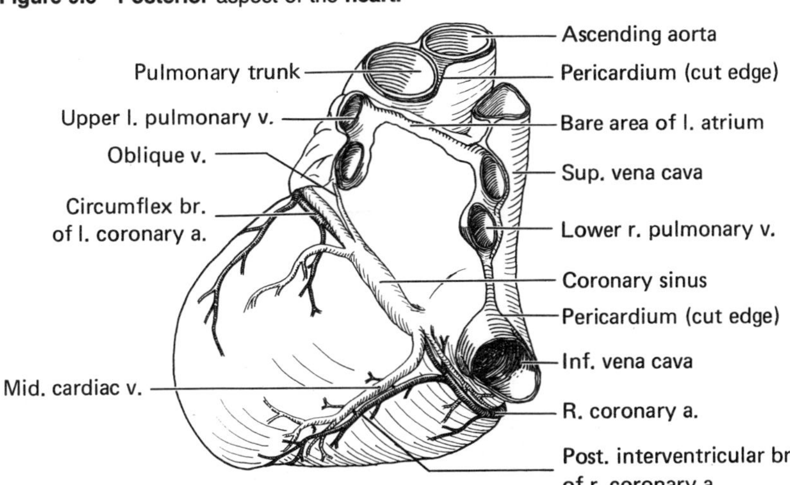

enters the pericardial cavity, the line of reflection from the visceral to the parietal pericardium runs uninterrupted downward along the right side of the **right pulmonary veins** and the **inferior vena cava,** around the latter and up along its left side and the left side of the **right pulmonary veins,** then across the posterior aspect of the upper part of the **left atrium,** down on the right side of the **left pulmonary veins,** upward again along their left side, then to the right along the posterior wall of the **transverse sinus,** and finally, across the front of the superior vena cava to reach the starting point. Notice that the transverse sinus lies between the arterial and venous pericardial reflections and marks the site of the obliterated **dorsal mesocardium** (dorsal mesentery) of the embryonic heart.

HEART

Now direct your attention to the anterior or **sternocostal surface of** the **heart** (Fig. 9.5). It is formed principally by the **right ventricle,** but all four chambers of the heart contribute to it. Its right margin is formed by the **right atrium,** the **auricle** of which will be seen as a pointed appendage projecting upward and farther to the left than does the main part of the atrium. The **right atrium** is separated from the **right ventricle** by the **coronary** (**atrioventricular**) **sulcus,** which crosses the anterior surface of the heart, running downward and slightly to the right.

The **sulci** on the external surface of the heart are grooves or furrows in its muscular wall. In the undissected heart, however, they do not ordinarily appear as grooves since they are so filled by **epicardial fat** that the visceral pericardium covering them is not indented. Usually they can be recognized by the presence of this fat and by the fact that the **coronary arteries** and their larger branches are lodged in them.

The **right ventricle** forms about two-thirds of the **sternocostal surface** of the heart. It is widest inferiorly, just above the diaphragm. Superiorly, it narrows and becomes continuous with the **pulmonary trunk.** The left extremity of the anterior surface is formed by the **left ventricle.** It is separated from the right ventricle by the interventricular septum, the position of which is indicated on the sternocostal surface of the heart by the **anterior interventricular sulcus,** which runs downward and to the left. At the left of the base of the pulmonary trunk, the **auricle of** the **left atrium** forms a small part of the sternocostal surface.

The relationship of the anterior surface of the **heart** to the **anterior thoracic wall** is of importance and can be studied by replacing the portion of the sternum and its attached ribs that was previously removed. The exact outline of the heart as projected against the chest wall varies somewhat in individual cases but on the average is about as follows (Fig. 9.7). Beginning at a point corresponding to the lower border of the second left costal cartilage about 1.5 cm to the left of the edge of the sternum, the left border follows a line somewhat convex to the left, running down to the fifth intercostal space about 9 cm from the midline. From here, the inferior border follows a nearly straight line across to the sixth right costal cartilage about 1.5 cm from the junction of this cartilage with the sternum. From here, the right margin, somewhat convex to the right, runs upward to the upper border of the third right costal cartilage about 1.5 cm from the sternum. The upper border, which corresponds to the junction of the superior vena cava with the right atrium and the junction of the right ventricle with the pulmonary trunk, lies behind a line running from the upper border of the third right cartilage about 1.5 cm to the right of the sternum to the lower border of the second left cartilage about 1.5 cm to the left of the sternum.

The heart may be moved about in the pericardial cavity to observe its other surfaces. The **right lateral surface** is formed entirely by the **right atrium** and is in relation, through the fibrous and parietal pericardium, with the right phrenic nerve and the right mediastinal pleura. The inferior or **diaphragmatic surface** is separated from the sternocostal surface by the sharp inferior border, the **acute margin.** This surface rests against the dia-

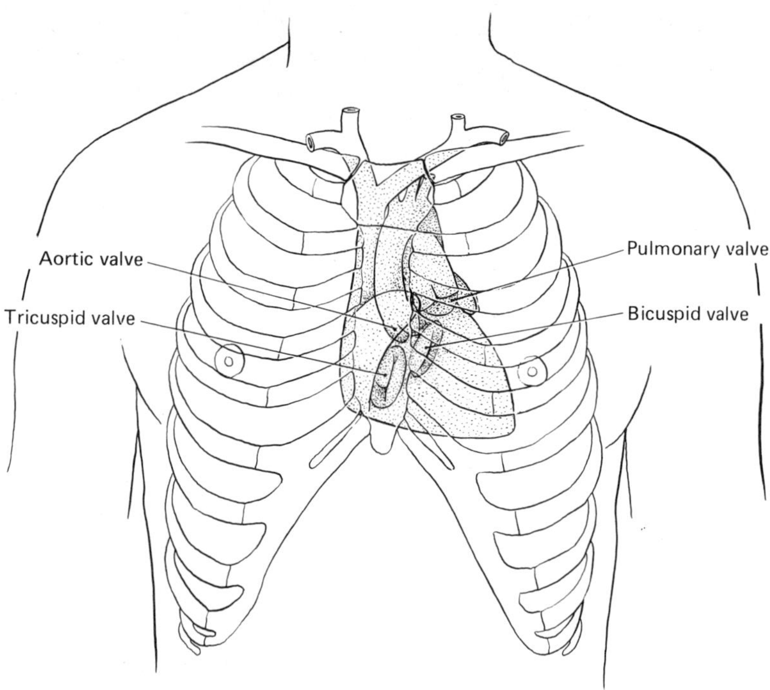

Figure 9.7 Surface **projection of** the **heart** and its **valves.**

phragm, from which it is separated only by the diaphragmatic portion of the parietal pericardium. It is crossed by the **posterior interventricular sulcus,** which indicates the separation of the **right ventricle** from the **left ventricle,** each forming about half of the diaphragmatic surface.

The **coronary (atrioventricular) sulcus** completely encircles the heart, separating the two **atria** from the two **ventricles.** The **anterior** and **posterior interventricular sulci** begin at the **coronary sulcus** on the anterior and posterior surfaces of the heart, respectively, and meet near the left extremity of the **acute margin.**

The left side of the heart has a more rounded border, the **obtuse margin,** which is formed entirely by the **left ventricle** and is interposed between the sternocostal and diaphragmatic surfaces. The heart projects farthest to the left and inferiorly to its **apex,** which is also formed entirely by the left ventricle.

The **posterior surface** corresponds to the **base of** the **heart,** to which the vessels are attached. Its only free portion is the surface of the left atrium, which forms the anterior wall of the **oblique sinus.**

For the most part, the interior of the heart can be studied more effectively after the organ has been removed from the body. It is advisable, however, to open the **right atrium** while the heart is still *in situ*. Before doing this, however, extend the opening in the pericardium, if necessary. *Then open the right atrium by three incisions (Fig. 9.8). Make a longitudinal incision through the wall of the atrium beginning slightly below the tip of the auricle and running down to the inferior border of the atrium a little to the right of the coronary sulcus. From each end of this longitudinal incision, make a transverse incision backward to the posterior border of the atrium. The upper incision will cross the atrium just below the termination of the superior vena cava, and the lower one will cross just above the termination of the inferior*

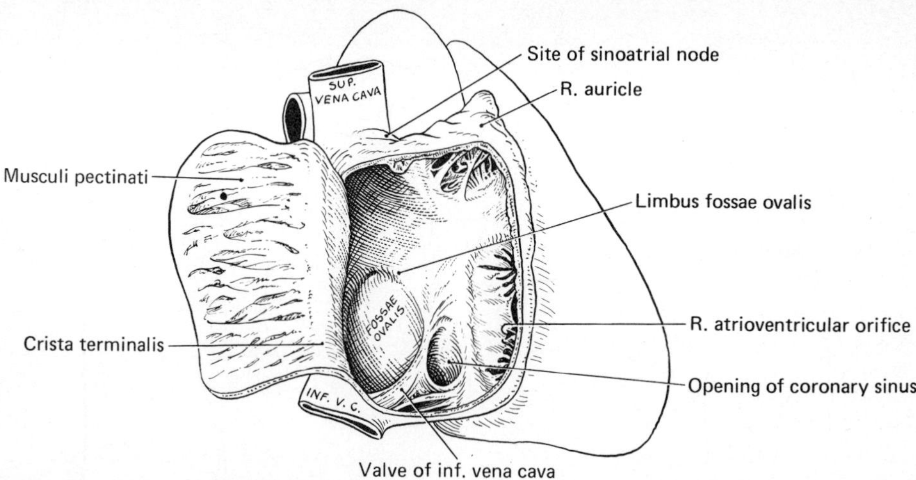

Figure 9.8 The interior of the **right atrium.**

vena cava. Turn the flap thus marked out to the right and backward, thereby exposing the interior of the atrium. The cavity is usually filled with coagulated blood; remove it and clean the wall of the atrium as thoroughly as possible.

The inner surface of the right atrium, like all the chambers of the heart, is lined with thin, smooth epithelium, the **endocardium,** which is continuous with the **endothelium** of the blood vessels. Through the endocardium the muscular layer, or **myocardium,** which forms the main thickness of the atrial wall, can be seen. The myocardium of the posterior wall of the right atrium, into which the veins open, is smooth. This portion of the atrium is known as the **sinus venarum.** It is marked off from the roughened anterior part by the **crista terminalis,** a longitudinal muscular ridge running from the inferior vena cava to the superior vena cava on the inner surface of the right wall of the atrium (externally it appears as a groove, the sulcus terminalis) (Fig. 9.8). Running forward from the crista terminalis on the inner surface of the anterior atrial wall are smaller transverse muscular ridges, the **musculi pectinati.** They are particularly well developed in the auricle.

The **superior vena cava** opens into the highest part of the **sinus venarum.** Its opening has no valve. The large opening of the inferior vena cava is below and posterior. Running in front and to the left side of this opening is an endocardial fold, the **valve of** the **inferior vena cava.** It is almost always rudimentary. To the left of the caval orifice is another opening in the lower posterior wall of the atrium for the **coronary sinus,** a vein that is lodged in the posterior part of the coronary sulcus. This opening also is guarded by a rudimentary valvular fold. Anteriorly, inferiorly, and toward the left, the right atrium communicates with the right ventricle through the very large **right atrioventricular orifice.** The position of this opening corresponds to that of the lower and right portion of the coronary sulcus on the exterior of the heart. It lies toward the right behind the body of the sternum at about the level of the fourth intercostal space (Fig. 9.7). It is guarded by the **tricuspid** or **right atrioventricular valve.** Other minute orifices may be seen scattered over the atrial wall that represent the openings of the **venae cordis minimae,** small veins that carry blood from the heart wall.

The posteromedial wall of the right atrium is formed by the **interatrial septum,** which separates it from the left atrium. Note a shallow oval depression on this wall. This, the **fossa ovalis,** indicates the position of the **foramen ovale,** through which blood passed from the right atrium directly into the left atrium in the fetal heart. The fossa ovalis is bounded superiorly and to the left by a low, semicircular ridge, the **limbus fossae ovalis,** which is usually continuous below with the valve of the inferior vena cava.

In many cases, a valvular passageway (patent foramen ovale) through the interatrial septum persists in the adult, running from the upper part of the fossa ovalis behind the limbus to open into the left atrium.

When study of the right atrium is completed, remove the heart from the body. An excellent opportunity is now afforded for reviewing the lines of **pericardial reflection,** since the heart will be removed by cutting through the vessels along the reflections. First cut through the ascending aorta and the pulmonary trunk just inferior to the level at which the pericardium is reflected from them. Pull these cut vessels forward so that the **transverse sinus** can be opened and the continuity of the **coronary sulcus** along its lower border can be demonstrated. Next, cut the superior vena cava transversely just below its entrance into the pericardial cavity, the inferior vena cava just above the diaphragm, and the four pulmonary veins near their entrance into the heart. The **visceral pericardium** covering these veins will necessarily be cut at the same time as the vessels, and, if the knife is carried through the pericardium along the line of reflection connecting the veins, the heart will be freed from the pericardial wall and can be removed from the body. Observe that the only portion of the external surface of the heart that is devoid of a visceral pericardial covering is a narrow area running transversely across the upper posterior aspect of the organ between the **upper right pulmonary vein** and the **upper left pulmonary vein** (Fig. 9.6). This **bare area,** which lies between the transverse sinus and the upper end of the oblique sinus, is formed by the upper border of the left atrium. When the heart is in position, the bare area is in direct relation with the inferior surface of the right branch of the pulmonary trunk.

The **ascending aorta** takes origin from the **left ventricle** behind the left side of the sternum at the level of the third intercostal space (Fig. 9.7). Posterior to the sternal angle, it becomes continuous with the arch of the aorta. At its origin, the ascending aorta is overlapped anteriorly and to the left by the pulmonary trunk, which should be separated from it to expose the aortic sinuses. The **aortic sinuses** are marked by three swellings or dilatations at the base of the **ascending aorta.** They correspond in position to the cusps of the aortic valve, which lie within the ascending aorta and which will be seen somewhat later. The names used to describe the sinuses and the valves do not correspond to their actual position in the body. The terms used are "right," "left," and "posterior." Observe that the **right aortic sinus** is actually anterior in position, the **left sinus** lies posteriorly and to the left, and the **posterior sinus** is posterior and to the right (Fig. 9.10).

The only branches of the ascending aorta are the **right** and **left coronary arteries.** They are the arteries that supply the heart itself with blood and should now be cleaned and studied. The coronary arteries and their larger branches are lodged in the sulci on the external surface of the heart. Cleaning them sometimes involves removing the **epicardial fat** in which they are embedded. The **cardiac veins,** which carry blood back to the right atrium from the heart wall, will be encountered at the same time. Nerve filaments will also be found in association with the vessels; they belong to the **coronary plexus** of nerves and represent branches of distribution of the **cardiac plexus.** Note them and then remove them to facilitate cleaning the vessels (Figs. 9.5 and 9.6).

The **right coronary artery** arises from the **right aortic sinus** behind the right border of the pulmonary trunk. It runs downward and to the right in the **coronary sulcus** and then in the posterior part of the coronary sulcus where it terminates by anastomosing with the **circumflex branch of** the **left coronary artery.** At the upper end of the posterior interventricular sulcus, the right coronary artery gives off a large **posterior interventricular**

branch that runs in the sulcus giving branches that run downward over the wall of the ventricle and smaller branches that run upward in the wall of the right atrium. A large **right marginal branch** arises from it near the acute margin. The **right coronary artery** carries blood mainly to the walls of the right atrium and right ventricle and, through its posterior interventricular branch, to the posterior half of the interventricular septum.

The **left coronary artery** arises from the left aortic sinus and passes to the left, behind the pulmonary trunk in that portion of the coronary sulcus that lies in the **transverse sinus of** the **pericardium.** As it emerges from the left end of the transverse sinus, it is overlapped by the auricle of the left atrium and here divides into its two main branches, the **anterior interventricular artery** and the **circumflex artery**. The **anterior interventricular branch** runs downward and forward in the **anterior interventricular sulcus,** giving numerous small branches to the sternocostal surface of the heart. The **circumflex branch** passes to the left and posteriorly in the **coronary sulcus** to anastomose with the terminal part of the right coronary artery. From it arise numerous branches to the left atrium and left ventricle. A **left marginal branch** is distributed to the left obtuse margin. The left coronary artery supplies most of the walls of the left atrium and left ventricle and the anterior half of the interventricular septum.

Blood carried to the heart wall by the coronary arteries is returned to the right atrium by the **cardiac veins** (Figs. 9.5 and 9.6). The largest is the **coronary sinus,** which is lodged in the posterior part of the coronary sulcus. It runs downward and to the right to terminate in the right atrium at the orifice that has already been seen in the interior of the atrium. The **great cardiac vein** runs upward in the **anterior interventricular sulcus** and then around the left margin of the heart in the coronary sulcus to terminate in the coronary sinus, which actually may be regarded as its direct continuation. The **middle cardiac vein** ascends in the **posterior interventricular sulcus** to join the coronary sinus near the termination of the latter; it is sometimes larger than the great cardiac vein. The **small cardiac vein** winds around the right margin of the heart in the coronary sulcus, to join the coronary sinus near its termination. The **anterior cardiac veins** are small veins that run upward on the right side of the anterior surface of the right ventricle. They join the small cardiac vein or enter the right atrium directly. The **oblique vein** of the left atrium is a small channel that runs downward and to the right on the posterior surface of the left atrium to join the coronary sinus. It cannot always be demonstrated, but is of interest because it represents a remnant of the left common cardinal vein of the embryo.

When you have completed the study of the blood vessels supplying the heart wall open the **right ventricle** (Fig. 9.9). *Beginning at the cut edge of the pulmonary trunk, make an incision running downward through the anterior wall of the pulmonary trunk and the right ventricle to the acute margin; this incision should run about 1.5 cm to the right and parallel to the anterior interventricular sulcus. From the lower end of this incision, carry another incision to the right, parallel to and just above the acute inferior margin, to within 1 cm of the coronary sulcus. By this means the right ventricle and the pulmonary trunk will be fully opened. Wash out any blood that fills them.*

The walls of the **right ventricle** are anterior, inferior, and medial. The **anterior wall** corresponds to the sternocostal surface of the heart and the **inferior wall** to the diaphragmatic surface. The **medial wall,** which is actually posteromedial in position, is formed by the **interventricular septum** and separates the right and left ventricles. This wall bulges anteriorly and to the right, giving the cavity of the right ventricle a semilunar shape in transverse section. Almost the entire inner surface of the ventricle is thrown into irregular muscular ridges and bands, the **trabeculae carneae.** The cavity of the right ventricle narrows superiorly to become continuous with the **pulmonary trunk.** The narrow superior portion of the right ventricle just below the pulmonary trunk is known as the **conus arteriosus** (infundibulum). The conus, which is relatively free of trabeculae carneae, is

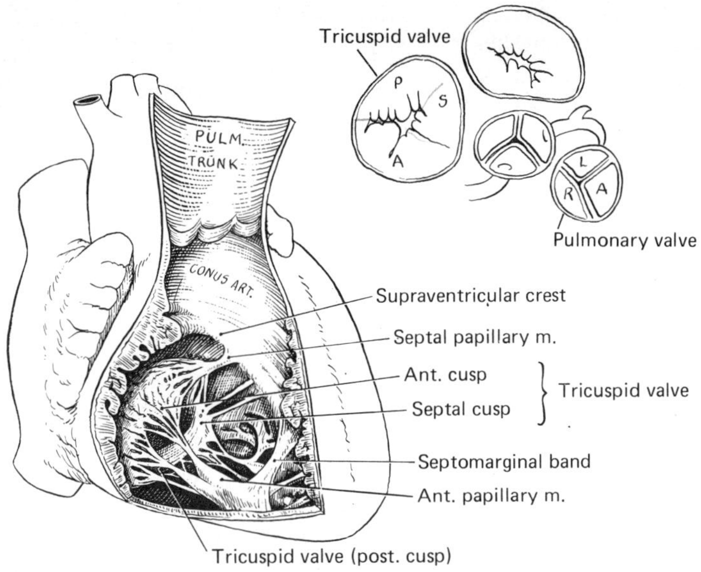

Figure 9.9 The interior of the **right ventricle.** In the upper right corner the valves are diagrammatically represented in the same relative positions as they would appear in this view of the heart.

marked off from the main ventricular cavity by the **supraventricular crest,** a transverse muscular ridge on the septal wall of the ventricle.

Posteriorly and to the right, the ventricle communicates with the right atrium through the **right atrioventricular orifice.** It is surrounded by a ring of fibrous tissue, the **right anulus fibrosus,** which forms part of the heart skeleton over which cardiac muscle is placed. The muscle fibers in the wall of the atrium are not continuous through this ring with the muscle fibers of the ventricular wall, but this fact cannot be demonstrated very well in the ordinary dissection. The **tricuspid** or **right atrioventricular valve** is attached to the inner margin of the anulus fibrosus.

The **tricuspid valve** is an annular sheet of fibrous tissue, covered on each of its surfaces by a layer of endocardium; it is attached peripherally to the **anulus fibrosus** and has a free edge projecting into the cavity of the ventricle. It is incompletely divided into **three cusps** by three notches in the free margin (Fig 9.9). The position of the cusps is usually as follows: the **anterior cusp** is in relation to the anterior sternocostal wall of the ventricle; the **posterior (inferior) cusp,** to the diaphragmatic wall; and the **septal (medial) cusp,** to the interventricular septum. Observe that all three cusps are continuous with one another toward the anulus fibrosus and separate only near the free margin. Occasionally four cusps may be present. The projection of the tricuspid valve on the anterior thoracic wall is at the middle of the sternum at the level of the fourth intercostal space (Fig. 9.7).

Small fibrous strands, the **chordae tendineae,** run from the wall of the ventricle to attach to the free margin and to the ventricular surface of the tricuspid valve. Their attachment to the ventricular wall is at the **papillary muscles,** conical projections of the ventricular wall myocardium. The positions of the papillary muscles of the right ventricle are not entirely constant. There is usually one large **anterior papillary muscle** projecting into the ventricle from the anterior wall. From it, **chordae tendineae** run to the adjacent margins of the anterior and posterior cusps of the valve. There is usually a single, small **septal papillary muscle** on the posterior wall of the conus arteriosus just to the left of the supraventricular crest; it gives chordae tendineae to the anterior and septal cusps.

Sometimes a large **posterior papillary muscle** is found projecting from the diaphragmatic wall, but more frequently this is represented by a group of smaller posterior papillary muscles, from which chordae tendineae run to the septal and posterior cusps of the valve. The function of the tricuspid valve is to prevent the backflow of blood from the ventricle into the right atrium.

When blood enters the ventricle from the atrium, the valve is forced open against the ventricular wall. During ventricular contraction (systole) blood attempts to flow back through this opening, but the pressure forces the free edges of the three cusps together, closing the atrioventricular orifice. Simultaneous contraction of the papillary muscles maintain tension on the chordae tendineae to keep the cusps of the tricuspid valve from being forced backward into the atrium during the ventricular contraction.

The pulmonary trunk orifice lies behind the left edge of the sternum at about the level of the upper border of the left third costal cartilage (Fig. 9.7). It is guarded by the **valve of** the **pulmonary trunk,** which should now be examined. The valve is formed by three **semilunar cusps,** the **anterior, right,** and **left,** which together completely surround the pulmonary orifice internally. Observe that the anterior cusp actually lies anteriorly and to the left, the right cusp anteriorly and to the right, and the left cusp posteriorly. The anterior cusp will probably have been injured when the ventricle was opened, but the structure of all three is similar. Each consists of a semilunar fold of fibrous tissue covered on both surfaces by an endothelial layer. One margin of a cusp is attached to the wall of the pulmonary trunk along a line convex toward the cavity of the ventricle. The other margin is free and projects into the lumen of the artery. At the middle of each free margin is a small, fibrocartilaginous body, the **nodule.**

When blood flows from the ventricle into the artery, the cusps are forced upward against the walls of the vessel. During ventricular relaxation, blood attempts to flow back from the artery into the ventricle, but the valves bulge into the lumen of the pulmonary trunk, and the three free margins meet, closing the orifice. When the valve is closed, the three nodules meet at the center of the lumen.

Open the **left atrium** next by making two incisions in its posterior wall. *The first should run from side to side across the posterior wall parallel to and just above the coronary sulcus. The other should be carried upward from the middle of the first to the upper border of the atrium; it will cut the posterior wall of the atrium longitudinally about halfway between the right and the left pulmonary veins. If it seems desirable to open the atrium more widely, a third incision can be made transversely across the upper border of the atrium between the two upper pulmonary veins. Clean the atrial cavity.*

The wall of the left atrium is smooth throughout, except in the auricle, where musculi pectinati are apparent. The auricle communicates with the main cavity of the atrium at its upper left side, just in front of the opening of the upper left pulmonary vein. The four **pulmonary veins** open directly into the atrium without valves. Below and to the left, the atrium opens into the left ventricle by the **left atrioventricular orifice,** which is somewhat smaller than the right atrioventricular orifice.

To the right and anteriorly, the wall of the left atrium is formed by the **atrial septum.** At the anterior part of this wall, a shallow semilunar depression will be seen, bounded posteriorly by a low ridge that corresponds in position to the **fossa ovalis** in the right atrium. Attempt to pass a blunt probe from the fossa ovalis of the right atrium forward and to the left through the atrial septum into the left atrium.

In about 25 percent of cases, a narrow passageway remains anatomically patent in this location in the adult, a remnant of the **foramen ovale** of the fetus. Such a passage is not necessarily physiologically patent or attended by any symptoms of disease during life, since the pressure of the blood in the two atria keeps its walls in apposition.

Go on now to the **left ventricle.** It and the ascending aorta can be opened by a single incision (Fig. 9.10). *Enter the scalpel just below the cor-*

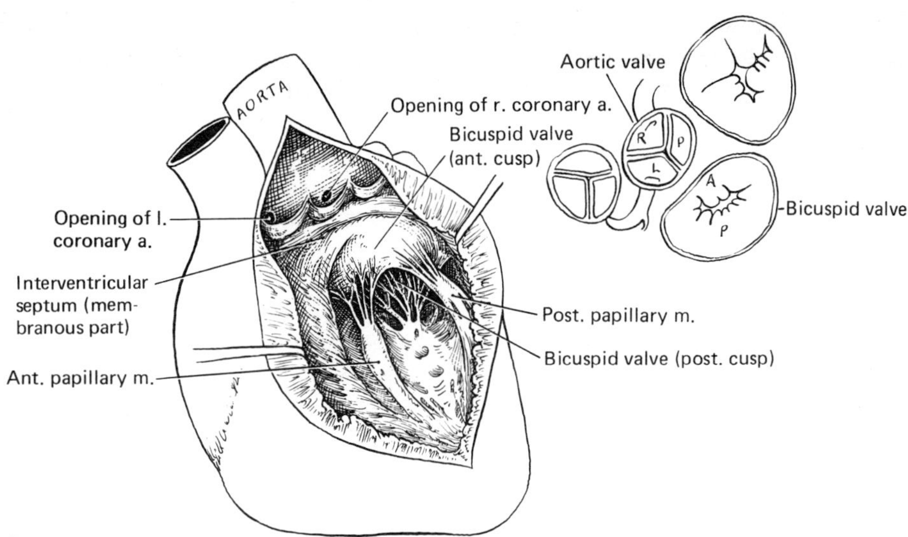

Figure 9.10 The interior of the **left ventricle.** In the upper right corner the valves are diagrammatically represented in the same position as they would appear in this view of the heart.

onary sulcus and carry it downward through the wall of the left ventricle along a line slightly to the left of the anterior interventricular sulcus to the apex of the heart. The same incision should be continued upward from the point at which it was begun, through the coronary sulcus and the wall of the ascending aorta. This incision will cut the circumflex branch of the left coronary artery near its origin, where it lies in the coronary sulcus; it will pass upward through the base of the ascending aorta just behind the origin of the left coronary artery and then straight upward to the cut end of the aorta. The ascending aorta and the left ventricle can then be spread open, cleaned of blood, and studied.

Observe that the **wall of** the **left ventricle,** except at the apex, is much thicker than that of the right. The cavity of the ventricle is roughly conical in outline; the apex of the cone is represented by the apex of the heart, and its base by the atrioventricular and aortic orifices, the latter lying in front and slightly to the right of the former. The ventricular wall is covered throughout by **trabeculae carneae,** except in its upper anterior part, which leads to the aortic orifice. This smooth area is known as the **aortic vestibule.** The anterior and right portion of the wall is formed by the **interventricular septum,** so that the left ventricle lies not only to the left of but also posterior to the right ventricle.

The **left atrioventricular orifice** lies posterior to the left side of the sternum at about the level of the fourth costal cartilage (Fig. 9.7). Like the right orifice, it is surrounded by a fibrous ring, the **left anulus fibrosus,** which provides a physical separation between the atrial and the ventricular musculatures. The orifice is guarded by the **bicuspid (mitral) valve,** which is similar to the tricuspid valve in structure except that it ordinarily has only two cusps. These **cusps** are **anterior** and **posterior** in position (Fig. 9.10). Like the cusps of the tricuspid valve, they are prevented from being forced into the atrium by **chordae tendineae,** which run from the papillary muscles to the free margins and ventricular surfaces of the cusps. In most cases, two very large papillary muscles will be found in the left ventricle. One of these, the **anterior papillary muscle,** springs from the lower part of the septal wall of the ventricle and the other, the **posterior papillary muscle,** arises from the diaphragmatic wall; from each of them chordae tendineae pass to both cusps of the valve. Note that while a considerable portion of the right ventricular cavity intervenes between the right atrioventricular and the pulmonary orifices, the only structure separating the left atrioventricular orifice from the aortic orifice is the **anterior cusp of** the **bicuspid valve.**

The **aortic orifice** lies behind the left side of the sternum at about the level of the third intercostal space (Fig. 9.7). It leads from the upper anterior part of the **left ventricle** into the **ascending aorta** and is posterior to the conus arteriosus of the right ventricle. It is guarded by the **aortic valve,** which is formed by **three semilunar cusps.** In details of structure, these cusps are similar to those of the pulmonary valve already examined, but it should be observed that the aortic cusps are much stronger. In position they correspond to the aortic sinuses and are similarly named. One of the cusps may have been cut in opening the ventricle. Above the **right cusp** on the inner wall of the aorta find the orifice of the right coronary artery; above the **left cusp** is the orifice of the left coronary artery. The **posterior cusp** is in close relation to the anterior cusp of the bicuspid valve (Fig. 9.10).

Certain features of the **interventricular septum** deserve particular attention. The septum is for the most part **thick and muscular.** However, a small portion, the **membranous part of** the **interventricular septum,** is thin. This is the upper, posterior part of the septum, and, in the left ventricle, it lies just below and between the right and the posterior aortic semilunar cusps. The membranous part of the septum is not entirely interventricular. Inferiorly, it separates the left and the right ventricles. However, since the peripheral attachment of the septal cusp of the tricuspid valve crosses its right side, its highest part lies between the left ventricle and the right atrium.

The myocardium of the atria is not continuous with that of the ventricles but is interrupted by the anuli fibrosi. Conduction of impulses from the atrial musculature to the ventricular musculature, therefore, is accomplished by the **atrioventricular bundle,** a branched bundle of **cardiac muscle** that is specialized to conduct electrical impulses. The central point or **atrioventricular node** of this bundle lies in the wall of the right atrium near the coronary sinus orifice. It receives strands of **specialized muscle fibers from** the **walls of both atria.** From the node, the atrioventricular bundle courses along the lower margin of the membranous part of the interventricular septum. Once in the septum, the bundle divides, giving a branch to each ventricle. The bundle as a whole cannot be satisfactorily demonstrated in the ordinary cadaver heart, but the left branch can frequently be seen subjacent to the endocardium, spreading downward over the septal wall of the left ventricle. Individual strands from this branch, covered only by a layer of endocardium, sometimes bridge the lower part of the cavity of the ventricle to reach the posterior papillary muscle. They have been called the **false chordae tendineae,** since they resemble the chordae in appearance, though not in structure or function. The septomarginal trabecula (''moderator band''), one of the more visible false chordae tendineae, is located at the apical end of the right ventricle, extending from the interventricular septum to the base of the anterior papillary muscle. Although heart muscle fibers can contract autonomously, the rhythmic and synchronous contraction of the heart musculature is regulated by the **sinoatrial node,** ''the pacemaker,'' which is located in the wall of the right atrium where the superior vena cava meets the sulcus terminalis.

TRACHEA, BRONCHI, AND LUNGS

The next step in the dissection is to study the **trachea** and to remove the lower part of the trachea, the two **lungs,** and the **pleurae** from the body. First strip the pericardium remaining on the cut ends of the aorta, the pulmonary trunk, and the superior vena cava; remove all the pericardium above the level of the upper pulmonary veins. The superior vena cava should then be turned to the right, and the arch of the aorta turned to the left. To do this, it is necessary to cut the brachiocephalic artery slightly above its origin; it can then be left in place against the trachea and the arch of the aorta. Now swing the left common carotid and the left subclavian arteries to the left side with the aortic arch, thus exposing the lower part of the trachea and the right pulmonary artery (Fig. 9.11).

The **trachea** divides into the **right** and **left principal bronchi** at the **carina,** at about the level of the fifth thoracic vertebra. Each bronchus then passes downward and laterally into the root of the corresponding lung. The **pulmonary trunk** divides into **right** and **left pulmonary arteries** in front of the **left bronchus.** Replace the aortic arch in position in order to demonstrate that the left bronchus and the right pulmonary artery lie under the arch. The **deep cardiac plexus** lies in the bifurcation of the trachea posterior to the right pulmonary artery. Cleaning the lower part of the trachea and the bronchi, you will find groups of large **tracheal** and **bronchial lymph nodes.** They are usually blackened by the deposition in them of carbon particles removed from the air in the lungs. Remove them, once their position has been noted. Observe that the **left bronchus** makes a sharper angle with the trachea than does the right. The right pulmonary artery may be cut near its

Figure 9.11 The **thoracic cavity** after removal of the heart. The arch of the aorta has been turned to the left and the superior vena cava to the right.

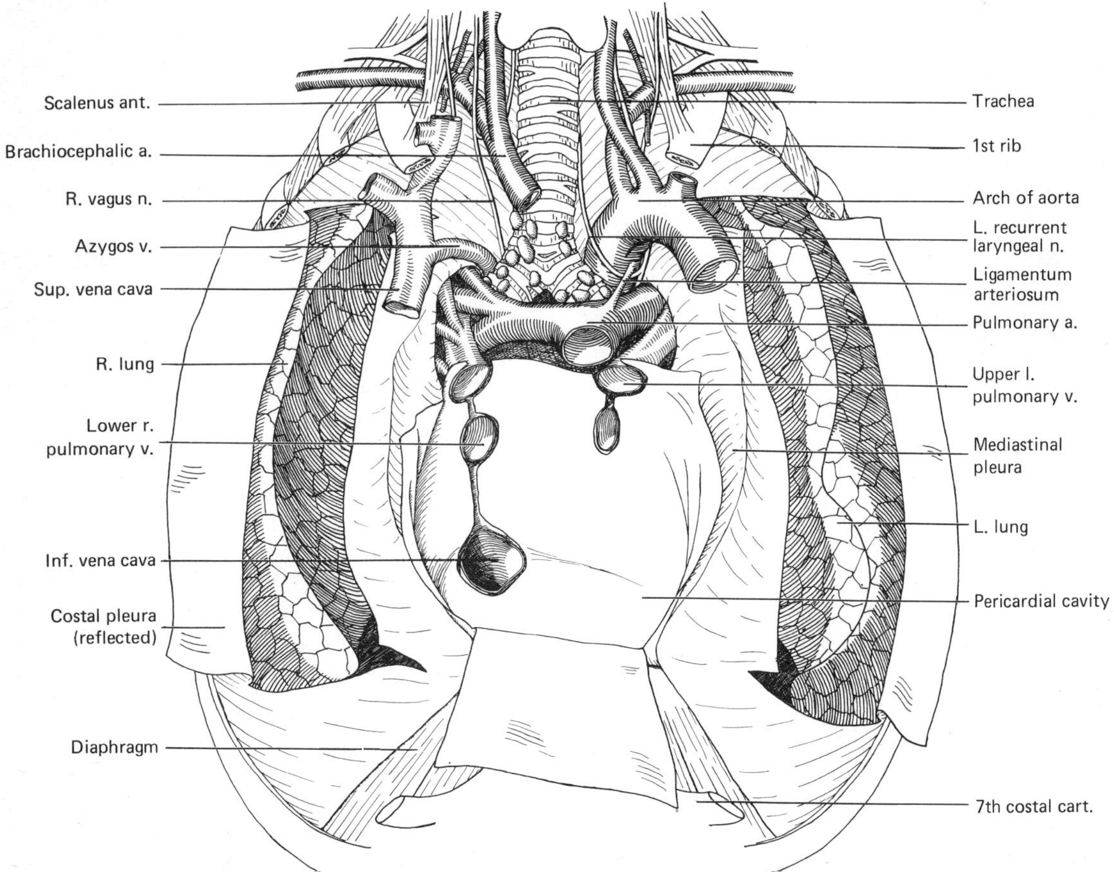

origin from the main trunk if the extrapulmonary portions of the bronchi cannot be satisfactorily cleaned while the pulmonary trunk is intact.

Attempt to identify the **bronchial vessels** before the lungs and trachea are removed. The origin, course, and distribution of these vessels are described subsequently.

The two lungs, together with the lower part of the trachea, the pulmonary trunk and its branches, the pulmonary veins, and the remnants of the pleurae are now to be removed as one unit. First cut through the **ligamentum arteriosum,** which connects the pulmonary trunk to the undersurface of the arch of the aorta. The **recurrent laryngeal branch of** the **left vagus nerve** turns upward behind this ligament on the inner surface of the aortic arch to reach the groove between the trachea and the esophagus; be careful not to damage it. Cut through the trachea transversely about 5 cm above its bifurcation. Do not cut the **esophagus** lying immediately behind the trachea, to which it is loosely attached by areolar tissue. Pull the lower cut portion of the trachea forward and separate its posterior surface from the anterior surface of the esophagus. Next, free the cut ends of the **pulmonary veins** from the pericardium. This can be done either by stripping the pericardium from them or by cutting through each of the veins just external to the pericardium. Next, separate the parietal pleura completely from the thoracic wall wherever it is still attached. In most places, it will strip off very readily except in the case of the diaphragmatic pleura. This can be left in place and separated from the remainder of the parietal pleura by cutting it with the knife. The trachea, bronchi, lungs, pulmonary arteries and veins, and pleurae are held in place only by a little areolar tissue. Remove the entire complex from the body. In separating the **left bronchus** from the posterior part of the arch and the beginning of the descending aorta, be careful not to injure the **left vagus nerve,** which runs downward behind the bronchus to come into relation with the esophagus. Behind the **right bronchus,** the **right vagus nerve** and the **azygos vein** are apt to be injured if care is not taken. Cut the left bronchus and left pulmonary vessels transversely to separate the lungs.

Remove the parietal pleura and study the lungs. The surfaces of each lung are **costal, mediastinal,** and **diaphragmatic.** A sharp **inferior border** separates the diaphragmatic surface from the costal and mediastinal surfaces. Anteriorly, the costal and mediastinal surfaces are separated by a sharp **anterior border.** Posteriorly, there is no distinct border between the mediastinal and the costal surfaces. The portion of the costal surface that lies immediately posterior to the mediastinal surface is in relation, not to the ribs, but to the sides of the bodies of the vertebrae. The remainder of the costal surface is very extensive and is in relation to the ribs and intercostal spaces. The greatest posterior extent of the lung, as well as its greatest convexity, is on this surface along a vertical line corresponding to the angles of the successive ribs. The mediastinal surface of each lung is related, through the mediastinal pleura, to the various structures of the mediastinum, and it shows characteristic grooves and ridges corresponding to the mediastinal structures adjacent to it. The anterior margin of the left lung is indented by a wide **cardiac notch** corresponding to the protrusion of the apex of the heart to the left side. Each lung is marked anteriorly a little below its apex by a groove caused by the **subclavian artery.**

The **lungs** are divided into **lobes** by **interlobar fissures.** These fissures cut through the substance of the lung from the periphery almost to the root. The visceral pleura follows the contours of the fissures. Unfortunately, the fissures are often difficult to demonstrate in the cadaver, since adhesions between the opposing surfaces of the lobes partially or wholly obliterate the fissures. The **primary (oblique) fissure** of each lung lies in an oblique plane running inferiorly and anteriorly from the posterior aspect a little below the apex to the anterior part of the diaphragmatic surface. The **left lung** has only **two lobes, upper** and **lower,** separated by this fissure. The anterior inferior portion of the upper lobe is usually referred to as the **lingula.** In the **right lung,** there is a

second (horizontal) fissure that runs horizontally posteriorly and laterally from the anterior border at about the level of the fourth chondrosternal junction to meet the oblique fissure. The **right lung** is thus divided into three lobes, **upper, middle,** and **lower;** the upper and middle lobes together correspond to the upper lobe of the left lung. Alternatively, the lingula may be considered the homologue of the middle lobe of the right lung.

The **hilum of** the **lung** is the region on its mediastinal aspect where the structures comprising the **root of** the **lung** enter. The principal structures entering the hilum of each lung are the **bronchus,** the **pulmonary artery,** and the **pulmonary veins.** Observe that the pulmonary veins are the most anterior in position and the bronchus is most posterior. Follow the bronchi and the vessels into the lungs by dissecting away the lung substance.

Each **principal (primary) bronchus** is continued downward and laterally to the base of the lung. From the principal bronchus arises a series of **lobar (secondary) branches** that are distributed to the various lobes. The lobar bronchi divide into **segmental bronchi** for the various bronchopulmonary segments. The bronchopulmonary segments are independent subunits of the lobes, each having its own segmental bronchus and pulmonary artery.

They are the smallest entities that can be surgically dissected from the lung. The names and locations of the **bronchopulmonary segments** (Fig. 9.12) should be studied, since they are of importance in diagnosis and surgery of various diseases of the lungs.

Near the hilum, the pulmonary artery crosses the principal bronchus anteriorly to reach a position posterolateral to the bronchus, a position it retains throughout the rest of its course. The first lobar branch of the **right principal bronchus** is known as the **eparterial bronchus,** since it arises **above** the point at which the right pulmonary artery

Figure 9.12 Anterior view of the larger branches of the **bronchi** and **pulmonary arteries,** shown in relation to the **lobes** and **bronchopulmonary segments** of the right and left lungs.

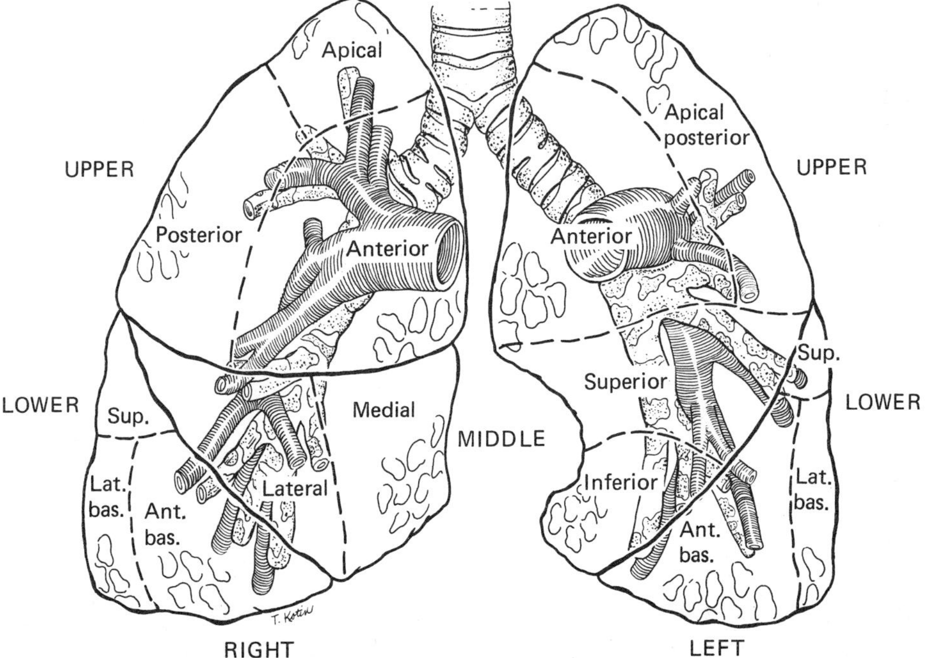

crosses the bronchus. The eparterial bronchus is distributed to the **upper lobe of** the **right lung** and is accompanied by a branch of the right pulmonary artery and a tributary of the right superior pulmonary vein. The remaining branches of the right bronchus are known as **hyparterial bronchi,** since they arise **below** the crossing of the pulmonary artery. The larger ones arise alternately and run anteriorly or posteriorly from the principal bronchus. The **first hyparterial bronchus** is anterior and is distributed to the **middle lobe;** it is acccompanied by a branch of the artery and a tributary of the upper right pulmonary vein. The **remaining hyparterial branches** are distributed to the **lower lobe** and are accompanied by branches of the artery and tributaries of the lower vein.

There is no eparterial bronchus in the **left lung.** The first hyparterial bronchus is quite large; it is distributed to the **upper lobe** and is accompanied by a branch of the left pulmonary artery and the upper left pulmonary vein. The remaining branches of the principal bronchus are distributed to the **lower lobe,** accompanied by branches of the artery and tributaries of the lower left vein.

The **pulmonary artery** carries **venous blood** to the lungs for aeration, after which it is returned to the heart by the **pulmonary veins.** The **bronchial arteries** supply **arterial blood** to the lung substance itself. Look for them on the posterior aspect of the bronchi, the ramifications of which they follow in their distribution to the lungs. There are usually **two bronchial arteries** in the **left lung** and **one** in the **right lung.** The origin of the bronchial arteries will, of course, have been torn away in removing the lungs. The **left** ones arise from the upper part of the **descending thoracic aorta;** the **right** one may arise from the **descending thoracic aorta** or from one of its **upper right intercostal branches,** or from the **subclavian** or **internal thoracic arteries.**

POSTERIOR MEDIASTINUM

Now study the **posterior mediastinum** and the deeper structures of the superior mediastinum. Cut through the azygos vein at its termination in the superior vena cava and remove the remnants of the superior vena cava and the brachiocephalic veins. Remove any parietal pleura that remains adhered to the thoracic wall, with the exception of the diaphragmatic pleura, which may be left on the diaphragm. The entire pericardium except its diaphragmatic portion should also be removed. By removing the portion of pericardial sac that formed the posterior wall of the oblique sinus, you will expose the lower part of the esophagus. Clean the **esophagus** and expose, but do not injure, the **esophageal plexus;** this plexus of nerves is derived from the **two vagi** and is in intimate relation to the external surface of the esophagus (Fig. 9.13).

The **esophagus** is flattened to present anterior and posterior surfaces. It enters the thorax through the **superior thoracic aperture.** In the superior mediastinum, it lies posterior to the trachea and anterior to the bodies of the vertebrae. In the upper part of the posterior mediastinum, the descending thoracic aorta lies to its left side and slightly posterior to it. More inferiorly, the esophagus inclines slightly forward and toward the left so that it comes to lie in front of the aorta; it leaves the thoracic cavity by passing through an aperture, the esophageal hiatus, in the **muscular part of** the **diaphragm** at about the level of the tenth thoracic vertebra.

Trace the course of the two vagi in the posterior mediastinum (Fig. 9.13). After descending behind the left bronchus, the **left vagus** crosses in front of the descending aorta to reach the anterior surface of the esophagus, where it ramifies to form the **anterior part of** the **esophageal plexus.** The **right vagus** passes downward across the medial aspect of the arch of the azygos vein to reach the posterior surface of the esophagus, where it splits into several branches to form the **posterior part of** the **esophageal plexus.** The anterior and posterior parts of the plexus communicate freely around the borders of the esophagus. A short distance above the diaphragm the plexus is usually resolved again into **two main trunks,** the **anterior**

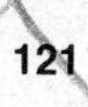

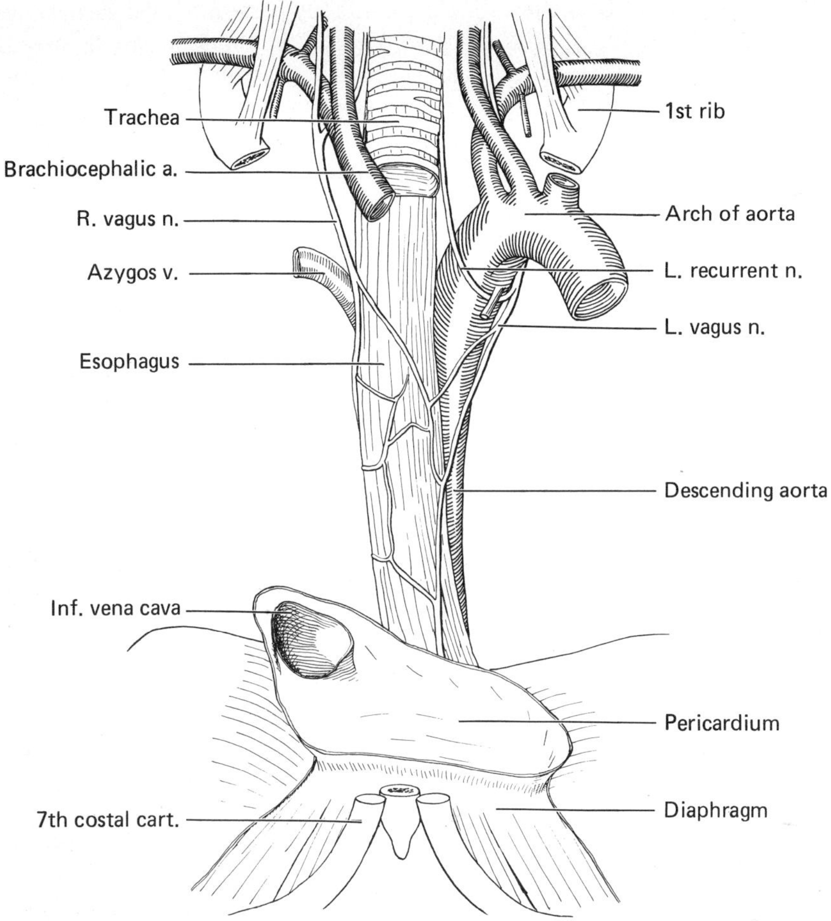

Figure 9.13 Semidiagrammatic representation of the anterior structures of the **posterior mediastinum.** The arch of the aorta has been turned to the left.

and **posterior vagal trunks.** As they pass through the **esophageal hiatus of** the **diaphragm,** the anterior vagal trunk divides and spreads over the anterior aspect of the stomach, and the posterior vagal trunk ramifies over the posterior surface of the stomach.

Make a longitudinal incision through the anterior wall of the esophagus and observe that the lumen appears, in cross section, as a slitlike aperture, corresponding to the anteroposterior flattening of the organ.

Then free and elevate the esophagus from the underlying structures.

Clean and study the **thoracic part of** the **descending aorta.** It begins at the left side of the intervertebral disk between the fourth and fifth thoracic vertebrae as a continuation of the arch of the aorta and lies entirely in the **posterior mediastinum.** As it descends through the posterior mediastinum, the aorta inclines slightly forward and to the right and leaves the thorax through the **aortic hiatus of** the **diaphragm,** which lies in the median plane in front of the twelfth thoracic vertebra. The only branches arising from its anterior aspect are the **bronchial arteries,** of which mention has already been made, and a variable number of small **esophageal** and **mediastinal branches.** If the descending aorta is pulled forward, a series of paired **posterior intercostal arteries** will be seen arising from its posterior aspect. There are usually nine pairs of posterior intercostals, one for each pair of intercostal spaces beginning with the third. The paired **subcostal arteries** run below the twelfth ribs but otherwise are similar to the intercostals.

The posterior intercostal arteries, the azygos system of veins, the proximal portions of the intercostal nerves, and the thoracic portions of the sympathetic nerve trunks should now be studied together. Free and elevate the left common carotid artery, the left subclavian artery, and the arch of the aorta. Then clean the sympathetic trunks (Fig. 9.14).

Each **sympathetic trunk** begins in the **neck** and is continued through the **thorax** into the **abdomen** and **pelvis.** It will be found passing through the superior thoracic aperture anterior to the head of the first rib and running downward through the thorax in the areolar tissue just external to the parietal pleura anterior to the heads of the ribs. In the lower part of the thorax, it inclines slightly forward, coming to lie against the sides of the bodies of the vertebrae. Each trunk leaves the thorax by passing behind the diaphragm. A series of **ganglionic enlargements** occurs along its course. These ganglia generally lie against the heads of the ribs; the first thoracic ganglion is sometimes fused with the lowest cervical ganglion to form a large **stellate ganglion.** Identify the **greater splanchnic nerve.** This large nerve arises from the sympathetic trunk by a series of roots, usually from the fifth through the ninth thoracic ganglia, that pass forward and downward along the sides of the vertebrae. The roots join to form the greater splanchnic nerve, which passes downward and pierces the crus of the diaphragm. The **lesser splanchnic nerve,** usually formed by roots from the tenth and eleventh thoracic ganglia, runs forward and downward from the sympathetic trunk at a lower level; it also passes through the diaphragm slightly posterior to the greater splanchnic nerve. Each of the **thoracic ganglia** usually communicates with the corresponding **intercostal nerve** by two small posteriorly directed branches, the **gray** and **white rami communicantes.** Although it is nearly impossible to distinguish between the rami in a gross dissection, you should demonstrate that at least two nerve bundles, the rami, connect each ganglion with the corresponding ventral ramus of the spinal nerve.

The **intercostal nerves** are the ventral rami of the first 11 pairs of the thoracic spinal nerves; one is found in each **intercostal space** emerging from the posterior aspect of the bodies of the vertebrae between the heads of the adjacent ribs. Follow them laterally in the intercostal spaces and observe that they lie on the internal surfaces of the external intercostal muscles, which extend as far medially as the heads of the ribs. Note that the **internal intercostal muscles** extend medially only as far as the angles of the ribs and that the intercostal nerves pass out of sight here by continuing laterally between the internal and innermost intercostal muscles. Each intercostal nerve is accompanied by an **intercostal vein** and an **intercostal artery** throughout its course; the nerve is usually the most inferior in position and the vein the most superior of the three structures (Fig. 9.14).

The **posterior intercostal arteries** of the first two intercostal spaces are usually derived from the **supreme intercostal artery,** which is a branch of the costocervical trunk of the subclavian artery. The supreme intercostal artery will be found descending anterior to the neck of the first rib; it gives a branch to the first intercostal space and usually continues downward over the neck of the second rib to end as the intercostal artery of the second space. The posterior intercostal arteries of the lower spaces are branches of the **descending aorta.** Observe that the more superior posterior intercostals run upward as well as laterally across the bodies of the vertebrae to reach the spaces they supply. As they cross the bodies of the vertebrae and the heads of the ribs, the right posterior in-

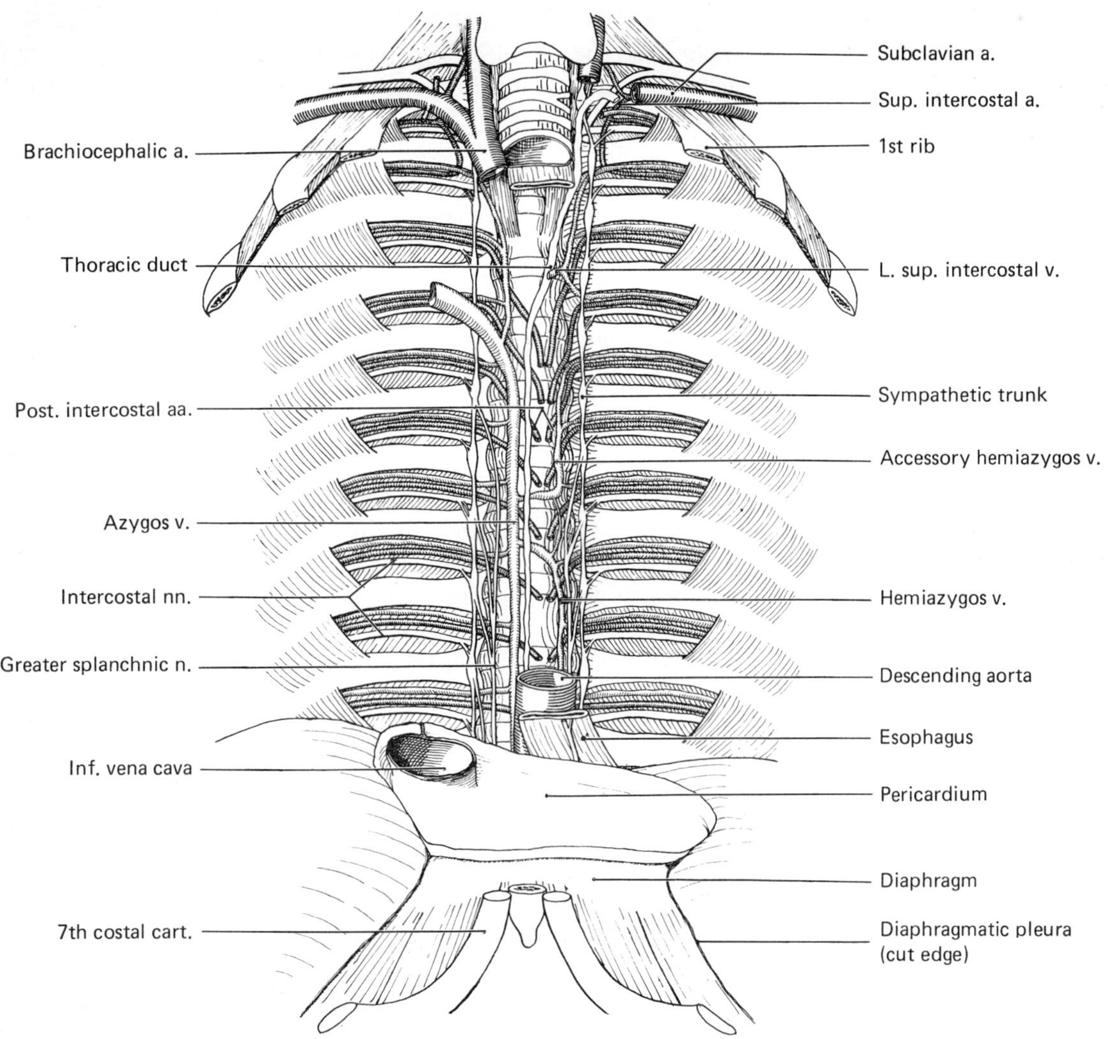

Figure 9.14 The **posterior thoracic wall** and deep structures of the posterior mediastinum.

tercostals cross the posterior aspects of the thoracic duct, azygos vein, and right sympathetic trunk; the left intercostals have a similar relation to the hemiazygos or accessory hemiazygos vein and the left sympathetic trunk.

The thoracic duct and azygos system of veins should be studied next. Dissect the descending aorta free from the surrounding connective tissue and retract it outward, cutting, if necessary, some of the intercostal arteries to facilitate the retraction of the aorta. Then clean the thoracic duct.

The **thoracic duct,** which drains all the lymph from the inferior extremities, pelvis, abdomen, thorax, left upper extremity, and left side of the head, is a small, very thin-walled vessel, usually white or gray. It enters the thorax through the **aortic hiatus of** the **diaphragm,** lying posterior to and to the right of the aorta. It ascends in the midline through the **posterior mediastinum,** where it lies in front of the bodies of the vertebrae and right posterior intercostal arteries and posterior to the esophagus (Fig. 9.14). In the **superior mediastinum,** it bends to the left, emerging from behind the left side of the esophagus to come into relation with the left pleura; it continues upward into the root of the neck, where it arches across the dome of the pleura to terminate in the origin of the **left brachiocephalic vein** or in the termination of the **left subclavian** or **left internal jugular vein.**

The azygos system of veins consists of the azygos, hemiazygos, and accessory hemiazygos veins, the longitudinal channels into which most of the intercostal veins drain. The **azygos vein** is a continuation of the **right ascending lumbar vein** of the abdomen; it enters the thorax through the aortic hiatus, where it lies to the right of and behind the aorta, and to the right of the thoracic duct. It ascends through the **posterior mediastinum** along the right side of the anterior aspects of the bodies of the vertebrae to about the level of the fourth thoracic vertebra, where it arches forward over the root of the right lung to enter the **superior vena cava.** It receives all the right intercostal veins except the first. The veins from the second, third, and fourth spaces, however, usually do not enter the azygos directly but unite to form a common trunk known as the **right superior intercostal vein,** which descends along the bodies of the upper vertebrae to reach the azygos. The intercostal vein of the first space usually drains into the brachiocephalic vein of its own side or into one of the tributaries of the brachiocephalic.

The drainage of the intercostal spaces of the left side is subject to a great deal of minor variation, and no precise description can be given to fit all cases. In the majority of cases, the **left superior intercostal vein,** the terminal part of which was seen at an earlier stage of the dissection crossing the left side of the arch of the aorta to terminate in the left brachiocephalic vein, receives the intercostal veins of the second, third, and fourth spaces. The **hemiazygos vein** is a continuation of the **left ascending lumbar vein;** it enters the thorax by passing through the muscular substance of the **diaphragm** and will be found ascending in the **posterior mediastinum** in front of the left sides of the lower thoracic vertebrae and behind the left side of the aorta to about the level of the eighth thoracic vertebra. Here it turns to the right behind the aorta and thoracic duct to enter the **azygos;** it receives the intercostal veins of the lower four or five spaces. The veins from the spaces between those drained by the **hemiazygos** and those drained by the **left superior intercostal vein** are drained by the **accessory hemiazygos.** This is a longitudinal channel in line with the hemiazygos but at a higher level. Superiorly, it frequently communicates with the **left superior intercostal vein;** inferiorly, it may join the **hemiazygos** or may cross the vertebral column to join the **azygos** independently of the hemiazygos.

Chapter 10

Abdominal Wall

SURFACE ANATOMY

Before dissecting the anterior abdominal wall, you should observe its surface landmarks and bony frame. A glance at a skeleton will make it apparent that the **bony wall of** the **abdominal cavity** is not as complete as that of the thoracic cavity. Superiorly, due to the domelike shape of the diaphragm, the abdominal cavity is protected by the **lower ribs;** inferiorly, the **coxal (hip) bones** help form its wall. In the intermediate region, however, the only skeletal support of the abdominal wall is given posteriorly by the **lumbar vertebrae.**

The **costal arch,** corresponding to the lower borders of the seventh to tenth costal cartilages on each side, can usually be seen and felt. The costal arches join in the midline to form the **infrasternal angle.** The depression on the surface of the body, at the apex of the arch, corresponds to the **xiphoid process of** the **sternum.** Below, on each coxal bone, identify the **anterior superior iliac spine.** Palpate the **iliac crest,** which runs backward and somewhat upward from the spine. Inferiorly, in the midline, feel the **pubic symphysis;** it is usually covered by a fairly thick pad of fat. A little lateral to the pubic symphysis on each side, locate a sharp bony projection, the **pubic tubercle.** Stretching between the pubic tubercle and the anterior superior iliac spine and separating the abdomen from the thigh, a curved linear depression is usually apparent. It corresponds to the **inguinal ligament.** Another linear depression, corresponding to the **linea alba,** stretches downward in the midline from the xiphoid process toward the pubis. The **umbilicus** lies on this line, nearer to the pubis than to the sternum at the level of the fourth lumbar vertebra. In well-developed subjects, another surface depression can be seen on

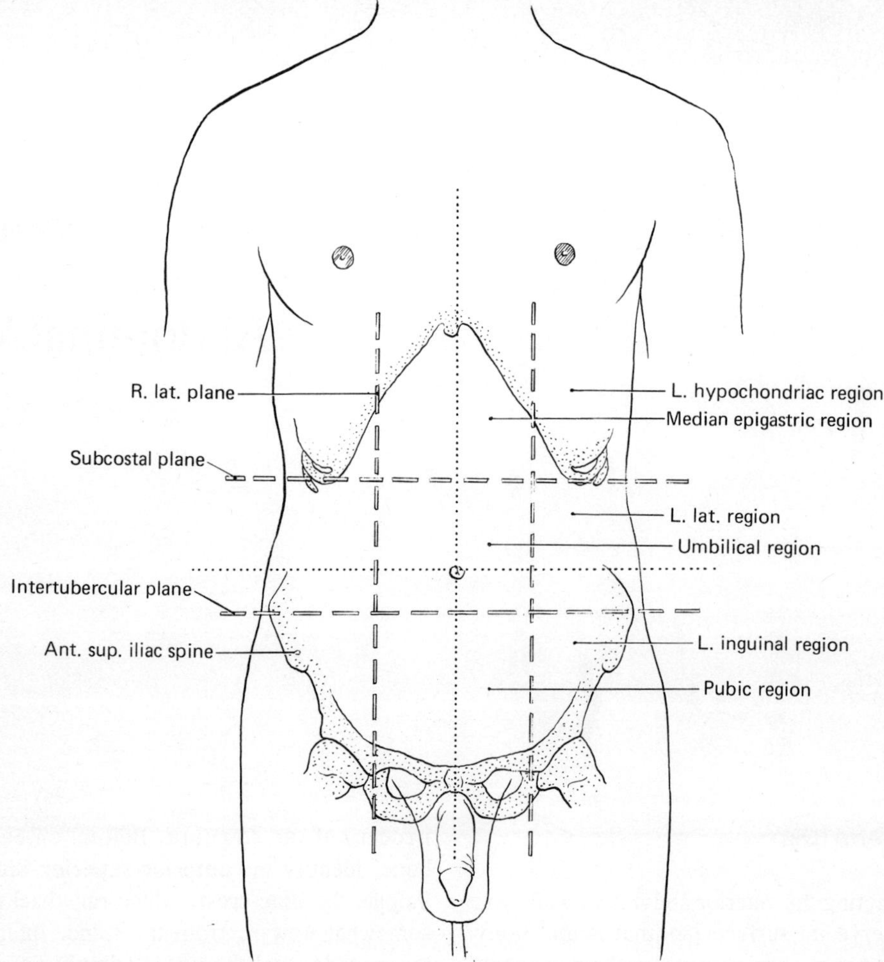

Figure 10.1 Topographical subdivision of the abdomen. The quadrants are partitioned by the dotted lines, and the nine regions by the dashed lines.

each side, 7 to 10 cm lateral and parallel to the linea alba superiorly but turning medially below. This indicates the position of the **linea semilunaris,** the lateral border of the rectus abdominis muscle. You may also find three transverse grooves, the **tendinous intersections**, running from one linea semilunaris to the other.

An appendectomy scar will typically be located at McBurney's point, one-third of the distance from the anterior superior iliac spine to the umbilicus.

TOPOGRAPHICAL REGIONS

The abdomen is theoretically divided into regions for purposes of making reference to pain and internal structure. Among the many ways of subdividing the abdomen, the easiest and most constant is to divide it into **quadrants** by imaginary vertical and horizontal planes through the umbilicus (Fig. 10.1). Alternatively, a **nine-region** subdivision is often used; for it, two transverse and two vertical planes are drawn (Fig. 10.1). The upper transverse

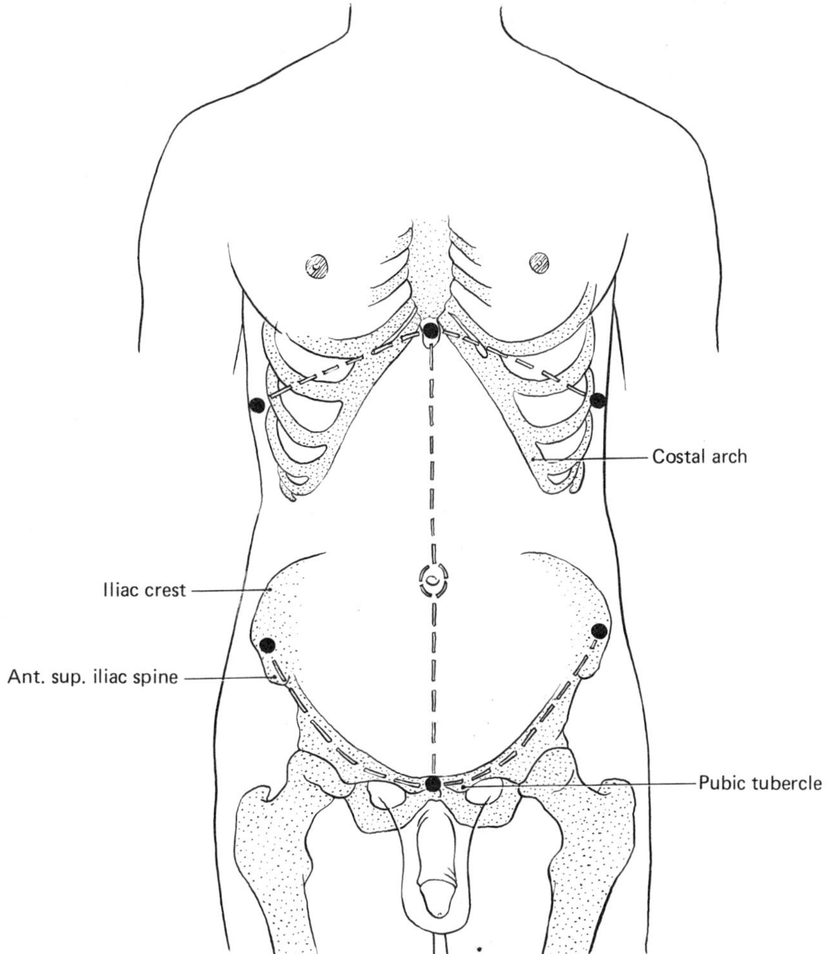

Figure 10.2 Surface landmarks and skin incisions on the abdomen.

plane, the **subcostal plane,** passes through the lowest portion of the tenth costal cartilages, and the lower transverse plane, the **intertubercular plane,** is at the level of the iliac tubercles. The vertical planes are the **right** and **left lateral planes.** They pass through the midpoint between the anterior superior iliac spine and the pubic symphysis on each side. The subdivisions of the abdomen created by these planes are, above the upper transverse plane, a **right** and a **left hypochondriac** and a **median epigastric region;** between the two transverse planes, a **right** and a **left lateral** and an **umbilical region;** below the inferior transverse plane, a **right** and a **left inguinal** and a **pubic region.** Be advised that slightly different planes are sometimes used to create the nine-region subdivision.

ABDOMINAL MUSCLES AND COMPANION STRUCTURES

Now make the following incisions through the skin as shown in Fig. 10.2: (1) in the midline, from the xiphisternal junction downward to the pubic symphysis (encircling the edge of the umbilicus), (2) from the upper end of the first incision, one on each side laterally and slightly downward across the body wall to the posterior axillary line, (3) from the lower end of the first incision, one on each side laterally along the pubic crest to the pubic tubercle and then upward along the line of the inguinal ligament extending for about 5 cm along the line of the iliac crest. Reflect laterally the large quadrilateral flaps of skin thus mapped out to expose the superficial fascia of the abdominal wall.

On its external aspect, the **superficial fascia** of the anterior abdominal wall does not differ appreciably from the same layer in other parts of the body, except that in obese subjects it is extremely thick. Dissect within the fascia and identify the **superficial epigastric, superficial circumflex iliac, umbilical,** and **thoracoepigastric veins.** The size and course of these superficial veins vary, but as a general rule, they connect the superficial veins of the inguinal region with those around the umbilicus and with the intercostal and axillary veins (Fig. 10.3).

If the main venous channels within the abdomen are occluded, some or all of these veins become enlarged to serve as collateral pathways for the return of venous blood around the site of occlusion. Varicose umbilical veins radiating from the umbilicus create a characteristic sign (referred to as "caput medusae"

Figure 10.3 The **subcutaneous vessels of** the anterior **abdominal wall.**

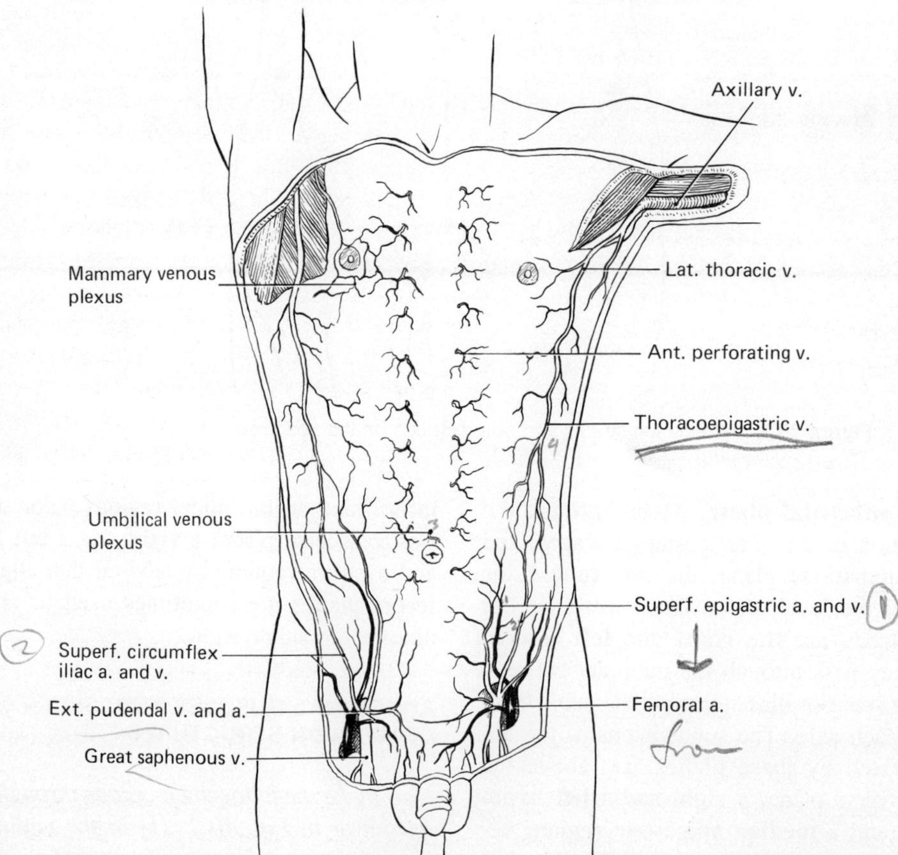

after the mythologic Medusa), which is sometimes associated with portal hypertension.

Cut through the superficial fascia in a straight line from one anterior superior iliac spine to the other. While making the incision, be careful not to cut through the **aponeurosis of** the **external abdominal oblique muscle** or the **sheath of** the **rectus abdominis muscle,** which lie immediately deep to the superficial fascia; they can be recognized by their light, glistening appearance. Remove all the superficial fascia above the transverse incision to expose the upper part of the rectus sheath and the external oblique muscle. As you remove the fascia, watch for the cutaneous nerves and vessels that supply the anterior abdominal wall. The continuations of the seventh to the eleventh intercostal nerves into the abdomen are called the **thoracoabdominal nerves.** The twelfth thoracic spinal nerve, the **subcostal nerve,** has a similar distribution. The **anterior cutaneous nerves** and **vessels** are the terminal portions of the thoracoabdominal nerves and superior epigastric artery, which pierce the rectus sheath in series from above downward about 2.5 cm lateral to the linea alba. The **lateral cutaneous branches** are derived from the same nerves and from the lower intercostal, subcostal, and lumbar arteries; they run downward and forward over the lateral part of the external oblique muscle.

The dermatome pattern of the abdominal wall is easy to learn if you remember that the belt of skin at the level of the umbilicus is innervated by the tenth thoracoabdominal nerve and that the others are evenly distributed above and below it down to the suprapubic region, which is innervated by the first lumbar segment.

The superficial fascia on the lower part of the anterior abdominal wall, where it still remains in place, is peculiar in that it may be separated into superficial and deep layers. (Many anatomists and physicians do not subscribe to this concept, but you should be aware of it since some do.) The **superficial layer,** known as the **fascia of Camper,** is the thicker of the two; it has the usual characteristics of fatty subcutaneous tissue and is directly continuous below the line of the inguinal ligament with the superficial fascia of the thigh. The **deeper layer,** the **fascia of Scarpa,** which lies just external to the lower part of the aponeurosis of the external oblique muscle, is more **membranous** and ends immediately below the inguinal ligament by fusing with the deep fascia (fascia lata) of the thigh. Medial to the pubic tubercle, it continues downward over the scrotum and posteriorly over the perineum.

Make a median vertical incision down to the pubic symphysis, through the superficial fascia on the lower part of the abdominal wall. Reflect downward and laterally toward the inguinal ligament the triangular flaps of fascia thus marked out on each side. Scarpa's and Camper's fasciae should be reflected as a single layer. Identify Scarpa's fascia on the deep surface of the reflected flap. The reflection can be continued only a short distance inferior to the inguinal ligament, because the fascia blends with the fascia lata. By removing the fascia, you will completely expose the **external oblique muscle** and the **rectus sheath.** Caution is advised because at the same time, the **superficial inguinal ring** and a portion of the **spermatic cord** (round ligament in the female) will be uncovered. In series with the cutaneous nerves already exposed on the upper part of the abdominal wall, look for the terminal **cutaneous portions of** the **iliohypogastric** and the **ilioinguinal nerves;** both are derived from the first lumbar nerve. The iliohypogastric nerve pierces the aponeurosis of the external oblique, often as two separate branches, laterally a short distance above the inguinal ligament; the ilioinguinal nerve emerges through the superficial inguinal ring with the spermatic cord. In dissecting the ilioinguinal nerves, try not to damage the external spermatic fascia.

Observe the **linea alba,** a dense aponeurotic band running from the **xiphoid process** to the **pubic symphysis,** that intervenes between the two recti muscles. The recti at present are enclosed and hidden within the aponeurotic **rectus sheath.** The **linea semilunaris** is the line that marks the **lateral border of** the **rectus muscle** and the line along which the aponeuroses of the three muscles of the anterolateral abdominal wall fuse in the formation of the rectus sheath. Study the external oblique, the most superficial of these.

The **external abdominal oblique muscle** arises by fleshy slips from the outer surfaces of the **lower eight ribs** just lateral to their costochondral junctions. The upper slips interdigitate with the serratus anterior and the lower ones with the latissimus dorsi. Fibers that arise from the lower two or three ribs run downward to insert into the anterior third of the **outer lip of** the **iliac crest.** The remaining fibers are not inserted into bone but run inferiorly and anteriorly to end in the broad sheet of fascia known as the **aponeurosis of** the **external oblique.** The aponeurosis of the external oblique continues medial to the linea semilunaris as one of the constituents of the **anterior layer of** the **sheath of** the **rectus abdominis muscle.** In the midline, the aponeurosis entwines with the same layer on the opposite side to form the linea alba. Between the **anterior superior iliac spine** and the **pubic tubercle,** the free inferior border of the aponeurosis is thickened to form the **inguinal ligament.**

The lateral border of the external oblique helps form the lumbar triangle along with the iliac crest and the latissimus dorsi muscle.

Define the **superficial inguinal ring.** It is a potential opening in the aponeurosis of the external oblique above the medial end of the inguinal ligament just superolateral to the pubic tubercle; through it the **spermatic cord** (**round ligament** in the female) emerges from the inguinal canal. The superficial inguinal ring is not an actual opening in the aponeurosis of the external oblique until the fascia of the external oblique is dissected away. That fascia is the outermost covering of the spermatic cord, is continuous with it, and extends downward into the scrotum. The covering is a much thinner layer than the aponeurosis, with which it is continuous around the lips of the superficial inguinal ring (Fig. 10.4). The edges of the superficial inguinal ring are fairly thick and are known as the **medial crus** and the **lateral crus.** Just superior to the ring, note some fibers running at about a right angle to the course of the fibers in the crura. They are the **intercrural fibers** (Fig. 10.4). The **inguinal canal** is an oblique passageway through the lower part of the anterior abdominal wall; through it the spermatic cord (round ligament) passes from the interior of the abdominal cavity to the scrotum (labium majus).

Now study the rectus abdominis muscle. To open the rectus sheath, make a longitudinal incision through its exposed anterior portion, from a point just below the xiphoid process to a point just above the pubic symphysis, parallel and just lateral to the linea alba. From each end of this incision make a transverse incision laterally to the linea semilunaris. Observe that above the upper transverse incision the anterior part of the rectus sheath is much thinner and blends with the fascia of the pectoralis major muscle. Turn the flaps marked out by the three incisions laterally to expose the anterior surface of the rectus abdominis muscle.

First observe whether or not the **pyramidalis muscle** is present. This small triangular muscle, which is totally lacking in about one-fifth of all cases, lies in front of the lower part of the rectus. It arises from the upper border of the **body of** the **pubis** near the symphysis and inserts into the **linea alba** between the symphysis and the umbilicus.

Next study the **rectus abdominis,** a broad, flat muscle that arises from the **pubic crest** and the **anterior surface of** the **symphysis** and inserts into the anterior surfaces of the fifth, sixth, and seventh **costal cartilages** and the **xiphoid process.** Observe its **tendinous intersections.** They are irregular transverse tendinous bands, usually three in number that cross the muscle and are quite firmly attached to the anterior part of the sheath.

Detach the rectus from the linea alba. Elevate and transect the muscle by an incision at the level of the umbilicus, and turn the muscle laterally to expose the posterior layer of its sheath. Do this with care, since other structures enclosed within the posterior part of the sheath must be cleaned and studied as the muscle is being reflected. These structures include the terminal parts of the thora-

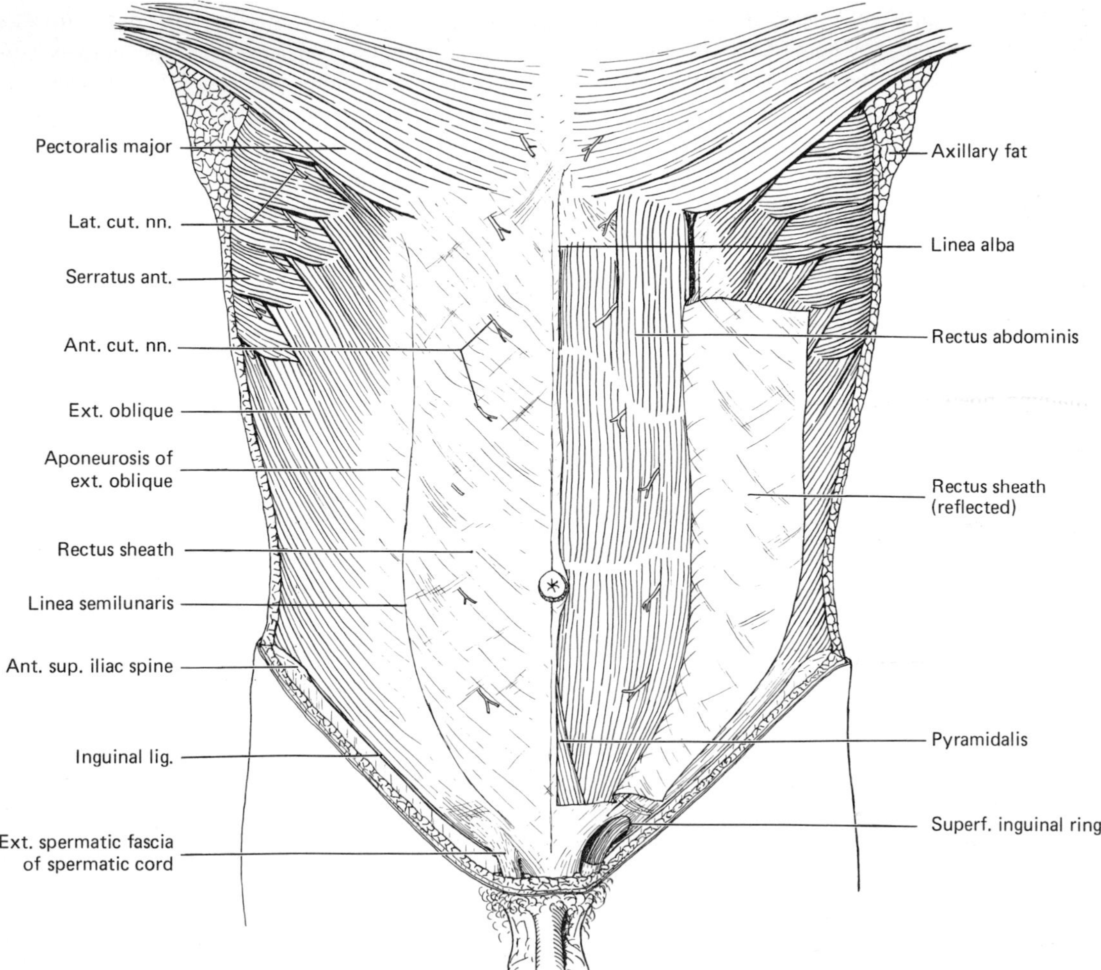

Figure 10.4 External **musculature of** the **abdominal wall.** On the left, the anterior part of the rectus sheath is reflected, and the external spermatic fascia has been removed to show the medial and lateral crural borders of the superficial inguinal ring. Note the intercrural fibers just superior to the ring.

coabdominal nerves and the superior and inferior epigastric arteries. The nerves pierce the posterior layer of the rectus sheath in longitudinal series near its lateral margin. They enter the deep surface of the rectus, which they supply, and finally pierce the anterior layer of the sheath, where they have already been seen as the **anterior cutaneous nerves of** the **abdominal wall.**

Surgical incisions through the anterior abdominal wall in the region of the rectus muscles are usually made in the midline to preserve the nerve supply to the rectus muscles, which enter laterally.

The **superior epigastric artery,** a terminal branch of the **internal thoracic artery,** enters the rectus sheath and the deep surface of the muscle by passing downward posterior to the seventh costal cartilage. The **inferior epigastic artery,** a branch of the **external iliac artery,** enters the lower lateral part of the rectus sheath, runs upward between the muscle and the posterior layer of the sheath, and finally enters the muscle to anastomose with the superior epigastric. Its origin will be seen later. Occasionally a continuous anastomosing channel may be found connecting the epigastric arteries on the deep surface of the rectus. Both arteries are accompanied by veins.

Observe that the **posterior layer of** the **rectus sheath** is thicker and tougher superiorly than it is inferiorly. In many cases, a **sharp inferior margin** can be seen about halfway between the umbilicus and the pubis, where the posterior layer of the sheath appears to stop. This is the **arcuate line (linea semicircularis).** Below this line, the rectus muscle rests posteriorly against the **transversalis fascia,** a thin fascial layer that lies just external to the extraperitoneal fat in the lower anterior abdominal wall. More frequently, a distinct line is not discernible, but the posterior layer of the sheath merely becomes gradually thinner in this region. The medial continuations of the internal oblique and transversus muscle aponeuroses cross from the posterior to the anterior layer of the sheath, causing the posterior layer to thin inferiorly.

The internal oblique and transversus muscles should be displayed completely on only one side. On the other side, do not dissect the anterior abdominal wall below a transverse line at the level of the anterior superior iliac spines. It will be done later when the inguinal canal and its relationship to inguinal hernia are studied.

Now reflect the external oblique muscle to expose the internal oblique. Care is necessary here, since the layers of muscle in the anterolateral abdominal wall are thin and are separated from each other by only thin layers of fascia. Detach the upper four slips of origin of the external oblique from the fifth to the eighth ribs. Then, in the interval between its fourth and fifth slips of origin, make a longitudinal incision through the muscle downward to the iliac crest. From the lower end of this incision, make a transverse cut through the muscle and its aponeurosis medially to the linea semilunaris. From the medial end of the transverse incision, make a third incision running downward through the aponeurosis to the upper border of the superficial inguinal ring. By these incisions, the external oblique muscle and its aponeurosis will be divided into three portions. First, reflect medially the large upper medial segment to the linea semilunaris. Observe that at this line the **external oblique aponeurosis** joins the **anterior layer of** the **rectus sheath.** Then turn the lower lateral triangular segment downward to the inguinal ligament (Fig. 10.5).

When this is done, you will have exposed the internal oblique muscle and will also have opened the medial portion of the inguinal canal. Clean and study the **internal abdominal oblique muscle.** It arises from the fused portion of the **thoracolumbar fascia** lateral to the erector spinae muscles, from the intermediate lip of the anterior two-thirds of the **iliac crest,** and from the **fascia of** the **iliopsoas muscle,** and is attached only loosely to the lateral half of the **inguinal ligament.** The highest fibers insert into the inferior borders of the **lower** three or four **ribs.** The remaining fibers, as they approach the linea semilunaris, terminate in an **aponeurosis** that joins the **rectus sheath. Superiorly,** the aponeurosis splits into **two parts,** some fibers join the **anterior** and some the **posterior layer of** the **sheath. Inferiorly,** however, the **entire aponeurosis of** the **internal oblique** passes **anterior to** the **rectus abdominis muscle.**

The **iliohypogastric nerve,** whose terminal part was seen piercing the external oblique, should now be traced back to where it pierces the lower portion of the internal oblique.

The **inguinal canal** has been partly opened by reflecting the external oblique aponeurosis. The canal which is an oblique passageway through the anterior abdominal wall, lies just above the medial third of the inguinal ligament. Its **anterior wall** is formed principally by the **aponeurosis of** the **external oblique.** Laterally, however, the **lower fibers of** the **internal oblique muscle** contribute to the anterior wall of the inguinal canal. Consequently, only the medial portion of the canal is presently open for inspection.

Observe that the **spermatic cord,** as it emerges into this part of the inguinal canal from behind the

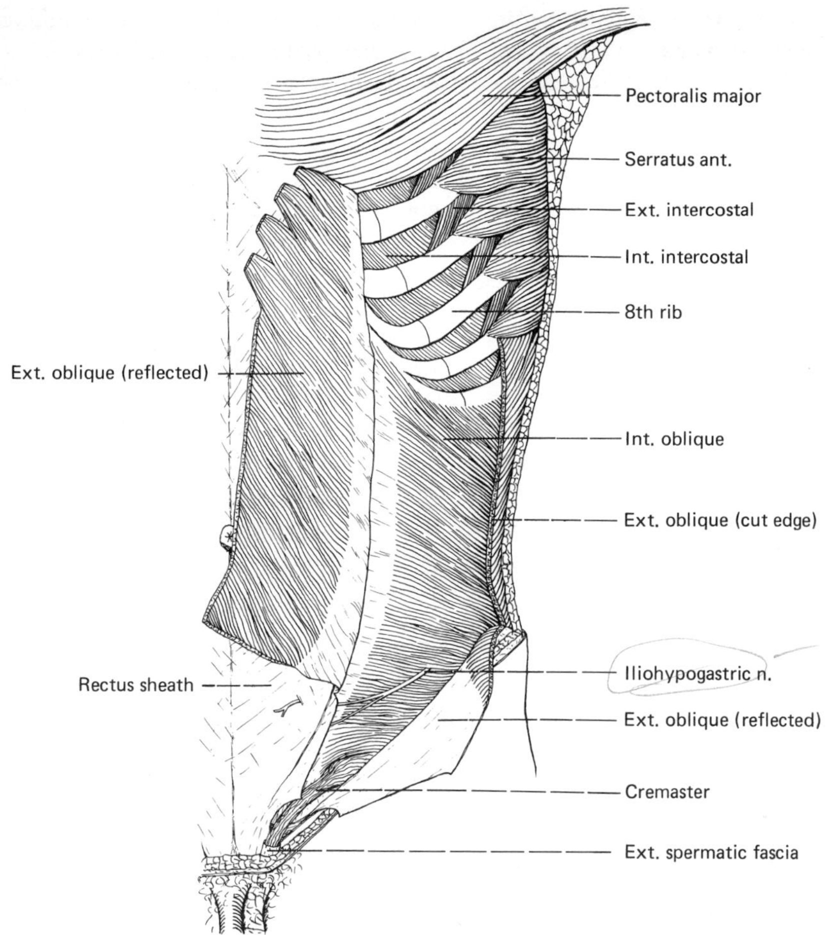

Figure 10.5 The left side of the anterior **abdominal wall** with the external oblique muscle reflected medially.

lower part of the internal oblique muscle, receives a covering known as the **cremasteric fascia** and **muscle.** The **cremaster muscle** is a thin layer of muscle fibers that runs downward around the **spermatic cord.** The fascia and muscle are derivatives of the internal oblique fascia and muscle. When the scrotum is dissected, you will find that some of these muscle fibers reach as far as the **testis,** which they encircle. After the cord has emerged through the superficial inguinal ring, the cremaster layer is covered externally by the external spermatic fascia (Fig. 10.5).

Observe the **lacunar ligament,** which stretches from the medial end of the **inguinal ligament** to the **pecten of** the **pubis.** For about 1.5 cm of its course, immediately internal to the superficial inguinal ring, the spermatic cord rests on the superior surface of the lacunar ligament. Consequently, the ligament is said to form the **floor** of the most medial part of the **inguinal canal.**

Now, as you prepare to reflect the internal oblique muscle, be careful not to cut the lower intercostal nerves, which cross its deep surface in the narrow interval between the internal oblique and transversus muscles. Make a longitudinal incision through the internal oblique in the same line as that previously made through the external oblique. Medial to this incision, detach the internal oblique from its attachments to the ribs superiorly, and to the iliac crest and the inguinal ligament inferiorly. The broad, flat medial portion of the muscle can then be reflected forward and medially to the linea semilunaris. In this manner you will expose the external surface of the transversus abdominis muscle and the vessels and nerves that lie between it and the internal oblique (Fig. 10.6). Elevate the dorsal part of the internal oblique, and note its connections to the thoracolumbar fascia.

The **thoracoabdominal** and the **subcostal** (twelfth thoracic) **nerves** run downward and forward across the external surface of the transversus muscle, supplying it and the internal and external oblique muscles. At the linea semilunaris, they enter the rectus sheath; their further distribution has been seen. The **iliohypogastric** and **ilioinguinal nerves,** branches of the ventral ramus of the first lumbar nerve, have a similar course across the lower part of the transversus. They do not, however, enter the rectus sheath. The iliohypogastric has already been seen piercing the internal oblique. The **ilioinguinal nerve** crosses the transversus just above the lateral part of the inguinal ligament and enters the **inguinal canal,** through which it accompanies the spermatic cord to the superficial inguinal ring.

Clean the exposed portion of the **deep circumflex iliac artery.** It pierces the transversus a short distance medial to the anterior superior iliac spine and runs posteriorly along the iliac crest between the transversus and the internal oblique. Just an-

Figure 10.6 The left side of the anterior **abdominal wall** with the external and internal oblique muscles reflected medially.

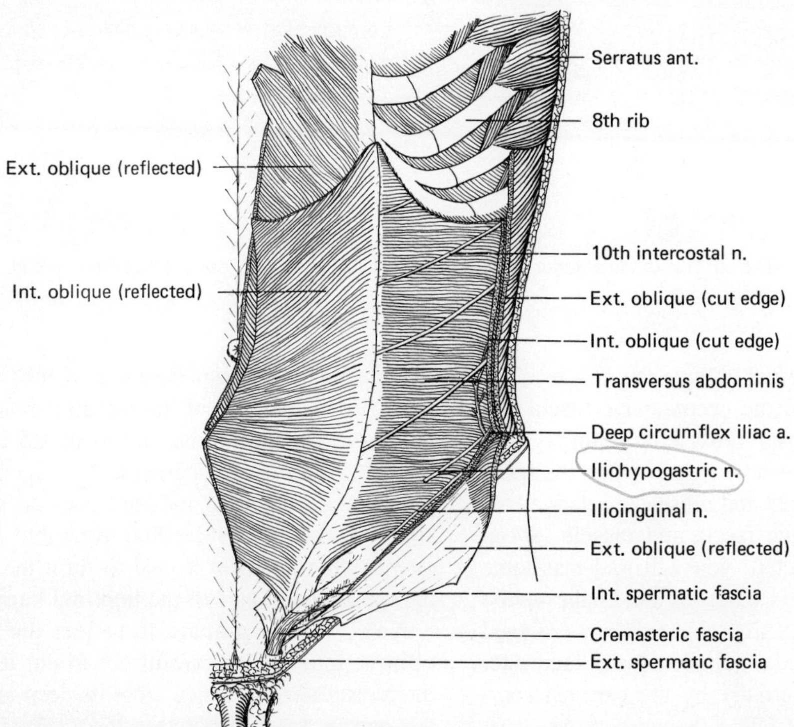

terior to the anterior superior iliac spine, it gives off a large branch that ascends on the transversus.

The **transversus abdominis** has a continuous origin from the inner surfaces of the **lower** six **costal cartilages,** the **thoracolumbar fascia,** the internal lip of the **iliac crest,** and the **fascia of** the **iliopsoas,** being attached only loosely by areolar tissue to the lateral third of the **inguinal ligament.** Its fibers cross the abdominal wall horizontally to end near the linea semilunaris in an **aponeurosis** that joins the **rectus sheath.** Throughout most of its extent, the aponeurosis of the transversus joins the **posterior layer of** the **rectus sheath; inferiorly,** however, it passes into the **anterior layer of** the **sheath.** The shifting of the transversus and internal oblique aponeuroses from the posterior to the anterior layers of the sheath is marked by the arcuate line. Observe that the most **inferior portion of** the **transversus aponeurosis** does not reach the rectus sheath at all but passes downward, lateral to the narrow inferior portion of the sheath, to attach directly to the **pecten of** the **pubis.** This portion of the aponeurosis of the transversus is known as the **falx inguinalis.** It is sometimes referred to as the **conjoined tendon** because it receives a few of the lowermost fibers of the internal oblique. Observe that the falx inguinalis lies immediately posterior to the portion of the spermatic cord that rests inferiorly on the lacunar ligament. Consequently, it is one of the constituents of the **posterior wall of** the **inguinal canal.**

The portion of the transversus that originates from the inguinal ligament and arches over the spermatic cord helps form, along with the internal oblique, the **roof of** the **inguinal canal.**

Internal to the transversus, you will expose the deepest layer of the anterior abdominal wall, the **transversalis fascia.** Aided by the conjoined tendon, it forms the **posterior wall of** the **inguinal canal** throughout the length of the canal.

At this point, you have removed the entire anterior wall of the inguinal canal. The internal opening, the **deep inguinal ring,** of the canal is thus exposed from the outside. It lies just above the middle of the inguinal ligament. It is described as an opening in the transversalis fascia, but from the outside it does not appear so, since the transversalis fascia is prolonged outward along the spermatic cord as the **internal spermatic fascia** (Fig. 10.6).

Chapter 11

Penis, Scrotum, and Testes

Direct your attention, in the male body, to the penis and scrotum. The **root of** the **penis** is situated in the perineum, firmly attached to the bone and fasciae of that region. Before skinning the **free portion** or **body of** the **penis,** observe that the skin near its end forms a free fold, the **prepuce** or foreskin, which covers the **glans penis,** the rounded extremity of the penis. The inner surface of the prepuce is covered with a layer of the epithelium that is continuous around the margin or **corona of** the **glans** with the epithelium covering the glans. Notice the **frenulum,** a fold of skin that attaches the prepuce to the underside of the glans.

Many cadavers will have been circumcised; this operation, which removes the prepuce, is usually done when the baby is two or three days old.

Make a longitudinal incision through the skin of the penis from the pubic symphysis to the tip of the glans. Then reflect the skin laterally to each side.

Define the **fundiform ligament of** the **penis.** Derived from the membranous layer of the superficial fascia, it extends from the linea alba, surrounds the penis, and ends in the scrotal septum. Deep to the fundiform ligament, find the **suspensory ligament of** the **penis.** It is a fibrous band that runs downward from the pubic symphysis and divides into two parts that are attached to the deep fascia on each side of the body of the penis.

Clean the vessels and nerves on the dorsum of the penis (anterior surface of the flaccid organ). Most superficially, in the midline, is the **superficial dorsal vein,** which should be dissected from the surrounding connective tissue and reflected laterally with the superficial fascia. In the **deep fascia** on the dorsum of the penis you will find the deep dorsal vein and the dorsal arteries and nerves, all of which enter the area by passing between the two parts of the suspensory ligament. The **deep dorsal vein** is in the midline. On each side of it are the **dorsal arteries,** and lateral to the artery on each side is the **dorsal nerve.** Numerous small branches arise from the artery and nerve as they approach the glans.

Attempt to separate the two main parts of the body of the penis—the **corpora cavernosa penis** and the **corpus spongiosum penis.** Observe that the **glans penis** is the expanded terminal portion of the corpus spongiosum penis. The corpora cavernosa cannot be separated because they are bound together by a tough connective tissue sheath called the **tunica albuginea.**

The **scrotum** is a sac made of skin and fascia that contains the lower ends of the spermatic cords and the testes and their coverings. The coverings of the testis are prolongations of the fascial coverings of the spermatic cord, which have already been observed. In addition, the testis has an innermost serous covering, the **tunica vaginalis,** which was originally continuous with the peritoneum and its adjacent layer of extraperitoneal connective tissue and fat.

On both sides, make a longitudinal incision through the skin of the scrotum from the region of the superficial inguinal ring down to the lower end of the scrotum; then reflect the skin from the anterior aspect of the scrotum. Observe that the skin is thin and rather firmly attached to the underlying superficial fascia.

The **superficial fascia of** the **scrotum** is known as the **dartos tunic.** It is devoid of fat and usually dark red because of the presence of smooth muscle fibers in it. In the midline, it is prolonged backward to form a **median scrotal septum** that divides the scrotal sac into two parts. Reflect the dartos tunic from the anterior aspect of the testis and free the spermatic cord and testis, together with their coverings, entirely from the scrotum. Note that the testis is attached to the scrotum by the **scrotal ligament,** which extends from the inferior aspect of the testis. Then study the spermatic cord between the superficial inguinal ring and the testis.

The reflection of each **fascial covering of** the **spermatic cord** is extremely difficult to achieve in most cases but should be attempted. The coverings are, from outside inward, the **external spermatic fascia** (derived from the external abdominal oblique fascia), the **cremaster muscle** and **fascia** (derived from the internal abdominal oblique muscle and fascia), and the **internal spermatic fascia** (derived from the transversalis fascia). When you have opened them, identify the various constituents of the spermatic cord proper; they lie within a layer of connective tissue that is continuous with the extraperitoneal tissue of the abdomen through the inguinal canal.

The **ductus (vas) deferens** can always be recognized tactilely by its hard, cordlike feel. Through it the spermatozoa pass from the testis to the urethra. It is usually the most posterior structure in the spermatic cord. Its small artery may be seen on its external surface. The **testicular artery** is the principal artery supplying the testis. It is surrounded by the **pampiniform plexus of veins,** which returns blood from the testis. The venous plexus converges to form the testicular vein at the deep inguinal ring. The **genital nerve** is a small nerve that supplies the **cremaster muscle.** It arises in the abdominal cavity as a branch of the genitofemoral nerve of the lumbar plexus. The spermatic cord also contains lymph channels that carry lymph away from the testis. Following the course of the testicular vessels, the lymph drains into preaortic nodes located at the level of the kidneys.

Metastasis of testicular carcinoma is difficult to detect at its onset because the lymph channels and nodes involved are deeply hidden in the abdomen.

The **tunica vaginalis** of the testis is a serous membrane that forms a completely enclosed sac akin to the pleural, peritoneal, and pericardial sacs. It is invaginated by the **testis** and **epididymis** so that it presents visceral and parietal portions. The **visceral tunica vaginalis** is closely applied to the superior, inferior, anterior, medial, and lateral aspects of the testis and epididymis. Posteriorly, the testis is not covered by the tunica vaginalis; here the visceral portion is reflected at each side to become continuous with the **parietal tunica vaginalis.** Between the visceral and parietal portions is a narrow cavity filled with a small amount of **serous fluid.** Open the cavity by making a longitudinal incision through the anterior part of the parietal tunica vaginalis. This exposes the testis and epididymis, covered by the visceral tunica vaginalis. Observe, however, that diseased testes with complete or partial obliteration of the cavity of the tunica vaginalis are fairly common in cadavers.

Excessive accumulation of serous fluid in the cavity is called a "hydrocele." It is usually drained with a needle passed through the wall of the scrotum.

The **testis** is an oval body, somewhat flattened at the sides. It normally lies free in the sac of the tunica vaginalis except posteriorly, where it is attached to the scrotal wall and to the epididymis. The **epididymis** is a curved, elongated structure applied to the posterolateral aspect of the testis. It is a reservoir for spermatozoa. The lower end, or **tail,** of the epididymis is held to the lower end of the testis by the visceral tunica vaginalis. Its enlarged upper end, the **head,** surmounts the upper end of the testis. The intervening **body** portion is partially separated from the testis by an inpocketing of the lateral part of the cavity of the tunica vaginalis. This cleftlike portion of the cavity is known as the **sinus of** the **epididymis.**

Free the body and tail of the epididymis from the testis by cutting through the tunica vaginalis along each side. Observe that the **ductus deferens** begins at the **tail of** the **epididymis** and then runs upward into the spermatic cord. Cut carefully through the visceral tunica vaginalis along its line of reflection from the upper end of the testis onto the head of the epididymis to demonstrate the **efferent ducts** of the testis. They are 15 to 20 small ducts that carry the spermatozoa from the upper end of the testis into the head of the epididymis. In the epididymis, all these ducts eventually unite to form a single duct, the **duct of** the **epididymis.** The body and tail of the epididymis consist of this single duct, which is tightly coiled.

Observe that the arteries and veins of the testis enter and leave its posterior border, where it is not covered by the tunica vaginalis. Section the **testis** transversely at about its middle to see its internal structure. Immediately internal to the tunica vaginalis is a heavy fibrous capsule, the **tunica albuginea.** Along the posterior border, where the vessels enter, this layer is thickened to form the **mediastinum testis.** From the mediastinum, fibrous partitions or septules radiate through the gland, dividing it into **lobules.** The **seminiferous tubules,** where the spermatozoa are formed, are contained within the lobules.

Sometimes during development the testis fails to descend into the scrotum and is found in the abdominal cavity or the inguinal canal. The condition is known as cryptorchidism. The testis must then be placed (by hormonal management or surgery) in the scrotum early in life if sterility is to be prevented.

Chapter 12

Inguinal Region

Make a transverse incision through the entire anterior abdominal wall, including the peritoneum, from a point a little above the anterior superior iliac spine on one side to the same point on the other side. Then draw the lower segment of the divided wall as far forward as possible and observe the disposition of the peritoneum on the inner surface of the lower part of the abdominal wall. The peritoneum does not form a perfectly smooth internal covering for the abdominal wall but projects backward into the abdominal cavity in the form of five folds or ridges on the internal surface of the wall.

In the midline, find the **median umbilical fold** running upward from the pubic symphysis to the umbilicus; it is a ridge that is created by the **median umbilical ligament** and its peritoneal covering. The ligament represents the adult remnant of the fetal **urachus,** which ascends from the apex of the bladder to the umbilical cord. Starting at the inferior limit of the anterior abdominal wall, a short distance lateral to the midline on either side, and running upward and medially to the umbilicus is another peritoneal ridge, the **medial umbilical fold.** It is caused by the presence of the **medial umbilical ligament,** a fibrous cord that represents the obliterated portion of the **fetal umbilical artery.** Still farther lateral is another peritoneal ridge caused by the **inferior epigastric artery** that runs upward and medially to enter the rectus sheath. It is called the **lateral umbilical fold** and is often not well marked. By means of these peritoneal folds, the peritoneum clothing the inner surface of the lower anterior abdominal wall is divided into three pairs of peritoneal fossae, which represent partial subdivisions of the general peritoneal cavity. Between the median and the medial umbilical folds on each side is the

supravesical fossa. Between the medial and the lateral folds is the **medial inguinal fossa.** The **lateral inguinal fossa** is lateral to the lateral umbilical fold.

From the transverse incision already made in the anterior abdominal wall, make a longitudinal incision just to the side of the midline down to the pubis. Then approach the intact inguinal canal from the interior of the abdominal cavity (Fig. 12.1).

With the **deep inguinal ring** as its center, carefully remove a circular piece of peritoneum and extraperitoneal tissue, about 5 cm in diameter, from the internal abdominal wall. The deep inguinal ring is located just superior to the midpoint of the inguinal ligament, lateral to the inferior epigastric artery. Its position can often be readily recognized while the peritoneum is still in place—the peritoneum usually dimples into it for a short distance.

The **transversalis fascia** stretches upward from the inguinal ligament. As seen from the inside, the deep inguinal ring appears as an opening in this fascia (just above the middle of the inguinal ligament). Observe that the **ductus deferens** enters the abdominal cavity at the **deep inguinal ring.** At the inguinal ligament, it turns downward and medially and crosses anterior to the external iliac vessels to run toward the brim of the pelvis immediately external to the peritoneum. In the **female,** its place is taken by the **round ligament of** the **uterus.**

The **external iliac artery** and **vein** are large vessels that run downward across the medial side of the present area of dissection to disappear behind the inguinal ligament. The artery is lateral to the vein. Lateral to the artery, above and behind the inguinal ligament, is the **iliac fascia,** a layer of fascia that covers the **psoas major** and **iliacus muscles.** In the male, the **testicular artery** and **vein** and the **genital branch of** the **genitofemoral nerve** run downward on the iliac fascia a short distance lateral to the external iliac artery to reach the deep inguinal ring. Clean the **inferior epigastric artery.** Observe that it arises from the **external iliac** just before the latter passes posterior to the inguinal ligament, that it is crossed internally near its origin by the ductus deferens, and that it runs upward in the anterior abdominal wall to pierce the transversalis fascia and enter the **rectus sheath.** In some cases, you will see another artery arising from the external iliac in common with the inferior epigastric but turning medially to cross the external iliac vein and the pelvic brim. It is the

Figure 12.1 The right **deep inguinal ring** from the inner surface of the abdominal wall.

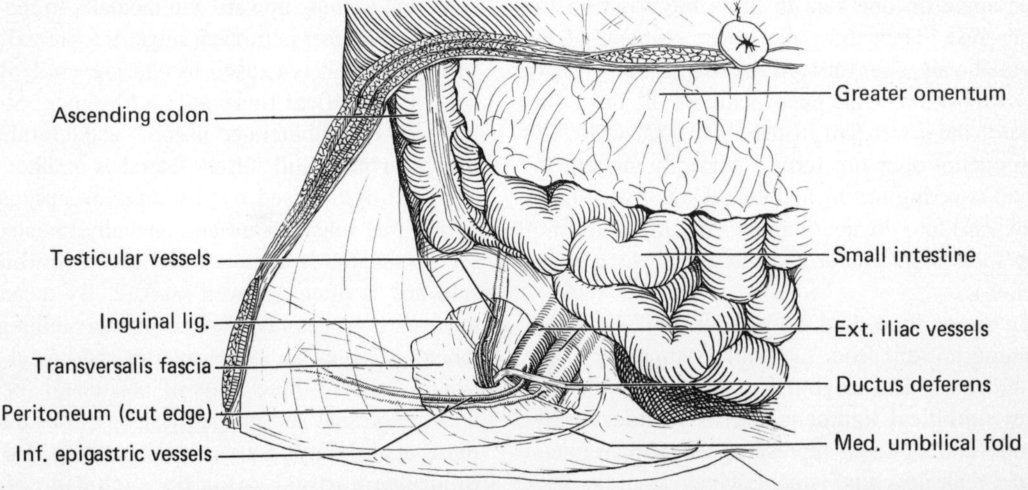

obturator artery, which most often arises within the pelvis as a branch of the internal iliac artery.

INGUINAL HERNIA

An **inguinal hernia** is the protrusion of a portion of the abdominal contents, usually a loop of intestine, into the inguinal canal. There are two principal types of inguinal hernia. An **indirect inguinal hernia** is one in which the herniating mass enters the **deep ring,** traverses the entire length of the **inguinal canal,** and emerges at the **superficial ring.** A **direct inguinal hernia** is one that pushes through the posterior wall of the canal at some point **medial to** the **deep ring,** traverses the **medial end of** the **canal,** and emerges at the **superficial ring.** Note the inguinal triangle; it is bounded by the lateral border of the rectus abdominis muscle medially, the inguinal ligament inferiorly, and the inferior epigastric artery laterally. All direct hernias pass through it. Any inguinal hernia will push before it, as the most internal of its coverings, a layer of peritoneum and extraperitoneal fat, but its outer coverings will differ according to the point at which it enters the inguinal canal.

If you introduce your little finger into the deep ring from within the abdominal cavity and push it through the inguinal canal to the superficial ring, the coverings of an indirect hernia will be readily demonstrated. They are the same as the normal coverings of the spermatic cord. As your finger emerges through the superficial ring, it is covered externally by internal spermatic fascia, cremaster muscle and fascia, and external spermatic fascia. If such a hernia reaches as far as the scrotum, it appears in the interval between the internal spermatic fascia and the parietal tunica vaginalis.

Observe that the **covering of** a **direct inguinal hernia** will not be the same in all cases. A direct hernia that enters the posterior wall of the canal just **medial to** the **deep ring** will push before it a covering of transversalis fascia, which will take the place of the internal spermatic fascia, and will appear **in** the **scrotum between** the **internal spermatic** and **cremaster muscles** and **fascia.** However, a direct hernia that enters the inguinal canal by pushing through the **medial end of** its **posterior wall** will receive neither internal spermatic fascia nor cremaster muscle and fascia but instead, coverings derived from the transversalis fascia and the falx inguinalis (or conjoined tendon), respectively. As the hernia passes through the superficial ring, it will lie internal to the external spermatic fascia and will appear **in** the **scrotum,** covered by peritoneum, extraperitoneal fat, transversalis fascia, and falx inguinalis, **in** the **interval between** the **external spermatic fascia** and the **cremasteric fascia.**

Inguinal hernia is more common in men than in women. Due in part to a partial or total persisting processus vaginalis, the indirect type occurs more frequently than the direct type.

Standard repairs for inguinal hernia consist of reducing the abdominal wall defect by suturing the lower edge of the muscle and fasciae to the pectineal ligament, which runs along the superior ramus of the pubis.

Chapter 13

Abdominal Cavity

The abdominal cavity has already been partially opened by a transverse and a lower vertical incision (page 139). Open the cavity completely by making a second vertical incision through the entire thickness of the wall to the left of the median line, running upward from the transverse incision to the costal arch. By doing this, you will have opened the **peritoneal cavity,** which is contained **within** the **abdominal cavity.**

The **peritoneum** is the great **serous membrane** of the abdominal cavity. Like the pleural and pericardial serous membranes, which enclose their respective cavities, it encloses the **peritoneal cavity** between its layers, the **parietal** and **visceral peritoneal layers.** In the **male,** the peritoneal cavity is completely closed and contains a film of serous fluid. In the **female,** the peritoneum is pierced by two small openings, the **mouths of** the **uterine tubes,** but elsewhere it completely encloses the peritoneal cavity. The arrangement of the peritoneum is extremely complex because it is invaginated by numerous abdominal organs whose outer serous coat is the peritoneum. Before proceeding to a detailed study of the peritoneum, identify the various abdominal organs that invaginate it.

Peritonitis, inflammation of the peritoneum, is a very serious disease and is often fatal. Perforated ulcers, a ruptured appendix, penetrating wounds of the abdomen, and bacterial infections are common causes of peritonitis.

If the lower ribs, costal cartilages, and xiphoid process prevent you from examining the liver and the adjacent viscera, cut the costal cartilages on the right side about 2.5 cm parallel and lateral to the xiphoid process and extend the cut into the anterior part of the diaphragm. Then laterally retract the two parts of the lower thoracic cage to each side.

INSPECTION OF VISCERA

The **liver** is a large, solid, brownish red organ occupying the right hypochondriac and parts of the epigastric and left hypochondriac regions. The **stomach** is continuous with the esophagus just below the diaphragm; it is in the epigastric and left hypochondriac regions, partially overlapped anteriorly by the liver. The appearance of the stomach varies greatly in different subjects. Its walls are often completely collapsed and contracted, so that its characteristic outline does not appear. The **spleen,** a solid organ similar in color to the liver, is posterior to the upper part of the stomach and just below the diaphragm in the left hypochondriac region. At its right extremity, behind the liver, the stomach narrows to the pylorus, which is continuous with the **duodenum,** the **first part of** the **small intestine.** You will see only the beginning of the duodenum now, passing to the right posterior to the liver and disappearing behind the posterior wall of the peritoneal cavity as it enters the retroperitoneal space.

Observe that the broad, convex anterior surface (which is actually anterosuperior in position) of the stomach is covered by the liver superiorly but is in contact with the lower anterior part of the diaphragm and the anterior abdominal wall inferiorly. The curved right and upper border of this surface is known as the **lesser curvature**; the much longer curved border formed by the left and inferior margin is known as the **greater curvature.**

Descending from the greater curvature is the **greater omentum,** a broad free fold of peritoneum that contains a considerable quantity of fat. The inferior extent of the greater omentum below the greater curvature varies in different subjects; in some cases it extends well into the pubic region, completely overlapping the coils of small intestine, which fill the lower part of the abdominal cavity. Turn the greater omentum upward and observe that its upper posterior border is attached to the **transverse colon,** the portion of large intestine that crosses the abdominal cavity from right to left.

Turn the transverse colon upward, together with the peritoneal fold (mesocolon) that attaches it to the posterior wall of the abdominal cavity, and identify the **duodenojejunal flexure.** At this point, which is slightly to the left of the midline in the upper part of the umbilical region, the terminal portion of the **duodenum** emerges through the posterior peritoneal wall to become continuous with the **jejunum,** the **second part of** the **small intestine.** The numerous coils of the jejunum and the **ileum** (the **third part of** the **small intestine**) fill the umbilical and pubic regions and also extend into the cavity of the pelvis minor. Draw them forward and observe that they are attached to the posterior wall by a broad, thick peritoneal fold, the **mesentery.**

In the right inguinal region, the ileum ends by joining the **cecum,** the **first part of** the **large intestine.** Identify the **vermiform appendix,** a fingerlike process that typically projects to the left from the cecum but may turn upward behind the cecum or otherwise vary in position. Find the **ascending colon** running upward through the right inguinal and lateral regions, closely applied to the posterior wall. The ascending colon is continuous with the **transverse colon** at the **right colic flexure,** which is under cover of the lower right border of the liver. At the **left colic flexure,** which is in the left hypochondriac region in relation to the lower part of the spleen, the transverse colon becomes continuous with the **descending colon.** It passes downward through the left lateral region to become continuous in the left inguinal region with the **sigmoid colon,** which crosses the left side of the pelvic brim to enter the pelvis minor.

PERITONEUM

Now study the **peritoneum** in its entirety. It can be subdivided, on the basis of its relationship to other structures, into **visceral peritoneum,** i.e., peritoneum forming the **outer serous coat of** a **visceral organ;** and **parietal peritoneum,** i.e., peritoneum forming the **walls of** the **peritoneal cavity.** In addition, there are double folds of peritoneum called **peritoneal ligaments** and **mesen-**

teries that help hold the viscera in place and afford a passageway through which blood vessels and nerves reach the various intraperitoneal organs. They may represent the continuity of visceral with parietal peritoneum, or they may connect the visceral peritoneum of two or more organs. The parietal peritoneum is closely applied anteriorly and laterally to the inner surface of the abdominal wall, and superiorly to the inferior surface of the diaphragm. The posterior extent of the peritoneal cavity is not, however, as great as that of the abdominal cavity; at later stages of the dissection, you will find numerous **structures** that are within the abdominal cavity but **behind** the **posterior parietal peritoneum.** Such structures are described as being **retroperitoneal** (Fig. 13.1). **Organs** that **project** freely **into** the **peritoneum** and

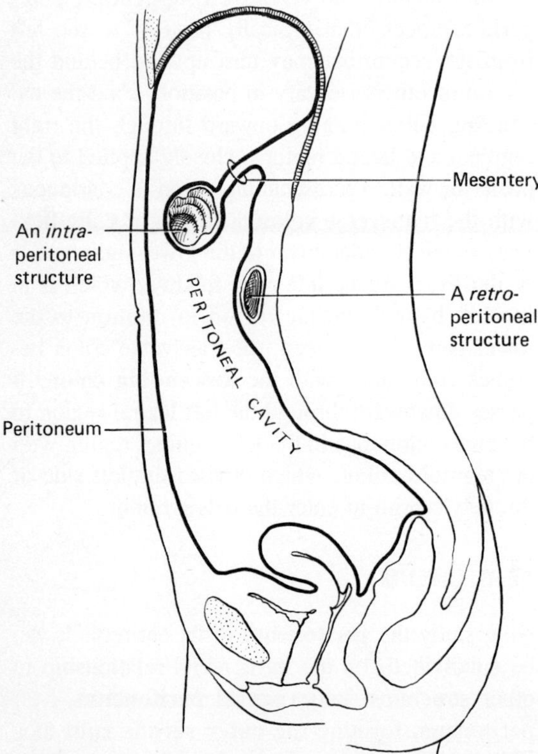

Figure 13.1 Diagrammatic representation of the **peritoneal cavity,** an **intraperitoneal structure,** and a **retroperitoneal structure.**

thus receive a coat of visceral peritoneum are described as being **intraperitoneal.** However, such organs **are not within** the **peritoneal cavity** as the term intraperitoneal might suggest, since they are separated from the peritoneal cavity by their visceral covering of peritoneum. Inferiorly, the peritoneum descends below the pelvic brim, where you will observe its disposition when the pelvis is studied.

Observe the **falciform ligament of** the **liver.** It is a fold of peritoneum that connects the **parietal peritoneum of** the **anterior abdominal wall** with the **visceral peritoneum** clothing the anterior surface **of** the **liver.** Classically, the attachment of the falciform ligament to the liver marked the division of the organ into right and left lobes, but today that is not considered accurate (see page 154). Inferiorly, it presents a free margin running downward and forward from the lower border of the liver toward the umbilicus. The **round ligament of** the **liver (ligamentum teres hepatis),** a cordlike structure representing the **obliterated umbilical vein** of the fetus, lies within the free margin.

Pass your hand upward over the right side of the liver and identify the anterior layer of the **coronary ligament.** This is a broad **peritoneal reflection** from the upper surface of the liver to the undersurface of the **diaphragm.** The posterior layer of the coronary ligament passes from the posterior surface of the liver to the diaphragm. The sharp, right free margin of the coronary ligament is known as the **right triangular ligament.** To the far left, the **left triangular ligament** is located on the upper surface of the left lobe.

Draw the left lobe of the liver forward and observe the **lesser omentum.** It is a flat peritoneal ligament that runs from the **lesser curvature of** the **stomach** (hepatogastric ligament) and the upper border of the first part of the **duodenum** (hepatoduodenal ligament) to the inferior surface of the **liver.** It is composed of **two layers of peritoneum,** anterior and posterior, that are closely applied to each other except near the right free margin, which runs from the duodenum to the lower part of the inferior surface of the liver. Around this margin the two layers are continuous with each other and the lesser omentum is thick, due to the presence within it of the **hepatic artery,** the **portal vein,** and the **common bile duct.** At the lesser curvature, the peritoneum comprising the lesser omentum becomes continuous with the visceral peritoneum clothing the anterior and posterior surfaces of the stomach. It becomes continuous with the visceral peritoneum on the inferior surface of the liver (Figs. 13.2 to 13.4).

The falciform ligament, the coronary and right and left triangular ligaments of the liver, and the lesser omentum are derived from the **ventral mesentery of** the **embryonic gut.** The derivatives in the adult of the **embryonic dorsal mesentery** are the greater omentum (the gastrophrenic, gastrocolic, and gastrolienal ligaments), the lienorenal ligament, the phrenicocolic ligament, the transverse mesocolon, the mesentery of the jejunum and ileum, and the sigmoid mesocolon. Now carefully investigate them (Fig. 13.2 to 13.6).

The **gastrophrenic ligament** is a short peritoneal fold running from the upper part of the greater curvature to the peritoneum covering the diaphragm. The **gastrolienal ligament** is a fold of peritoneum joining the left portion of the greater curvature to the hilum of the spleen. The **lienorenal ligament** runs posteriorly from the hilum of the spleen to the parietal peritoneum on the posterior body wall, just anterior to the left kidney (hence its name).

Figure 13.2 Diagrammatic midsagittal section through the abdominal cavity showing the **disposition of** the **peritoneum.** In this figure, and in the four succeeding ones, the body wall is represented by diagonal shading, the organs by vertical shading, and the peritoneum by the broken line.

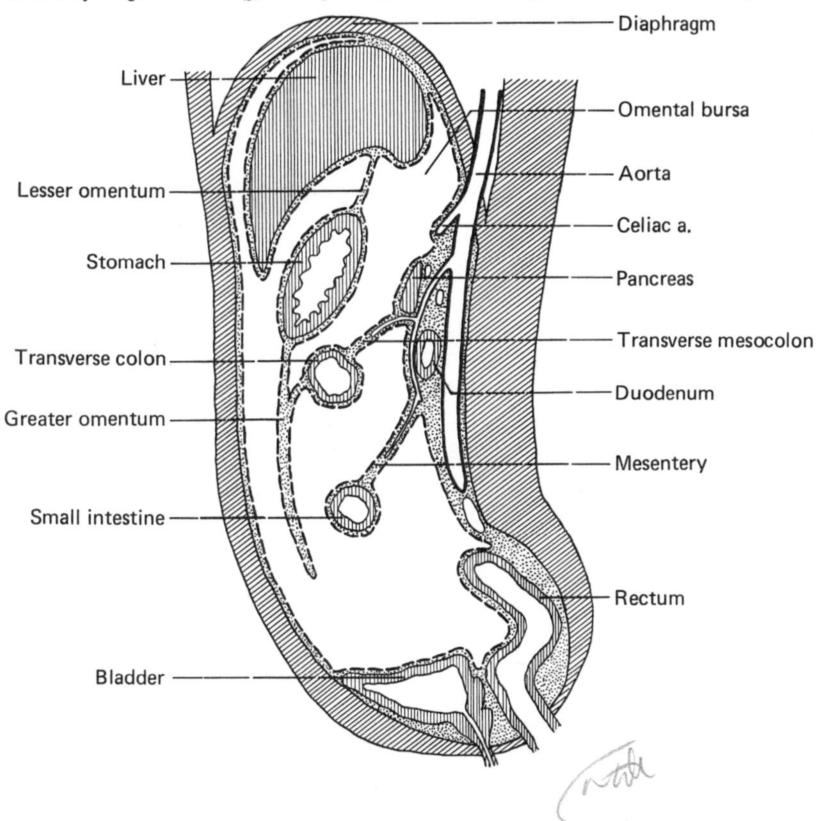

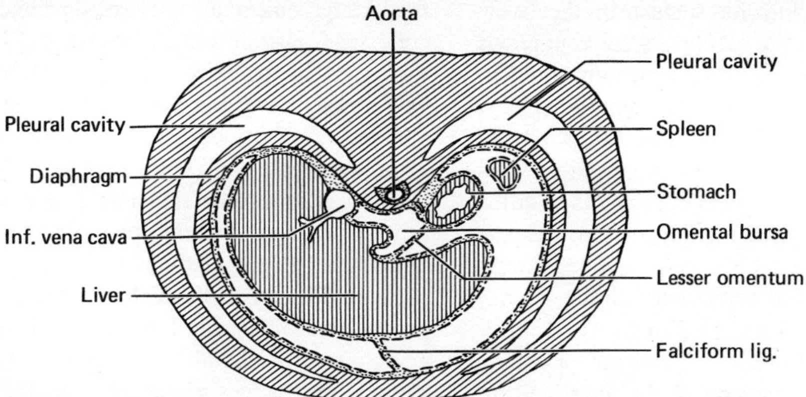

Figure 13.3 Transverse section through the **abdominal cavity** at the level of the superior recess of the omental bursa. The **peritoneum** is represented by the broken line.

The **transverse mesocolon** is a broad peritoneal ligament that runs upward and backward from the posterior surface of the transverse colon to the posterior wall of the peritoneal cavity. The posterior layer of the transverse mesocolon is continuous with the posterior parietal peritoneum below the line of attachment of the transverse mesocolon. It is referred to as the **descending layer of** the **transverse mesocolon,** and inferiorly is continuous with the anterior layer of the mesentery.

The **mesentery** is the double-layer **peritoneal ligament** that supports the **jejunum** and **ileum.** Posteriorly, it is continuous with the posterior parietal peritoneum along an oblique line running from the duodenojejunal flexure downward and to the right to the ileocecal junction; anteriorly, it is continuous with the visceral peritoneum clothing the jejunum and ileum. Its intestinal attachment is necessarily much longer than its parietal attachment, giving the entire mesentery the form of a frill.

The complex arrangement of peritoneal reflections and folds sometimes creates fossae or blind peritoneal pouches. Peritoneal fossae are common near the duo-

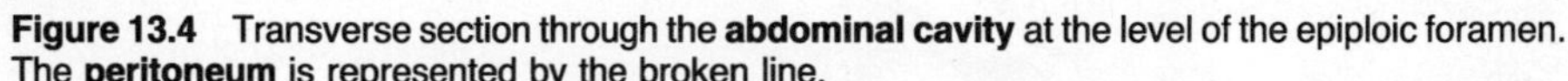

Figure 13.4 Transverse section through the **abdominal cavity** at the level of the epiploic foramen. The **peritoneum** is represented by the broken line.

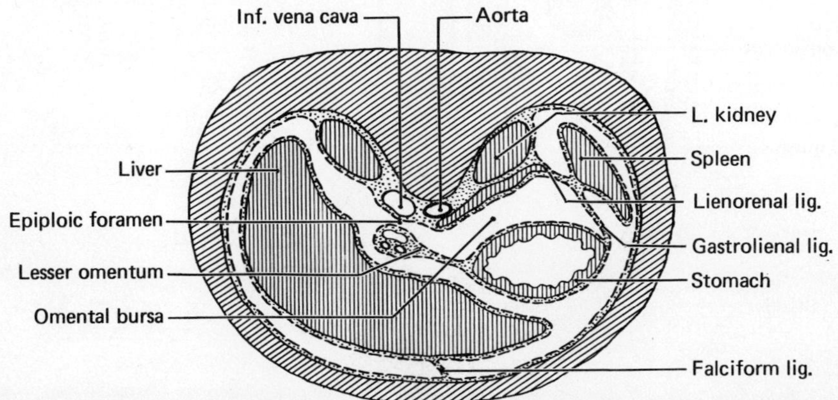

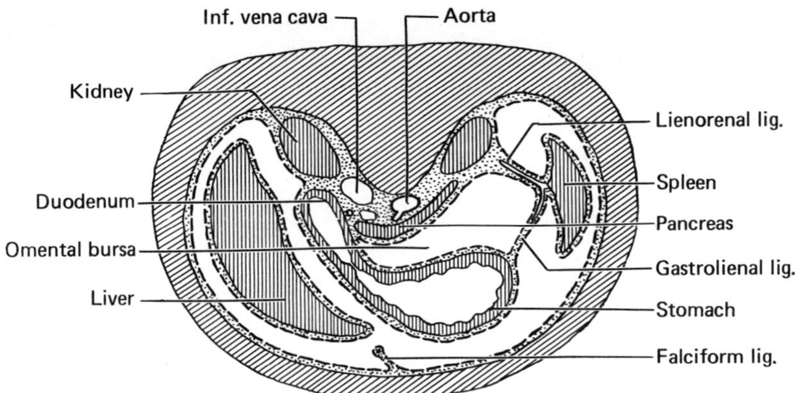

Figure 13.5 Transverse section through the **abdominal cavity** at a level slightly below the epiploic foramen. The **peritoneum** is represented by the broken line.

denojejunal and ileocecal junctions. They are potential sites of intraperitoneal hernias because a segment of intestine can become lodged in them.

The **ascending** and **descending colons** have no mesenteries and therefore, are retroperitoneal. The **cecum** is usually attached to the posterior wall by a short **mesocecum;** the **vermiform appendix** is usually also supported by a peritoneal fold, the **mesoappendix.** The **sigmoid colon** is suspended from the parietal peritoneum of the left iliac fossa by a peritoneal fold, the **sigmoid mesocolon,** which crosses the pelvic brim to enter the pelvis.

The **phrenicocolic ligament** is a small, transverse, shelflike fold of peritoneum stretching from the lateral aspect of the upper part of the descending colon to the lower left portion of the diaphragm; the lower tip of the spleen usually rests on its upper surface.

The portion of the peritoneal cavity that you have investigated so far is known as the **greater peritoneal sac.** There is another subdivision of the cavity, the **lesser peritoneal sac,** or **omental bursa,** to which you should now turn your attention. The omental bursa lies posterior to the lesser

Figure 13.6 Transverse section through the **abdominal cavity** at the level of the umbilical region. The **peritoneum** is represented by the broken line.

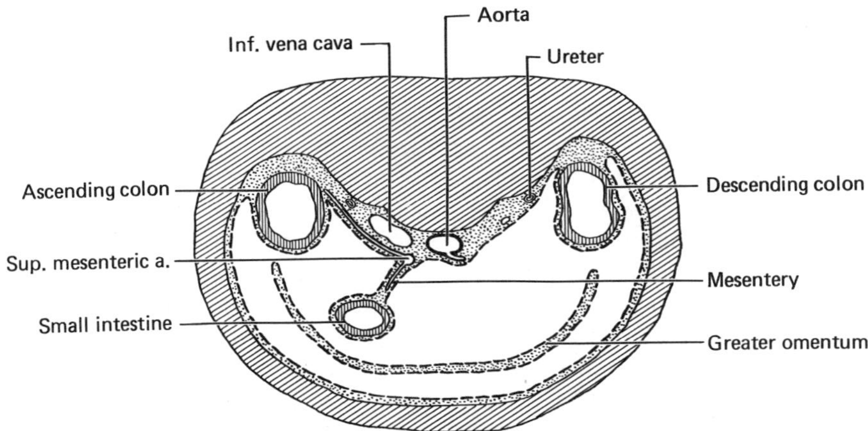

omentum, the stomach, and the upper anterior part of the great omentum (Figs. 13.2 to 13.5). Its only **communication with** the **greater sac** is through the **epiploic foramen,** an opening that lies immediately posterior to the right free margin of the lesser omentum. Push your finger upward and to the left along the inferior surface of the right lobe of the liver and behind the lesser omentum; it will pass through the epiploic foramen and enter the omental bursa. The epiploic foramen is bounded superiorly by peritoneum on the inferior surface of the liver, anteriorly by the posterior layer of the lesser omentum, inferiorly by the peritoneum on the first part of the duodenum, and posteriorly by parietal peritoneum that covers the inferior vena cava.

Open the omental bursa inferiorly by making an incision through the greater omentum parallel to and about 1.5 cm below the greater curvature of the stomach; do not make the incision too far to the left and upward or else it will sever the gastrolienal ligament. The boundaries of the omental bursa can be explored through this opening.

The **pancreas** can usually be seen through the **ascending layer of** the **transverse mesocolon,** crossing the posterior abdominal wall just above the attachment of the transverse mesocolon.

Occasionally, the omental bursa extends downward within the greater omentum to its lower border. Usually, however, the anterior and posterior layers of the greater omentum are firmly fused and therefore, the omental bursa cannot extend below the lower border of the transverse colon (Fig. 13.2).

The most superior portion of the **omental bursa** is known as its **superior recess.** Observe that a small portion of the posterior surface of the right lobe of the liver projects into the superior recess. This, the **caudate lobe of** the **liver,** is the only part of the liver that bulges into the wall of the omental bursa.

In some cases you will be able to study the stomach simply by pulling the liver upward out of the way. In other cases, however, it will be helpful for you to remove the left lobe of the liver. *This may be facilitated by making an incision on the left side through the lower costal cartilages and into the peripheral part of the diaphragm, retracting the costal cartilages laterally. Make an incision through the left lobe, starting anteriorly just to the left of the attachment of the falciform ligament and running straight backward to emerge just to the left of the attachment of the lesser omentum. To detach the left lobe from the diaphragm, you must cut the left triangular ligament.*

Dissect the peritoneum along the lesser and greater curvatures of the stomach and clean the vessels that supply blood to the stomach. The origins of these vessels will be seen somewhat later.

The **left gastric artery** reaches the upper end of the lesser curvature by passing through the left gastropancreatic fold (Fig. 13.7). It runs downward and to the right along the **lesser curvature** to anastomose with the **right gastric artery.** Find the **right gastroepiploic artery** at the right end of the **greater curvature** and trace it to the left, where it anastomoses with the **left gastroepiploic artery.** The left gastroepiploic reaches the left side of the greater curvature by passing forward within the gastrolienal ligament; it then runs downward and to the right along the greater curvature. The **short gastric arteries,** which also reach the stomach through the gastrolienal ligament, supply the upper part of the greater curvature. All these vessels give branches to both surfaces of the stomach. The **left gastric artery** sends branches upward to the esophagus.

Remove the anterior layer of peritoneum from the right portion of the lesser omentum anterior to the epiploic foramen, and clean the structures within it. The **common hepatic artery** passes through the right gastropancreatic fold and then upward within the lesser omentum, where it terminates by dividing into the **proper hepatic** and **gastroduodenal arteries.** The gastroduodenal artery passes downward behind the first part of the duodenum. The proper hepatic artery usually first

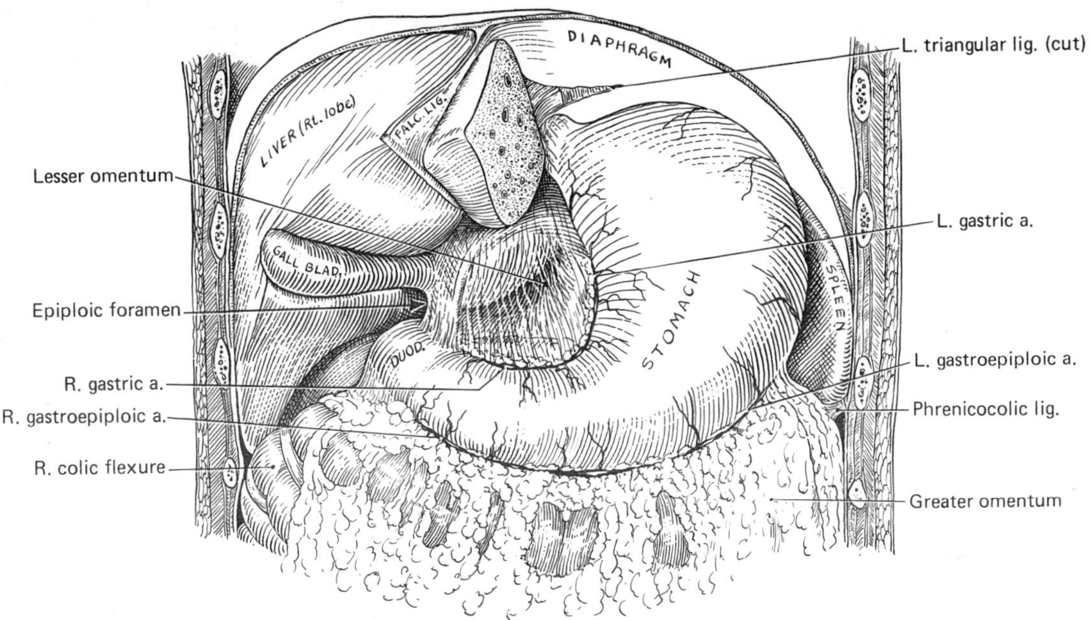

Figure 13.7 Anterior view of the **structures in** the upper part of the **abdominal cavity.** The left lobe of the liver has been removed.

gives off the **right gastric artery** and then, continuing upward in the omentum, ends by dividing into the **right** and **left hepatic arteries,** which enter the right and left lobes of the liver.

The **common bile duct,** which lies to the right of the proper hepatic artery, is formed in the lesser omentum by the junction of the **cystic duct** and the **common hepatic duct.** The **cystic duct** is the narrowed continuation of the **gallbladder** (Fig. 13.8). It is accompanied by the **cystic artery,** a branch of the **right hepatic artery.** The **common hepatic duct** is formed by the junction of **right** and **left hepatic ducts** from the respective lobes of the liver. The common bile duct leaves the lesser omentum by descending posterior to the first part of the duodenum.

The **portal vein** is a wide channel that lies posterior to the proper hepatic artery and the bile duct. It enters the lesser omentum from behind the first part of the duodenum. In the omentum, it divides into **right** and **left lobar branches,** which enter the **lobes of** the **liver.** Before its division, it usually receives the **left gastric vein,** which enters the omentum through the right gastropancreatic fold. (The left gastric vein is sometimes called the **coronary vein of** the **stomach** because of its circular course along the lesser curvature of the stomach to the left and then back to the right along the posterior abdominal wall.)

Trace the **common hepatic artery** back through the right gastropancreatic fold to its origin from the **celiac trunk.** Clean the celiac trunk (Fig. 13.8). It is a short, thick artery that runs forward from the **abdominal aorta** at the level of the twelfth thoracic vertebra just inferior to the aortic hiatus of the diaphragm. It is covered by peritoneum on the posterior wall of the omental bursa and is entangled in a dense network of nerve fibers and ganglia called the **celiac plexus.** This plexus and others like it, associated with branches of the abdominal aorta, represent the autonomic nerve supply to the viscera; the nerve fibers form peri-

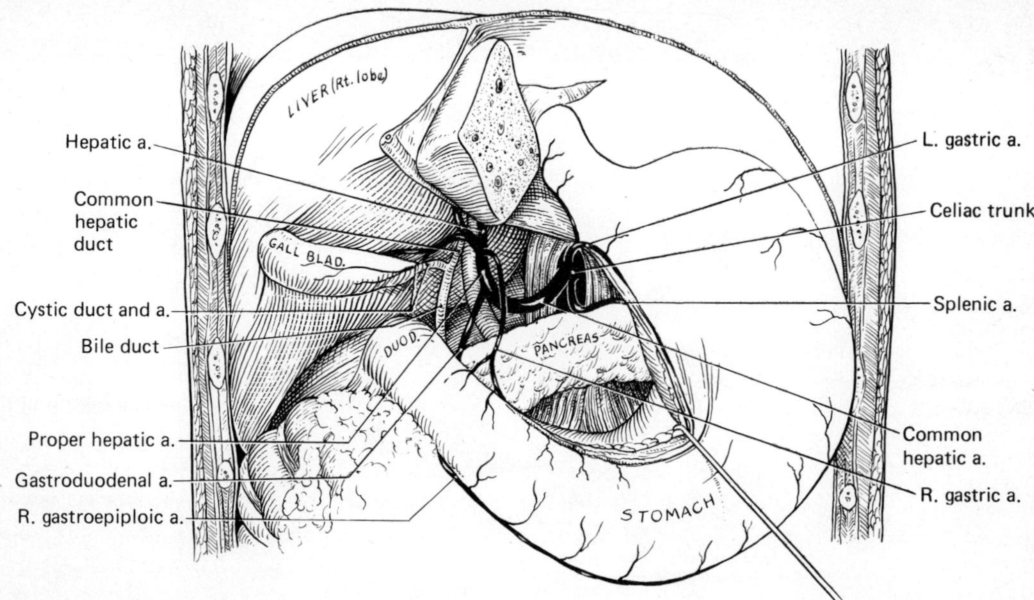

Figure 13.8 The **structures in** the right margin of the **lesser omentum** and the **stomach bed.**

vascular plexuses and are carried to their destinations along the blood vessels. The fibers of the celiac plexus are distributed to the viscera that receive their blood supply from branches of the celiac trunk. The three branches are the **common hepatic,** the **left gastric,** and the **splenic arteries.** Trace the left gastric artery through the left gastropancreatic fold to the point at which it reaches the stomach. Clean the beginning of the splenic artery and observe that it runs to the left along the upper border of the pancreas, behind the peritoneum on the posterior wall of the omental bursa (Fig. 13.9).

Free and elevate the duodenum just beyond its junction with the pylorus. Turn the pyloric end of the stomach to the left, and trace the **gastroduodenal artery** downward posterior to the first part of the duodenum, where it ends by dividing into the **right gastroepiploic** and the **superior pancreaticoduodenal arteries.** Follow the right gastroepiploic to the greater curvature. The superior pancreaticoduodenal artery will be traced later downward along the medial border of the duodenum.

STOMACH

The stomach presents anterior and posterior surfaces that face into the greater and lesser peritoneal sacs, respectively. Its borders, as already noted, are the greater and lesser curvatures. The stomach is divided into the **cardia,** the **fundus,** the **body,** and the **pylorus.** The cardiac portion is where the esophagus empties into the stomach. The fundus is the expanded upper portion above a horizontal plane passing through the esophageal orifice. The cardia is continuous inferiorly with the body, which is separated from the narrow pylorus by a notch, called the **angular notch,** in the lesser curvature. The pyloric portion is continuous with the **duodenum.**

Free and elevate the stomach. Then make an incision through its wall along the greater curvature, extending through the pyloric canal and into the superior part of the duodenum. Retract the cut edges of the stomach and duodenum and remove the food contents.

Observe that the gastric **mucous membrane** is pitted by **minute depressions** that are more numerous toward the pylorus than at the fundus. Observe the projecting folds, **rugae,** of the mucous membrane. In a distended stomach they are obliterated, but they appear with contraction of the muscular wall, since the mucous membrane does not contract with the muscle.

Gastric ulcer, one type of peptic ulceration, is a common cause of upper gastrointestinal tract bleeding. In this case, the bleeding is usually from the right and/or left gastric arteries.

The stomach opens into the pylorus through the **pyloric antrum,** which is the first section just to the right of the angular notch. The **pyloric canal** is the narrowed right end of the pylorus, leading to the **pyloric orifice,** the opening into the duodenum. Study the **pyloric sphincter,** the thick, circular ring of smooth muscle by which the pyloric orifice is kept closed, except when food is passing from the stomach to the duodenum.

Study the **stomach bed,** the complex of structures on which the posterior surface of the stomach rests (Fig. 13.9). Observe that most inferiorly the stomach bed is formed by the **transverse colon.** Above this, the posterior surface of the stomach rests on the **transverse mesocolon,** through which it is related to coils of the **small intestine.** Above the parietal attachment of the transverse mesocolon, the stomach bed is formed to the right by the **parietal peritoneum** on the posterior wall of the omental bursa and to the left by the gastric surface of the **spleen.** The spleen is, however, separated from the stomach by the gastrolienal and lienorenal ligaments.

Remove the parietal peritoneum forming the upper right portion of the stomach bed, and expose the retroperitoneal structures that are contiguous with the posterior surface of the stomach. Crossing the posterior abdominal wall immediately above the attachment of the transverse mesocolon are the **body** and **tail of** the **pancreas.** Above the pancreas and immediately to the right of the spleen, a small portion of the anterior surface of the **left kidney** can be exposed; it is kept from contact

Figure 13.9 The **stomach bed** after removal of the stomach, liver, and posterior parietal peritoneum.

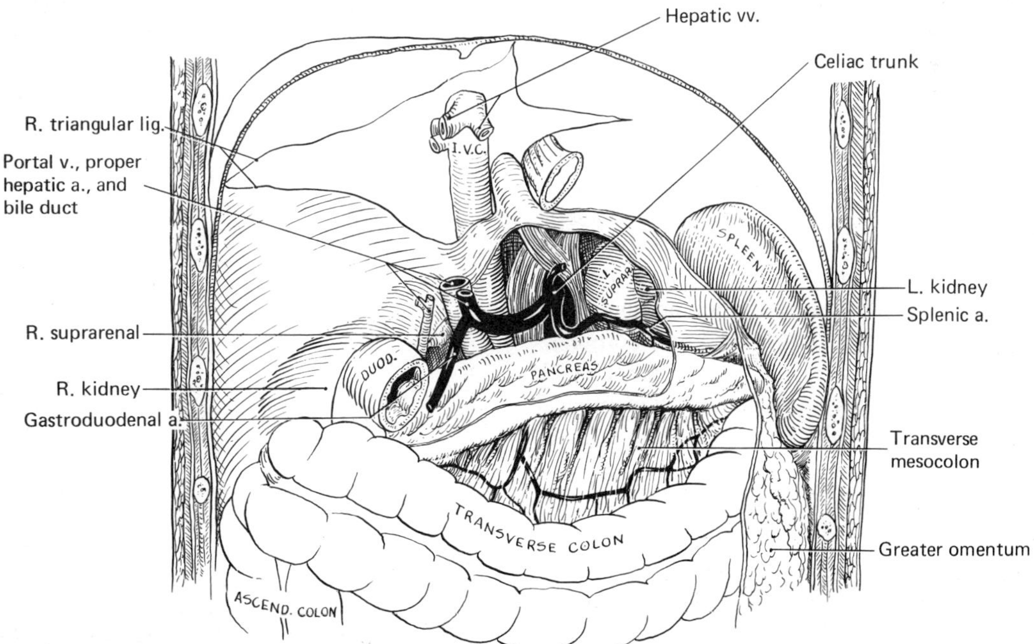

with the posterior surface of the stomach only by the parietal peritoneum and some extraperitoneal areolar tissue. To the right of the kidney, the **left suprarenal (adrenal) gland** takes part in forming the stomach bed. To the right of and superior to the suprarenal, the **left crus of** the **diaphragm** lies behind the highest part of the stomach.

Clean the entire **splenic artery,** which is quite tortuous. As it crosses the posterior abdominal wall above the pancreas, it gives off numerous small **pancreatic branches.** It passes between the two layers of the lienorenal ligament to reach the hilum of the spleen, where it terminates by dividing into three or four **splenic branches** and the **left gastroepiploic** and **short gastric arteries,** which pass forward through the gastrolienal ligament to reach the stomach.

SPLEEN AND LIVER

Study the **spleen.** This organ is completely clothed with visceral peritoneum, except at its **hilum,** where it is joined by the lienorenal and gastrolienal ligaments. Note that the tail of the pancreas extends as far as the hilum of the spleen. The proximity of the two organs is important and must be considered in surgical removal of the spleen. The spleen has two primary surfaces. The **diaphragmatic surface** is smooth and convex and abuts the upper left portion of the diaphragm. The **visceral surface** is subdivided into three smaller surfaces, all of which converge toward the hilum. The largest and most anterior is the **gastric surface,** which is somewhat concave and forms a portion of the stomach bed. The upper posterior portion is the **renal surface.** It is related to the upper portion of the anterior surface of the left kidney, from which it is separated by peritoneum and extraperitoneal areolar tissue. The **colic surface** is most inferior; it is in contact with the left colic flexure and the phrenicocolic ligament. Starting at the hilum, bisect the spleen and note its internal structure.

Rupture of the spleen, with intraabdominal hemorrhage, is one of the most common injuries to intraabdominal organs. It is usually caused by blunt trauma to the lower left rib cage such as would occur in automobile, bicycle, or motorcycle accidents.

Now remove the liver and study its surfaces. In some cases the left lobe will already have been removed. Cut through the falciform ligament from its free margin up to the point at which it joins the coronary ligament and the left triangular ligament. Cut the right triangular ligament along the liver surface and continue the incision to the left through the anterior layer of the coronary ligament to the point at which it joins the falciform ligament. If the left lobe is still intact, continue the incision through the left triangular ligament. The anterior and posterior layers of the coronary ligament diverge as they pass to the left from the right triangular ligament enclosing a broad **bare area** *on the posterior surface of the right lobe of the liver that is in direct contact with the diaphragm. Free this area from the diaphragm and cut through the posterior layer of the coronary ligament. Sever the proper hepatic artery and the portal vein just below their division into right and left branches; cut the common bile duct at the same level. Immediately to the left of the bare area on the posterior surface of the right lobe, the liver partly encircles the* **inferior vena cava.** *All you need to do before removing the liver is to detach this portion of its posterior surface from the inferior vena cava. To do this, sever the* **hepatic veins,** *three or four short trunks that pass from the substance of the liver directly into the vena cava. Remove the right lobe, reattach the left lobe to it, and study the organ as a whole.*

As an alternative, *after cutting the coronary ligament and the hepatic veins (see above), pull the liver downward and forward, leaving the proper hepatic artery, portal vein, and common bile duct intact. The liver can be rotated on these structures to study its surfaces and then replaced at any time to study its relationships to the other viscera.*

The **superior, anterior,** and **right lateral surfaces of** the **liver** are in contact with the **diaphragm** and present a rounded contour corresponding to the form of that structure. Near the median line, the inferior margin projects below the **costal arch,** bringing the lower part of the anterior surface into contact with the **anterior abdominal wall.**

The posterior surface of the liver is ordinarily described as including the bare area, the fossa for the vena cava, the caudate lobe, and a small upper right portion of the left lobe that is in contact with the esophagus (Fig. 13.10). The **bare area** is the large triangular area of the right lobe that is enclosed by the **coronary** and **right triangular ligaments.** Below and to the left, this area is in contact with the **right suprarenal gland,** which here intervenes between the diaphragm and the liver. Dissect in the region from which the bare area was removed and expose the anterior surface of the right suprarenal (Fig. 13.9). Occasionally, the uppermost portion of the anterior surface of the right kidney is also high enough to touch the bare area.

Note the **fossa for** the **inferior vena cava** immediately to the left of the bare area and the **hepatic veins** opening into it.

The **caudate lobe** lies between the fossa for the vena cava and the attachment of the lesser omentum. It is covered with visceral peritoneum and, as already observed, projects into the wall of the superior recess of the omental bursa.

The **inferior surface of** the **left lobe** is in contact with the lesser omentum and the upper part of the anterior surface of the **stomach.** The inferior surface of the **right lobe** is marked by impressions corresponding to the shapes of the adjoining structures.

The **gallbladder** is closely applied to the inferior surface of the right lobe. The visceral peritoneum covering the inferior surface of the liver is reflected over the gallbladder. The **cystic duct** runs to the left from the gallbladder into the lesser omentum.

Observe the attachment of the lesser omentum. Toward its right margin it widens to enclose the porta hepatis. The **porta hepatis** is the hilum of the liver, where the **portal vein** and **hepatic artery** enter it and the **hepatic ducts** leave it.

Anterior to the porta hepatis and to the left of the gallbladder is a quadrangular portion of the inferior surface of the right lobe called the **quadrate lobe.** It is in contact with the pylorus and the beginning of the duodenum. Immediately to the right of the constricted portion of the gallbladder is a **duodenal impression.** The part of the inferior

Figure 13.10 The posterior and inferior **surfaces of** the **liver.**

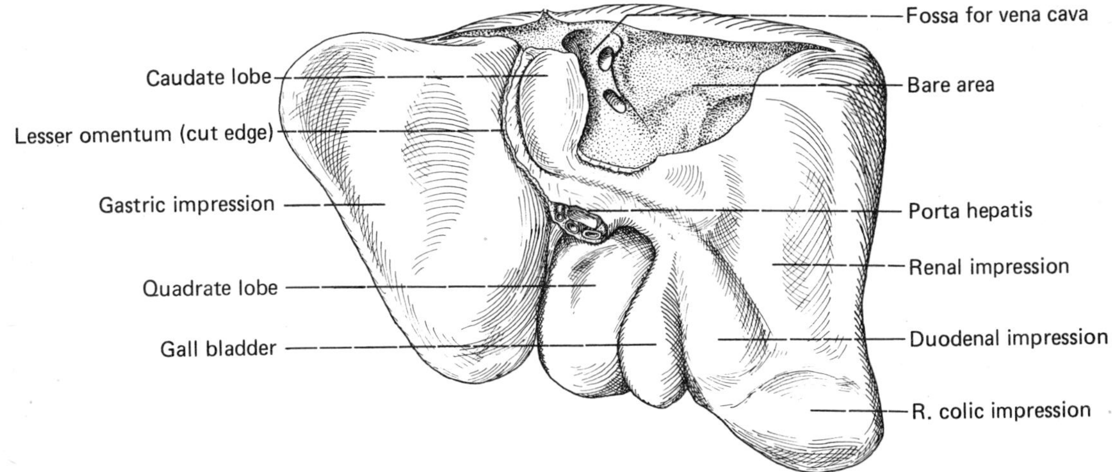

surface that is most anterior and farthest to the right exhibits a **colic impression** where the liver contacts the right colic flexure. The broad **renal impression** is above and behind the colic impression and occasionally extends onto the bare area. Here the right lobe of the liver is adjacent to the anterior surface of the right kidney but separated from it by a layer of parietal peritoneum.

Open the **gallbladder** by a longitudinal incision running from the fundus (expanded free segment) to the neck; examine its interior.

Gallstones may be present; their major constituents are bile pigments, calcium, and cholesterol.

The interior is stained dark green by **bile.** Observe that the lining membrane is ridged and that toward the neck the ridges take on a spiral form. This is the **spiral valve** of the gallbladder, which continues well into the **cystic duct.** Now dissect the gallbladder from the surface of the liver and identify the **cystic artery.**

Detach the left lobe of the liver once more and study the cut surface of the organ. The larger cut vessels are either branches of the **portal vein** or tributaries of the **hepatic veins.** These two sets of veins can always be distinguished from each other by the fact that each branch of the **portal vein** is accompanied by a branch of the **hepatic artery** and a tributary of the hepatic bile ducts. In addition, these three structures are enclosed in a fibrous sheath, constituting a **portal canal** (triad), while the hepatic veins, which have very thin walls, appear to be in direct contact with the liver substance.

Today, the most proper way of dividing the liver into lobes and segments is based on its biliary drainage or the divisions of its vascular supply. A vertical plane passing through the gallbladder and the inferior vena cava grossly approximates the division into right and left lobes. Accordingly, the falciform ligament more accurately divides the left lobe into medial and lateral segments. Review the segmentation of the liver from one of the standard texts.

LARGE AND SMALL INTESTINES

Now clean and study the superior mesenteric vessels. Turn the transverse colon and transverse mesocolon upward, and draw the coils of jejunum and ileum downward and to the left so that the right surface of the mesentery faces anteriorly. Remove as one large, continuous sheet of peritoneum the posterior layer of the transverse mesocolon, the right layer of the mesentery, and the parietal peritoneum of the posterior abdominal wall, which intervenes between these two mesenteries on the right side. By doing this, you will expose the anterior aspect of the terminal part of the duodenum and, enclosed within the bend of the duodenum, the lower part of the anterior surface of the head and neck of the pancreas (Fig. 13.11). Now make an incision through the parietal peritoneum just lateral to the ascending colon and a similar incision just lateral to the descending colon. By blunt dissection, free and reflect the ascending and descending colon toward the midline. This procedure, known as mobilization of the colon, simulates the primitive mesentery for the ascending and descending colon and exposes their blood supply. On the right side, the first part of the duodenum and part of the pancreas are visible, while on the left side, the terminal part of the duodenum and the remainder of the pancreas are exposed.

The **superior mesenteric artery** arises from the anterior aspect of the **abdominal aorta** a short distance below the celiac artery at the level of the first lumbar vertebra. It enters the present area of dissection by passing downward posterior to the neck of the pancreas and anterior to the lower part of the duodenum. From there the artery runs downward and to the right across the posterior abdominal wall along the root of the mesentery. Its terminal portion enters the mesentery to reach the lower part of the ileum. The **superior mesenteric vein** lies to the right of the artery and often overlaps it anteriorly. You may remove the tributaries of the vein, which correspond to the

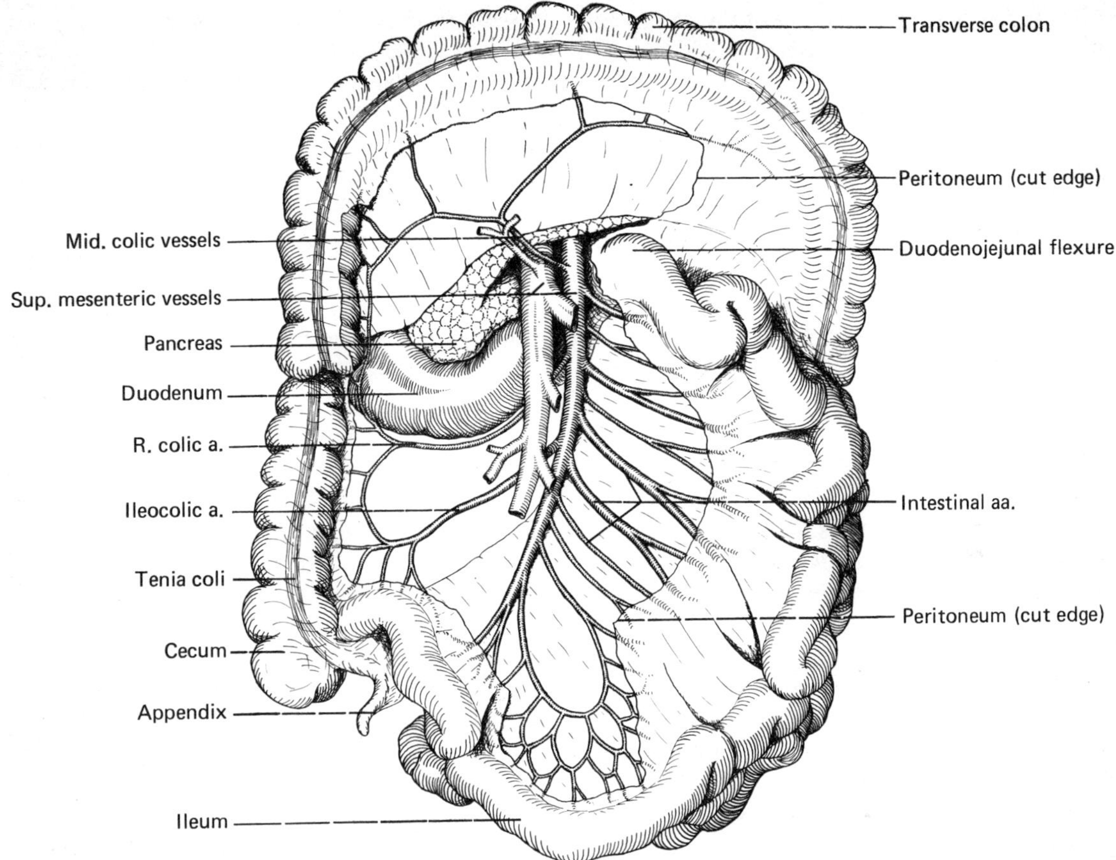

Figure 13.11 The **superior mesenteric artery** and its branches.

branches of the artery, when you clean the arteries, but retain the trunk of the vein.

Note the superior mesenteric plexus, which is continuous with the celiac plexus, surrounding the origin of the superior mesenteric artery. Sympathetic and parasympathetic nerve fibers are conveyed through the perivascular plexuses to the viscera supplied by the superior mesenteric artery.

The first branch of the superior mesenteric, the **inferior pancreaticoduodenal,** is at present hidden by the pancreas. Just below the pancreas, the superior mesenteric gives rise to the **middle colic artery.** It enters the transverse mesocolon, where it divides into **right** and **left branches,** which supply the transverse colon. Somewhat lower find the **right colic artery.** It crosses the right side of the posterior abdominal wall and divides into **ascending** and **descending branches,** which supply the **ascending colon;** the ascending branch anastomoses with the right branch of the middle colic artery. Arising usually somewhat below the right colic but sometimes by a common stem with it is the **ileocolic artery.** It runs downward and to the right across the posterior abdominal wall, giving branches to the **cecum, appendix,** and terminal part of the **ileum.** Its terminal branches anastomose with each other and with the descending branch of the right colic.

In its passage along the root of the mesentery, the **superior mesenteric artery** gives rise to a series of **intestinal arteries** that run forward through the mesentery to supply the **jejunum** and **ileum.** Each intestinal artery divides into two branches, which unite with similar branches from adjacent arteries to form a series of **arterial loops** or **arcades** in the mesentery. From these arcades other branches arise, which also unite to form smaller arches as they approach the intestine. Observe that these arterial arcades increase in number from the upper to the lower end of the mesentery. In the **upper part of** the **jejunal mesentery** there is usually only **one set of arterial arcades,** giving branches directly to the gut, while toward the **lower end of** the **ileum** there may be as many as **four** or **five sets of arcades.** Observe also that the amount of **fat** contained **within** the **mesentery** around the arterial arches **increases from above downward.** If the mesentery is held up to light, you will see large translucent areas within the arterial arches of the jejunal portion, while in the lower ileal portion the translucent areas are much smaller, due to the presence of a larger amount of fat.

Study the jejunum and ileum. Together they are about 6 to 7 m long in the living person. The division between jejunum and ileum is an arbitrary one, the **jejunum** being the **upper two-fifths** and the **ileum** the **lower three-fifths.** The difference is based on the fact that there is a gradual change in the character of the internal intestinal wall from the duodenojejunal flexure to the ileocecal junction, so that the characteristics of the lower end of the ileum differ considerably from those of the upper end of the jejunum.

Examine some of the more evident morphological differences. Section the jejunum about 3 cm below the duodenojejunal flexure; likewise, section the ileum about 3 cm from its junction with the cecum. Cut through the mesentery along the entire length of its intestinal attachment and remove the jejunum and ileum. Open the gut by longitudinal incisions in the wall at intervals along its length and compare the characteristics of its lining in different regions.

Observe that the **circular folds of** the **mucous membrane** are **larger** and closer together in the upper part of the **jejunum,** and almost entirely absent in the lower part of the ileum. In general, the **wall of** the **jejunum** is **thicker** than that of the ileum. Attempt to find some **solitary lymph nodules** or collections of **aggregated lymph nodules** in oval patches that may be as much as 5 to 6 cm long. They are **larger** and **more numerous** in the lower part of the **ileum.** In old age they seem to disappear entirely.

Observe the external characteristics of the **large intestine,** which comprises the cecum, colon, rectum, and anal canal. If in doubt, a surgeon, working in a circumscribed area in the abdominal cavity, cannot depend on diameter as a criterion for determining whether a bit of small or large intestine is being handled. Two features, however, are purely characteristic of the large intestine—the **teniae coli** and the **epiploic appendages.**

The **teniae coli** are **three separate longitudinal bands** of smooth muscle that **begin at** the **base of** the **vermiform process** and traverse the length of the large intestine. They terminate in the wall of the rectum. Between the teniae, the wall of the large intestine is thrown into three longitudinal series of **sacculations** called the **haustra.**

The **epiploic appendages** are small, fat-filled outpocketings of the **visceral peritoneum** covering the large intestine. They are found throughout its length, except along the rectum and anal canal.

The **cecum** is usually intraperitoneal, although in some cases the upper part of its posterior surface is not covered with peritoneum and is in direct contact with the abdominal wall. Open the cecum by an anterior longitudinal incision and observe the **ileocecal orifice.** This orifice, at which the ileum joins the cecum, appears as an anteroposterior slit in the medial wall of the cecum. It is bounded by a superior and an inferior lip, which constitute the **ileocecal valve** and represent a partial protrusion of the ileum into the cecum. Below the ileocecal orifice, identify the **orifice of** the **vermiform appendix,** which may be freely open or may be guarded by a fold of mucous membrane, the **valve of** the **vermiform appendix.**

The ascending colon is not covered posteriorly by peritoneum but is in direct contact with the extraperitoneal tissue of this portion of the abdominal wall. Observe, however, that the transverse mesocolon does not extend as far to the right as it does to the left. Consequently, the **first part of** the **transverse colon,** just to the left of the right colic flexure, **has no mesentery,** and its posterior surface touches the anterior surfaces of the **right kidney** and the descending portion of the **duodenum** as it crosses them.

DUODENUM AND PANCREAS

The **duodenum** is the **first part of** the **small intestine.** It is about 25 cm long and forms a C-shaped curve, encircling the **head of** the **pancreas.** It consists of superior, descending, inferior, and ascending portions. Except for the superior portion, which begins at the pylorus and is partly covered on its posterior surface by peritoneum, the duodenum is entirely retroperitoneal, covered only anteriorly by peritoneum. As noted above, its descending portion, where it is crossed anteriorly by the transverse colon, has no peritoneal covering whatever.

The **superior (first) part,** which is at the level of the first lumbar vertebra, runs upward and to the right from the pylorus for about 5 cm. The peritoneum on its upper border forms the lower boundary of the epiploic foramen. Below the right lobe of the liver, it turns downward as the **descending (second) part** and descends for about 7 or 10 cm in front of the medial portion of the anterior surface of the right kidney, the right renal vessels, and the right border of the inferior vena cava. Bending to the left as the **inferior (third) part,** which crosses the median plane, it turns upward to join the **ascending (fourth) segment.** This segment bends forward to join the jejunum at the **duodenojejunal flexure.** In addition to peritoneum, a band of retroperitoneal fibrous and muscular tissue extends from the right crus of the diaphragm to the duodenojejunal flexure to help suspend it in place. This is the **suspensory muscle of** the **duodenum (ligament of Treitz).** Observe that it is crossed anteriorly by the **superior mesenteric vessels** and usually by the root of the mesentery. Posteriorly, it is related to the inferior vena cava and the aorta.

The **pancreas** is an elongated gland consisting of head, neck, body, and tail. The **head** is the flattened portion that fills the concavity of the duodenal curve. Anteriorly, it is covered by peritoneum and crossed by the parietal attachment of the right end of the transverse mesocolon. Posteriorly, it rests against the inferior vena cava. Observe that the head's lower portion, the **uncinate process,** projects to the left behind the **superior mesenteric vessels** and superior to the inferior part of the duodenum. The **neck** is a short constricted portion, running upward and to the left from the upper part of the head to join the body. It rests posteriorly against the beginning of the portal vein.

The **body of** the **pancreas** runs to the left and somewhat upward across the posterior abdominal wall. The line of attachment of the transverse mesocolon usually follows the border separating anterior and inferior surfaces, so that the former faces into the omental bursa and is contiguous, through the peritoneum covering it, with the posterior surface of the stomach. The inferior surface of the pancreas faces downward into the greater sac. The posterior surface has no peritoneum and crosses the aorta and the upper part of the superior mesenteric artery; it is related also to the anterior surface of the left kidney. The **tail of** the **pancreas** is the narrowed left extremity of the body. It usually extends forward through the lienorenal ligament to come into contact with the **hilum of** the **spleen.**

Detach the tail, body, and neck of the pancreas from the posterior abdominal wall and turn them forward to expose the structures behind them. The

splenic vein is formed at the hilum of the spleen by the union of the **short gastric, left gastroepiploic,** and several small **splenic veins.** It traverses the lienorenal ligament and passes to the right across the posterior abdominal wall behind the upper border of the pancreas. Posterior to the neck of the pancreas, it joins the **superior mesenteric vein** to form the **portal vein,** which then passes upward behind the first part of the duodenum and into the lesser omentum. Clean the terminal portion of the **inferior mesenteric vein,** which generally ascends behind the pancreas to join the splenic vein. Occasionally, it lies farther to the right, opening into the termination of the superior mesenteric vein. Also notice the **left renal vein** behind the body of the pancreas; it crosses from the left kidney to the inferior vena cava by passing anterior to the aorta and behind the superior mesenteric artery (Fig. 13.12).

Portal hypertension as seen in cirrhosis of the liver is an excessive elevation of the portal venous blood pressure. The objective of surgical intervention is to divert portal blood flow away from the liver; such operations are referred to as portal-systemic shunts. One major type of shunt is the porta-caval anastomosis, in which the portal vein at its origin is sutured into the inferior vena cava. In another approach, the splenorenal anastomosis, the spleen is removed and the splenic vein is united to the left renal vein. These operations have numerous variations, but all are aimed at reducing portal venous flow.

Clean the **pancreaticoduodenal arteries.** The origin of the **superior pancreaticoduodenal** from the **gastroduodenal** has already been seen (see page 150). Trace it downward along the medial border of the descending part of the duodenum, where it gives branches to the duodenum and the head of the pancreas. The **inferior pancreaticoduodenal artery** arises from the **superior mesenteric** near the lower border of the pancreas. It runs to the right between the inferior part of the duodenum and the head of the pancreas, gives branches to both, and then turns upward to anastomose with the superior pancreaticoduodenal artery. The inferior pancreaticoduodenal occasionally arises from the first intestinal branch of the superior mesenteric.

The **common bile duct,** formed within the right margin of the lesser omentum by the junction of the **cystic** and **common hepatic ducts,** was last seen descending behind the first part of the duodenum. Now trace it downward between the descending part of the duodenum and the head of the pancreas to the point at which it enters the wall of the duodenum.

Dissect the pancreas and clean its ducts. The **pancreatic ducts** lie nearer to the posterior than the anterior surface of the gland and, consequently, can be more readily exposed from behind. They are small, thin-walled, and usually white or gray. The **main pancreatic duct** begins in the tail of the pancreas and passes to the right through the body; along its course it receives small ducts from the numerous lobules. It then passes downward and to the right through the neck and head and accompanies the **common bile duct** through the medial wall of the descending part of the duodenum. The **accessory pancreatic duct** is smaller; it begins in the lower part of the head and runs upward through the pancreas to open into the descending part of the duodenum above the main duct. The two ducts often communicate within the substance of the pancreas.

Open the **duodenum** and study its interior. Observe that the **circular folds of** the **mucosa** are large and numerous. Find the **greater duodenal papilla,** a small elevation at about the middle of the medial wall of the descending portion. At the summit of the papilla is the common orifice of the **main pancreatic** and **common bile ducts.** Just proximal to this narrow common opening, the lumen of the orifice may be dilated, forming the hepatopancreatic ampulla. The papilla is usually at the upper end of a longitudinal fold of the mucosa, the **longitudinal fold of** the **duodenum (plica longitudinalis).** Attempt to find the opening of the accessory duct, which, if present, is located more superior and anteromedial.

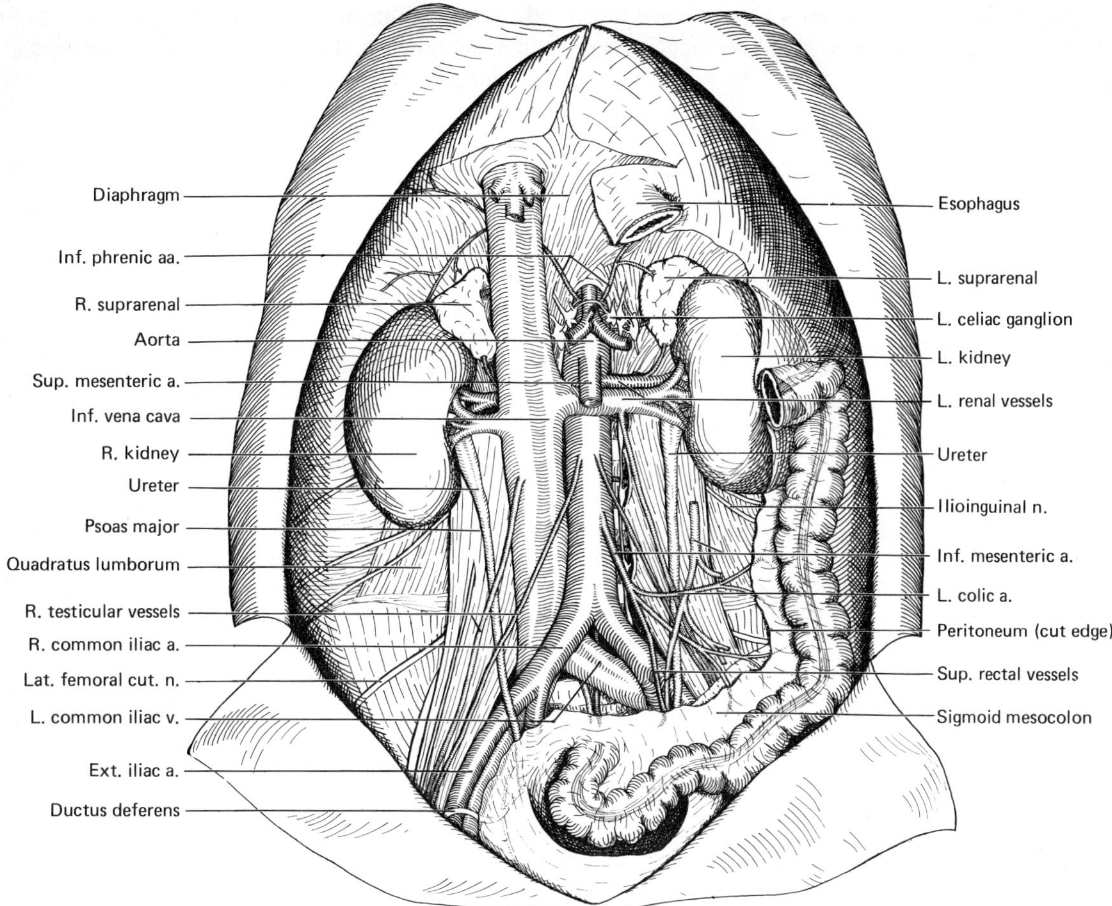

Figure 13.12 The retroperitoneal **structures on** the **posterior abdominal wall.**

Clean and study the inferior mesenteric vessels (Fig. 13.12). The **inferior mesenteric artery** is much smaller than the superior mesenteric. It arises from the front of the lower part of the **abdominal aorta** and runs downward and to the left, covered by the peritoneum on the posterior abdominal wall. Its first branch is the **left colic artery.** This vessel runs to the left behind the peritoneum and divides into **ascending** and **descending branches,** which supply the **descending colon;** the ascending branch anastomoses with the left branch of the middle colic artery. Below the left colic, several **sigmoid branches** arise from the inferior mesenteric. They pass forward in the sigmoid mesocolon to supply the **sigmoid colon.** They form anastomosing loops with one another, with the descending branch of the left colic, and with the superior rectal artery. The **superior rectal artery** is the direct continuation of the **inferior mesenteric;** it crosses the pelvic brim to enter the pelvis minor.

The series of anastomoses between the colic branches of the superior and inferior mesenteric arteries forms a distinct arcade, referred to as the ''marginal artery,'' around the edge of the large intestine from the ileum to the sigmoid colon. It provides an important collateral source of blood to a section of the colon whose main blood supply may be occluded.

The tributaries of the **inferior mesenteric vein** correspond to the branches of the artery. The trunk of the vein does not, however, accompany the artery but ascends retroperitoneally on the left side of the posterior abdominal wall deep to the pancreas to join the splenic vein or the superior mesenteric vein.

To study the subjacent structures, free and superiorly retract the spleen, pancreas, and duodenum. Later replace them to study their relationships to the adjacent organs.

SUPRARENALS AND KIDNEYS

The **suprarenal glands** are irregularly shaped and flattened anteroposteriorly. The **left suprarenal** is related anteriorly to the posterior surface of the stomach through the parietal peritoneum of the stomach bed; the lower part of its anterior surface often lies behind the pancreas. The anterior surface of the **right suprarenal** is overlapped on the left by the inferior vena cava but is elsewhere in contact with the liver.

The lower lateral portion of the posterior surface of each **suprarenal** is in direct contact with the upper medial part of the anterior surface of the corresponding **kidney;** above the kidney, each suprarenal rests posteriorly against the **diaphragm.** Make a tranverse incision through the middle of the suprarenal glands. Note the outer **cortical** and inner **medullary regions.**

The height to which the kidneys rise in the abdominal cavity is somewhat variable, a circumstance that can be readily understood from a knowledge of the embryology of these organs. In most cases, however, the lower pole of each kidney lies well above the iliac crest.

Examine the kidneys' position in relation to the adjoining structures. The anterior surface of the **right kidney** is in direct contact, near its medial border, with the descending portion of the **duodenum.** To the right of this, it presents a broad area that touches, through the parietal peritoneum, the inferior surface of the **liver.** Below the liver, this surface is in contact, without the intervention of any peritoneum, with the **right colic flexure.** The most inferomedial portion of the anterior surface of the right kidney abuts, through the peritoneum, on the coils of the **small intestine.** The **left kidney** is crossed anteriorly by the **pancreas.** Above the pancreas, it is related to the renal surface of the **spleen** and the posterior surface of the **stomach,** from both of which it is separated by parietal peritoneum. Below and to the right of the pancreas it is adjacent to coils of **small intestine;** to the left, it is related to the **left colic flexure.**

The **hilum of** each **kidney** is an oval area at the middle of its medial border, where the renal artery enters it and the renal vein, the lymphatics, and the ureter leave it. The **renal arteries** are branches of the abdominal aorta; the **renal veins** drain into the inferior vena cava. Near the hilum, the vein is usually the most anterior and the ureter the most posterior of the three structures. Observe that the **left renal vein** crosses **anterior to** the **aorta** and the **right renal artery** crosses **posterior to** the **vena cava.** It is not uncommon to find more than one renal artery on one or both sides. As it emerges from the hilum, the **ureter** is wide. Its diameter narrows, and it passes downward and medially across the posterior abdominal wall toward the pelvic brim.

Without severing the renal vessels or the ureter, make a longitudinal section through the kidney from the lateral border to the hilum and study the cut surfaces. Observe that the **kidney** has two parts, a cortex and a medulla. The **cortex** is the lighter-colored, peripheral portion. The inner, **medullary portion** is made up of a variable number of **renal pyramids,** which converge toward the center of the kidney and end there as rounded projections, the **renal papillae.** The excretory ducts empty into the minor calyxes at the apexes of the papillae. The minor calyxes coalesce into three or four major calyxes, which in turn join to form the renal pelvis, the dilated upper part of the ureter. The renal pelvis is in the renal sinus, the central cavity of the medial side of the kidney, along with fat and the renal vessels.

ABDOMINAL AORTA AND INFERIOR VENA CAVA

Clean and study the abdominal aorta and the inferior vena cava. As you do, notice the numerous fine nerve fibers that clothe the aorta and its primary branches. They constitute the **aortic plexus,** a **parasympathetic** and **sympathetic nerve net** that extends from the celiac plexus superiorly to the pelvic brim inferiorly. The aortic plexus is divisible into subordinate plexuses that are named according to the main arterial trunk with which each is associated, i.e., celiac, superior, and inferior mesenteric plexuses. Nerves that you dissect combine both sympathetic and parasympathetic efferent components as well as a visceral sensory component. They are conveyed along arteries in the form of perivascular plexuses to the viscera.

Once again, consider the **celiac plexus,** which is by now pretty much teased apart. It receives parasympathetic fibers from the **vagi** (anterior and posterior vagal trunks) and sympathetic fibers through the greater and lesser **splanchnic nerves.** The plexus consists of **celiac ganglia** (usually aggregated into two), their intercommunicating branches, and the branches of distribution. The left ganglion lies on the left crus of the diaphragm between the aorta and the left suprarenal. Carefully cut into the diaphragm to expose the left greater splanchnic nerve, which pierces the left crus to end in the ganglion. The right celiac ganglion occupies a similar position on the right side but is mostly covered by the inferior vena cava.

The other plexuses are extensions of the celiac plexus and are formed in a similar way. Parasympathetic innervation represented by the vagi distributes to viscera nourished by branches of the celiac trunk and the superior mesenteric artery; viscera supplied by the inferior mesenteric artery receive parasympathetic innervation from the second, third, and fourth sacral spinal cord segments. Keep in mind that a sensory component is also woven into the autonomic nervous system.

Observe the **superior hypogastric plexus** at the bifurcation of the aorta. It sends large nerve trunks, the right and left hypogastric nerves, over the sacral promontory along the common iliac arteries to join the **inferior hypogastric plexuses** within the pelvis.

The abdominal aorta begins at the **aortic hiatus of** the **diaphragm** as a continuation of the **thoracic aorta.** It descends in front of the bodies of the first four lumbar vertebrae to end, usually, in front of the **fourth lumbar vertebra,** by dividing into the **right** and **left common iliac arteries.** Anteriorly and to the left, it is related to the parietal peritoneum of the posterior abdominal wall, except where other structures intervene between it and the peritoneum. These structures are the pancreas, the inferior part of the duodenum, the splenic vein, the left renal vein, and portions of some of its own branches. To the right, it is related to the inferior vena cava, except most superiorly, where it is separated from the vena cava by the right crus of the diaphragm.

The **unpaired visceral branches** that arise from the anterior aspect of the aorta have already been studied. Investigate the **paired parietal branches** as they are described below.

The **inferior phrenic arteries** arise from the aorta between the two crura of the diaphragm. They pass upward and laterally across the inferior surface of the **diaphragm.** Observe that the right artery passes behind the inferior vena cava, and the left one passes behind the esophagus. One or both of the inferior phrenics may arise from the celiac trunk; the left inferior phrenic occasionally arises from the left gastric. Each inferior phrenic usually gives a **superior suprarenal artery** to the suprarenal gland.

The **middle suprarenal arteries** are small vessels, not always present, that arise from the lateral aspects of the aorta at about the same level as the origin of the superior mesenteric. They cross the crura of the diaphragm to reach the suprarenal glands.

The large **renal arteries** have already been observed. Before it reaches the hilum of the kidney, each renal artery usually gives an **inferior suprarenal artery** to the suprarenal gland. The right renal artery crosses behind the inferior vena cava.

The **testicular** or **ovarian arteries** arise from the front of the aorta a little below the origin of the superior mesenteric artery. They pass downward and laterally crossing over the ureter across the posterior abdominal wall. The testicular artery enters the deep inguinal ring, and the ovarian artery crosses in front of the common iliac artery to enter the pelvis minor.

The **common iliac arteries** are short, thick trunks that run downward and laterally from the termination of the **aorta** to end opposite the lumbosacral articulation by dividing into the **external iliac** and the **internal iliac arteries,** their only branches. Observe that the left common iliac artery is crossed anteriorly by the superior rectal vessels and also that each common iliac is crossed anteriorly by the ureter and, in the female, by the ovarian vessels.

In addition to the branches described above, four pairs of **lumbar arteries** and a single **middle sacral artery** arise from the **posterior aspect of** the **abdominal aorta.** The lumbar arteries can be more easily studied somewhat later; the **middle sacral artery** can be found now, emerging from behind the left common iliac vein and running downward in front of the body of the fifth lumbar vertebra into the pelvis.

The **inferior vena cava** is formed, to the right of the body of the **fifth lumbar vertebra** and behind the right common iliac artery, by the junction of the **right** and **left common iliac veins.** The common iliac veins are, at their origin, somewhat medial and posterior to the terminations of the common iliac arteries. Observe that the left common iliac vein is considerably longer than the right. It runs upward, medial to the left common iliac artery, to join the right vein behind the right common iliac artery; in its course it receives the middle sacral vein.

From its origin, the **inferior vena cava** ascends on the posterior abdominal wall to an orifice in the **tendinous portion of** the **diaphragm.** It lies in front of the right sides of the bodies of the lumbar vertebrae and the medial border of the right psoas major muscle. Its upper portion rests posteriorly against the diaphragm, and anteriorly, it is in contact with the liver, as previously observed. Below the liver, it is contiguous anteriorly and to the right with the parietal peritoneum, except where it is covered by the pancreas and duodenum. The largest tributaries of the inferior vena cava, above the common iliac veins, are the **renal veins.** Observe that while the **right suprarenal** and **right testicular** (or **ovarian**) **veins** drain directly into the vena cava, the **left suprarenal** and **left testicular** (or **ovarian**) **veins** join the **left renal vein.** The vena cava also receives the **inferior phrenic veins** and three or four **hepatic veins.**

Draw the vena cava forward and, dissecting carefully behind it, attempt to determine how many of the **lumbar veins** join it. There are four pairs of lumbar veins, corresponding to the lumbar arteries, but they do not always all join the vena cava. The upper ones usually drain into the right and left ascending lumbar veins, which pass through the diaphragm to join the **azygos** and **hemiazygos veins,** respectively.

Chapter 14

Diaphragm and Posterior Abdominal Wall

Study the **diaphragm,** the great domelike sheet of muscular and fibrous tissue that **separates** the **thoracic** and **abdominal cavities.** It consists of a **peripheral muscular portion** and a **central tendinous portion;** the muscle fibers take origin peripherally and insert into the central tendon. Anteriorly, the diaphragm originates by two small slips from the inside surface of the **xiphoid process,** then on each side by a series of six slips from the inner surfaces of the **cartilages of** the **lower** six **ribs,** which interdigitate with the slips of origin of the transversus abdominis. Posterolaterally between the cartilage of the twelfth rib and the vertebral column, the diaphragm takes origin from the **lateral** and **medial arcuate ligaments (lumbocostal arches)** (see below). Its most posterior portion arises from the lumbar vertebrae by means of the **right** and **left crura.**

The **posterior abdominal wall,** below the diaphragm and lateral to the vertebral column, is formed by the **psoas major** and **quadratus lumborum muscles.** The **arcuate ligaments** are not strictly ligaments, but are thickenings in the fascia covering the anterior surfaces of these muscles. They cannot always be seen as distinct structures, but the origin of the diaphragm from the quadratus and psoas fascia is constant. The **medial arcuate ligament** is a thickening of the fascia over the **psoas major** and extends from the body to the transverse process of the second lumbar vertebra; the **lateral arcuate ligament** is a fascial thickening over the **quadratus lumborum** from the same transverse process to the twelfth rib (Fig. 14.1).

The **crura** are the thickest and most fleshy portions of the diaphragm. The **right crus** is larger and descends lower than the left; it arises from the bodies of the first three lumbar vertebrae. The right crus splits to form the esophageal hiatus. The

left crus arises only from the first two lumbar vertebrae. The lowest portions of both crura are tendinous. As they ascend, the crura approach each other and their fibers cross-mingle anterior to the aorta to form the **aortic hiatus.** Observe that the **aortic hiatus** is not an actual opening in the diaphragm but a passage behind it at the level of the twelfth thoracic vertebra. When the diaphragm contracts, the aorta is protected from constriction by a fibrous arch, the **median arcuate ligament,** which connects the medial borders of the two crura and forms the actual border of the aortic hiatus.

Clean and study the psoas and quadratus muscles. While cleaning the psoas, watch for the **genitofemoral nerve,** which emerges through its substance and runs downward and laterally on its anterior surface. Similarly, while cleaning the quadratus, preserve the **subcostal, iliohypogastric,** and **ilioinguinal nerves,** all of which emerge from behind the lateral border of the psoas and cross the anterior surface of the quadratus.

First determine whether or not the **psoas minor** is present. This small muscle, often lacking on one or both sides, arises from the sides of the **bodies of** the **twelfth thoracic** and **first lumbar vertebrae.** Its fleshy body narrows to a flat tendon that passes downward on the anterior surface of the psoas major to insert on the **pecten of** the **pubis.**

The **psoas major** arises by a series of fleshy bundles from the **intervertebral disks** of all the lumbar vertebrae and from a series of **fibrous arches** that bridge the sides of the bodies of the lumbar vertebrae between the disks. Observe that the lumbar arteries pass around the sides of the bodies of the upper four lumbar vertebrae behind these fibrous arches. The psoas major also has a deep origin from the **transverse processes of** the **lumbar vertebrae.** The muscle fibers form a fusiform belly that crosses the ilium above the brim of the pelvis, where it lies lateral to the external iliac artery. It leaves the abdomen by passing behind the inguinal ligament into the thigh, where it inserts on the **lesser trochanter of** the **femur.**

The **quadratus lumborum** is a flat muscle lying lateral to the upper part of the psoas major between the twelfth rib and the iliac crest. It arises from the posterior part of the internal lip of the **iliac crest,** from the **iliolumbar ligament,** the **transverse processes of** the lower three or four **lumbar vertebrae,** and the deep surface of the **anterior lamella of** the **thoracolumbar fascia.** Some fibers pass upward to insert on the lower border of the **twelfth rib,** and others insert on the **transverse processes** of the upper two or three **lumbar vertebrae.**

Clean the **external iliac arteries.** Each arises opposite the lumbosacral articulation as one of the terminal branches of the **common iliac** and runs forward on the pelvic brim, at the medial border of the psoas major, to pass behind the medial part of the **inguinal ligament.** Beyond the inguinal ligament, it continues into the thigh as the **femoral artery.** It is crossed superiorly near the inguinal ligament by the ductus deferens (or the round ligament of the uterus). Just before it passes behind the inguinal ligament, it gives rise to its only branches, the **inferior epigastric** and **deep circumflex iliac arteries.** The full course of the inferior epigastric has already been traced. The **deep circumflex iliac artery** arises from the lateral side of the external iliac and runs laterally and upward along the line of fusion of the iliac fascia with the inguinal ligament. At the anterior superior iliac spine, it pierces the transversus muscle to run posteriorly along the iliac crest between the transversus and the internal oblique, where it has already been exposed. The **external iliac vein** begins behind the inguinal ligament as a continuation of the **femoral vein.** From this point to its termination in the common iliac vein, it lies just medial to the artery.

Below the iliac crest the posterolateral portion of the abdominal wall is formed by the **iliacus muscle,** a broad, flat muscle that fills the **iliac fossa,** from the bony surface of which it takes origin. Its fibers pass downward and medially behind the inguinal ligament to **join** the **tendon of** the **psoas major.** The iliacus is covered by a fairly dense fascial layer, the **iliac fascia,** which joins the inguinal ligament anteriorly. Remove the fascia to expose the muscle, but do not damage the **lateral femoral cutaneous nerve.** You will find it emerging from behind the psoas and running laterally across the iliacus. It enters the thigh behind the inguinal ligament just medial to the anterior superior iliac spine of the ilium. In the same area, find the **femoral nerve** emerging from the posterolateral side of the psoas (Fig. 14.1). Follow it along the lateral side of the psoas, in the groove between the psoas and the iliacus, to the point where it passes posterior to the inguinal ligament.

Clean and study the lumbar portions of the **sympathetic trunks.** Each sympathetic trunk enters the abdomen by passing under the medial arcuate ligament. It then runs downward on the ventrolateral surfaces of the bodies of the lumbar vertebrae just medial to the psoas major. Each trunk usually exhibits **four lumbar ganglia,** which send **rami communicantes** to the first four **lumbar nerves.**

Figure 14.1 The **posterior abdominal wall.** The psoas major has been removed on the right side to display the **lumbar plexus.**

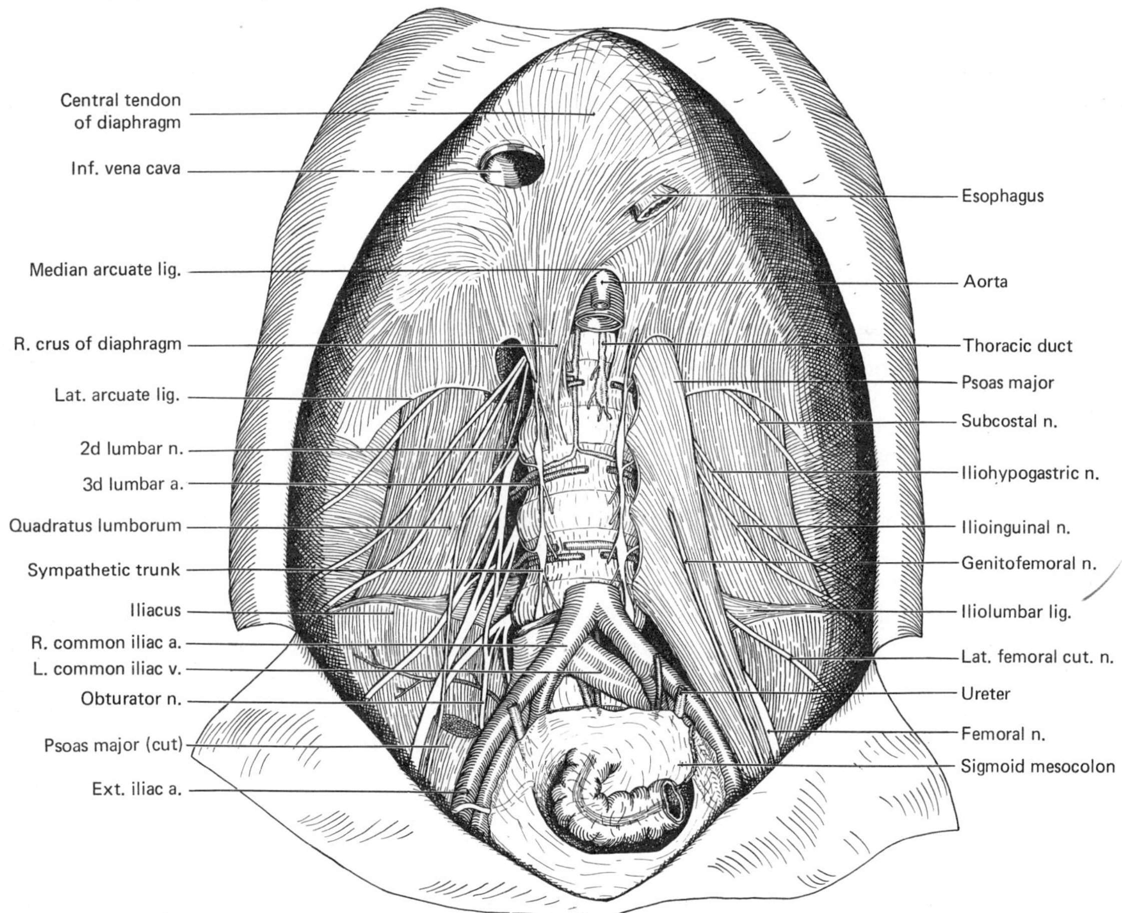

From the ganglia, branches pass forward to the **aortic plexus.** Inferiorly, the sympathetic trunks pass downward over the sacral promontory into the pelvis. Observe that the right trunk lies behind the inferior vena cava and the left one is crossed anteriorly by the left common iliac vessels.

Draw the aorta forward and display the four pairs of **lumbar arteries** arising from its posterior aspect. They pass backward and laterally around the bodies of the first four lumbar vertebrae, dorsal to the sympathetic trunks, and behind the psoas, which they supply. In their further course, they are usually behind the quadratus lumborum.

Attempt to display the **cisterna chyli,** the lower, expanded portion of the **thoracic duct.** It lies in the areolar tissue behind the aorta, and in front of the body of the second lumbar vertebra. Lymphatic vessels from all parts of the body **below the diaphragm** drain into it. From the cisterna, the thoracic duct ascends through the aortic hiatus into the posterior mediastinum of the thorax.

Portions of the **ilioinguinal, iliohypogastric, lateral femoral cutaneous, genitofemoral,** and **femoral nerves** have already been displayed in relation to the muscles of the posterior abdominal wall. All these nerves derive from the **lumbar plexus.** The distribution of the iliohypogastric and ilioinguinal nerves was followed in the dissection of the anterior abdominal wall. Now trace the **genitofemoral nerve** downward on the psoas; it terminates by dividing into two branches, the genital and the femoral. The **genital nerve** has already been traced into the deep inguinal ring as the nerve supply to the **cremaster muscle.** The **femoral branch** crosses the iliacus to pass behind the inguinal ligament into the thigh, where its cutaneous distribution will be seen later.

The **lumbar plexus** lies deeply within the substance of the **psoas major muscle.** You will have to cut away the psoas major carefully in order to display it. Start by following the genitofemoral nerve upward and posteriorly into the psoas muscle. Then remove the longitudinal strands of the muscle piecemeal to expose the lumbar plexus. When the plexus is exposed, you will see that it is derived from the **ventral rami** of the first four **lumbar nerves.** The branches that arise from the plexus are the iliohypogastric, ilioinguinal, femoral, genitofemoral, lateral femoral cutaneous, and obturator nerves. Some portion of each of these nerves, with the exception of the obturator, has already been seen. The **obturator nerve** arises within the psoas by three roots, which are derived from the ventral rami of the **second, third,** and **fourth lumbar nerves.** It emerges from the medial border of the psoas and enters the pelvis minor by passing downward behind the common iliac vessels (Fig. 14.1).

The **femoral nerve** is the largest branch of the lumbar plexus. It also is derived from the **second, third,** and **fourth lumbar nerves.** It emerges from the lateral border of the psoas, from which point its further abdominal course has already been seen; it gives **twigs** of supply **to** the **iliacus muscle.**

The **genitofemoral nerve** has two roots, which are derived from the **first** and **second lumbar nerves.** The **iliohypogastric** and **ilioinguinal nerves** are both derived from the **first lumbar nerve,** though they often also receive a communication from the last thoracic. Observe that, as they emerge from the lateral border of the psoas to cross the quadratus lumborum, these two nerves are contiguous with the posterior surface of the kidney. The **lateral femoral cutaneous nerve** is derived from the **second** and **third lumbars;** it is sometimes represented by two smaller nerves that cross the iliacus at some distance from each other.

In addition to these branches, the **four roots of** the **lumbar plexus** give **twigs** of supply directly **to** the **psoas** and **quadratus muscles.** From the **fourth** and **fifth lumbar nerves** a large branch **(lumbosacral trunk)** descends to join the sacral plexus. A small branch known as the **accessory obturator nerve** is sometimes found arising from the **third** and **fourth lumbar nerves;** it descends along the medial border of the psoas and enters the thigh by crossing over the pecten of the pubis. It innervates the pectineus muscle.

Chapter 15

Perineum

The **perineum** is a diamond-shaped area at the lower end of the trunk, between the thighs. It corresponds to the **inferior pelvic aperture** and is separated from the pelvic portion of the abdominopelvic cavity by the **pelvic diaphragm.** In the erect anatomical posture, the surface area of the perineum is reduced to a narrow groove running forward from the **coccyx** to the **pubis.**

Before starting the dissection, study an articulated bony pelvis, preferably one with the ligaments still in place (Fig. 15.1). Observe that the most anterior point of the perineum is represented in the skeleton by the lower end of the **pubic symphysis;** this bony surface is covered by the **arcuate pubic ligament.** Posteriorly, the perineum is limited by the coccyx. Its widest lateral extent is about midway between the pubic symphysis and the coccyx, and is limited on each side by the **ischial tuberosity.** Its anterolateral boundary is formed on each side by the **ischiopubic ramus.** Posterolaterally, the perineum is bounded by the **sacrotuberous ligament,** which stretches from the lower end of the sacrum and the coccyx to the ischial tuberosity. As the dissection proceeds, you will find that this ligament is covered externally by the lower part of the **gluteus maximus muscle,** so that the lower border of this muscle is sometimes regarded as forming, on each side, the posterolateral boundary of the perineum. The ischiopubic ramus, the ischial tuberosity, and the coccyx can be palpated from the surface and should be identified.

The diamond-shaped perineum is arbitrarily subdivided into two triangular regions by an imaginary transverse line running between the anterior portions of the two ischial tuberosities: an anterior **urogenital triangle** and a posterior **anal triangle.**

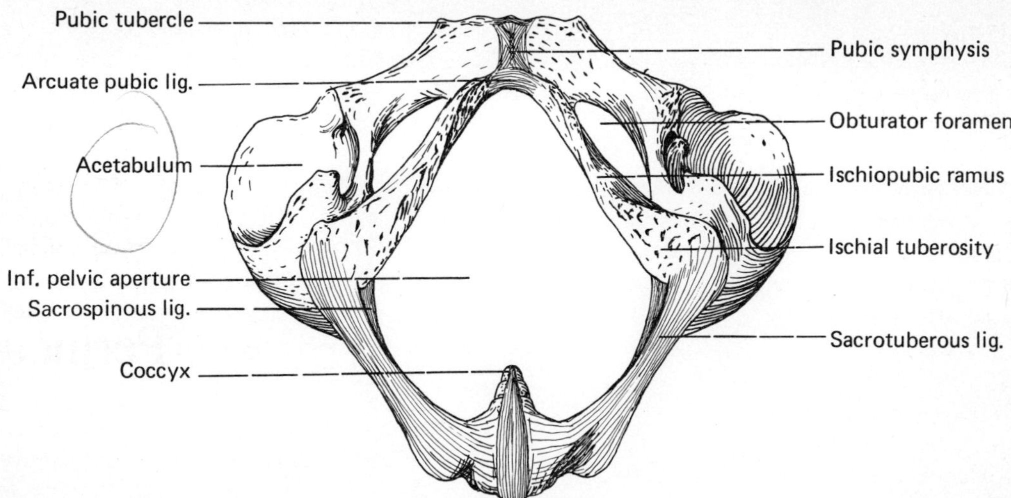

Figure 15.1 Inferior view of the **pelvic skeleton** with the ligaments in place.

To dissect the perineum, you will have to place the body in the lithotomy position, with the thighs widely spread and the inferior pelvic aperture facing upward. Throughout the dissection, you must bear in mind that with the body in this position structures that are anatomically superior or inferior will now appear to you in exactly the reverse positions.

The **urogenital triangle of** the **female** perineum contains the urethral orifice and the external genital organs, which should be studied before any dissection is done.

The **mons pubis** is an elevation of the skin in front of the pubic symphysis, which is caused by the presence of a thick layer of superficial adipose tissue. Extending downward and backward from the mons pubis on each side are the **labia majora,** folds of hair-bearing skin and fascia that diminish in size posteriorly and meet at the **posterior commissure,** a short distance in front of the **anus.** The narrow cleft between the two labia majora is the **urogenital (pudendal) fissure.** Overlapped by the labia majora are two much thinner integumental folds, the **labia minora,** which lie on each side of the **vaginal orifice.** Anteriorly, they converge, and each divides into two folds. The lower fold from each labium minus is attached to the undersurface of the **clitoris** to form the **frenulum of** the **clitoris.** The upper fold from each unites with the fold from the other side above the clitoris to form the **prepuce of** the **clitoris.** Between the frenulum and the prepuce, the **glans of** the **clitoris** is seen. The region between the labia minora is known as the **vestibule.** The vaginal orifice opens into the posterior part of the vestibule. It may or may not be partly guarded by a fold of mucous membrane, the **hymen.** Most often in sexually active women, only the ragged edges of the hymen, the **hymeneal caruncles,** remain. The **urethral orifice** is a small, slitlike opening in the wall of the vestibule slightly anterior to the vaginal orifice. On each side of the vaginal orifice, the minute opening of the **duct of** the **greater vestibular gland** may occasionally be seen.

Note the location of the anus in the anal triangle. Then make two incisions through the skin of the perineum as shown in Fig. 15.2: (1) a median longitudinal incision from the posterior part of the scrotum (or mons pubis) backward to a point about 2.5 cm above the tip of the coccyx (the incision must bifurcate to encircle the labia minora in the female and the anus in both sexes); and (2) a transverse incision passing in front of the anus from a point about 2.5 cm lateral to the ischial tuberosity on one side to a similar point on the other side. Four triangular flaps of skin will thus be marked out; reflect the two anterior ones forward and laterally and the two posterior ones backward and laterally.

The **subcutaneous connective tissue** of the perineum is now exposed. In the anal triangle, it is extremely thick with fat. In the urogenital triangle, however, it is thinner. The subcutaneous tissue over the urogenital triangle, like that over the lower abdominal wall, can be dissected into an outer fatty and an inner membranous layer.

The **superficial fatty layer** is continuous with the subcutaneous tissue of the thigh, anal triangle, and abdominal wall. In the female it contributes to the formation of the labia majora and is continuous with the fat of the mons pubis.

The **inner membranous layer** (commonly called Colles' fascia) is attached posteriorly to the posterior free margin of the urogenital diaphragm and laterally to the ischiopubic rami. Anteriorly, in the male, it is continuous with the dartos tunic of the scrotum and the superficial fascia of the penis. It is continuous around the sides of the penis and scrotum with the inner membranous layer over the ventral abdominal wall. The membranous fascia of the female urogenital triangle is the same as that of the male, except that it is divided into two lateral parts by the urogenital fissure.

A compartment exists between the membranous layer of the superficial fascia and the inferior fascial layer of the urogenital diaphragm. It is known as the **superficial perineal pouch.** This pouch contains primarily the structures that form the root of the penis (or clitoris) and their associated nerves and vessels.

Clinically, the pouch and its boundaries are important because the spread of urine extravasated through a perforation in the ventral wall of the penile urethra will be limited to the urogenital triangle, but may extend upward into the abdominal wall.

The anal triangle is similar in the male and female and is described first. The description of the urogenital triangle then follows, and because it differs slightly between the sexes, it is given separately for each sex (male, page 171; female, page 174).

Figure 15.2 Surface landmarks and skin incisions on the perineum.

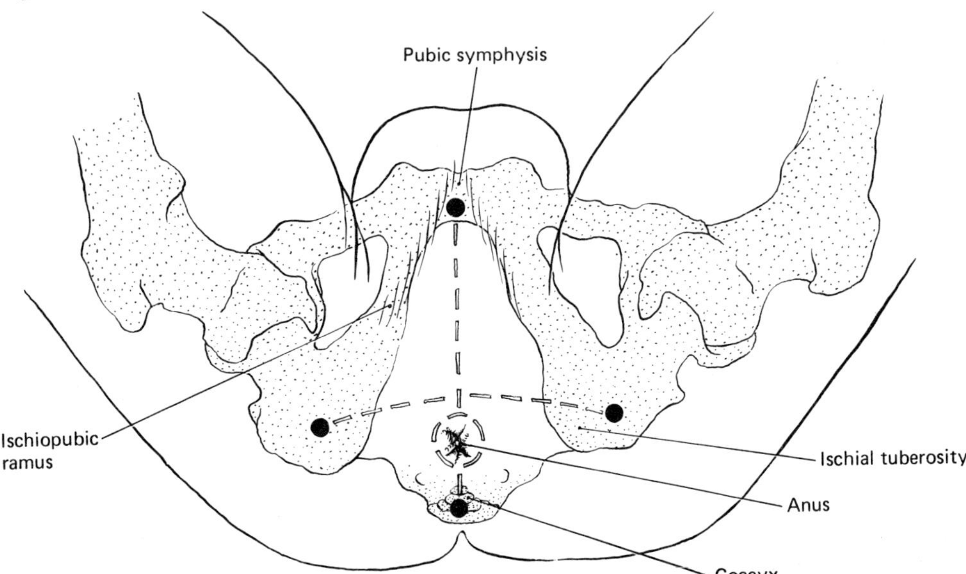

ANAL TRIANGLE

This dissection of the **anal triangle** consists principally of displaying the boundaries and contents of the two ischiorectal fossae. Each **ischiorectal fossa** is a potential space lying lateral to the lower end of the anal canal (Figs. 15.3 to 15.6). Its superomedial boundary is formed by the sloping inferior surface of the pelvic diaphragm and its fascia, which separates the fossa from the pelvic cavity. The lateral wall is formed by the obturator fascia, which clothes the inner surface of the obturator internus muscle; portions of this muscle are also seen in the pelvic and gluteal regions. Posteriorly, the ischiorectal fossa is bounded by the sacrotuberous ligament and the lower border of the gluteus maximus muscle. Its highest part, or roof, is formed by the line along which the pelvic diaphragm joins the obturator internus fascia. The fossa is filled by the **ischiorectal fat pad,** within which the inferior rectal nerves and vessels ramify as they pass from the lateral wall medially to the anal region. The internal pudendal artery and pudendal nerve, which are lodged in the lateral wall, will be freed later in the dissection.

Identify the **central tendon of** the **perineum** (gynecologically referred to as the **perineal body**). It is a tendinous septum in the midline of the perineum a short distance anterior to the anus. The bulbospongiosus, superficial transverse perineal, and external sphincter ani muscles all unite at the central tendon.

The central tendon marks the point at which surgical entrance (perineal approach) to the pelvic cavity is made.

In order to prevent vaginal or perineal tear during childbirth, the vaginal orifice is enlarged by a midline or a mediolateral diagonal incision (i.e., episiotomy) through the posterior vaginal wall and vulva. Following delivery the incision is sutured.

Clean the **external sphincter ani muscle.** It is a thick ring of muscle fibers (Figs. 15.3 to 15.6), running backward from the central tendon to the tip of the coccyx and encircling the anus. As you clean it, find small branches of the inferior rectal nerve and artery that emerge from the fat on each side to enter the muscle.

Insert the blade of a scalpel into the ischiorectal fat pad about midway between the anal orifice and the ischial tuberosity. Angle the blade tip slightly laterally and penetrate the fat pad to a depth of 5 cm. Then insert a finger into the opening made by the scalpel and attempt to palpate the inferior rectal vessels and nerves crossing from the lateral to the medial part of the fossa.

Now clean the lower border of the **gluteus maximus muscle** between the coccyx and the ischial tuberosity. By carefully probing with your finger or a blunt instrument in a medial to lateral direction to minimize tearing the inferior rectal nerves and vessels, remove the ischiorectal fat to display the walls of the fossa and the nerves and vessels. Do not damage the pelvic diaphragm, which forms the medial wall of the fossa; it is often very thin.

When the fossa is clean, you will see that the **inferior rectal vessels** and **nerves** emerge from the obturator fascia, run medially through the ischiorectal fossa, and ramify about the lower end of the **anal canal.** Emerging from the obturator fascia at the anterior end of the lateral wall of the ischiorectal fossa, the **perineal nerve** and **artery** may be identified. They pierce the obturator fascia, run forward for a short distance in the anterolateral angle of the ischiorectal fossa, and enter the superficial fascia of the urogenital triangle (Fig. 15.3).

The nerves and arteries so far exposed in the ischiorectal fossa are derived from the **pudendal nerve** and the **internal pudendal artery.** Before emerging into the fossa, they are lodged in a canal in the obturator fascia known as the **pudendal (Alcock's) canal.** This canal runs forward in the lateral wall of the ischiorectal fossa from the lesser sciatic foramen to the posterior edge of the urogenital diaphragm. To display the structures it contains, open it on one side as described below.

Make a cut through the fibers of the gluteus maximus, just anterior to the ischial tuberosity. Identify the sacrotuberous ligament (Figs. 15.3 and 15.5). Insert a finger dorsal to this ligament and palpate the sacrospinous ligament. Now follow the course of the pudendal nerve and the internal pudendal artery between these two ligaments and forward into the pudendal canal.

The **pudendal nerve** is derived from the sacral plexus. It usually divides into two terminal branches, the perineal nerve and the dorsal nerve of the penis (or clitoris), before entering the perineum. Consequently, these two nerves will be found separately in the canal. The **perineal nerve** usually lies below the internal pudendal artery and leaves the canal in company with the perineal branch of the artery. The **dorsal nerve of** the **penis** (or **clitoris**) lies above the artery. This nerve and the internal pudendal artery leave the anterior end of the canal by passing between the two fascial layers of the urogenital diaphragm. The inferior rectal nerves, which arise from the pudendal nerve, may enter the posterior end of the canal separately or may arise within it as branches of the pudendal nerve. The **inferior rectal vessels** are similarly derived and distributed.

The "pudendal nerve block" is one type of obstetrical anesthesia. It is done where the nerve courses through the pudendal canal. The resultant perineal analgesia allows for delivery by forceps but does not interfere with the sensations of uterine contraction.

MALE UROGENITAL TRIANGLE

Skin the remaining posterior part of the scrotum and carefully dissect the terminal branches of the **posterior scrotal vessels** and **nerves** (Fig. 15.3). Then divide the scrotum in the midline and reflect the testes and their coverings laterally on each

Figure 15.3 Male perineum; superficial. Arteries and nerves have been omitted on the right.

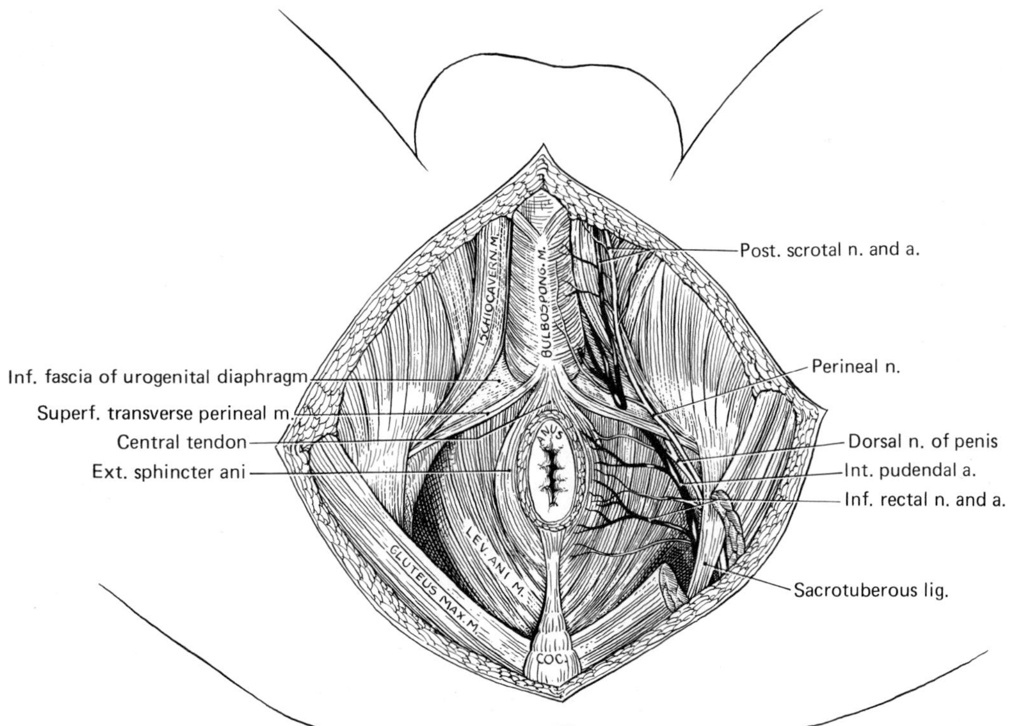

side. Carefully trace the nerves and vessels posteriorly through the fatty superficial fascia of the urogenital triangle to their origins. As you do, notice that the fatty layer of fascia is continuous laterally over the ischiopubic rami with the same layer of fascia on the medial aspect of the thigh and posteriorly in the anal triangle.

Traced anteriorly, the **perineal nerve** divides into superficial and deep branches. The **superficial branches** are the two or three posterior scrotal nerves that you have just found. They supply cutaneous innervation to the skin of the urogenital triangle and to the posterior part of the scrotum.

The **deep branches** supply the muscles of the superficial perineal pouch, which you should now clean. Observe that these nerves are all accompanied by branches of the **perineal artery.**

The **superficial transverse perineal muscle** is a small paired muscle, variable in size and degree of development and, consequently, often difficult to demonstrate. It arises from the inner surface of the anterior part of the ischial tuberosity and inserts into the central tendon of the perineum, where it blends with the external sphincter ani and the bulbospongiosus muscles.

The **ischiocavernosus** and **bulbospongiosus muscles** are thin sheets of muscle that cover the external surfaces of the structures forming the **root of** the **penis,** the **corpora cavernosa penis,** and the **corpus spongiosum penis,** respectively (Figs. 15.3 and 15.4). They are covered by a layer of **deep muscular fascia,** which continues anteriorly to surround the shaft of the penis as the **deep fascia of** the **penis.** The fascia is thin over the muscles but is thick over the shaft of the penis. The deep vessels and nerves of the penis are enclosed in the deep fascia. The suspensory ligament of the penis (see Chap. 11) attaches to the deep fascia.

The **bulbospongiosus muscle** arises from the central tendon of the perineum and from a median raphe running forward on the undersurface of the bulb. From here, its fibers diverge to surround the bulb and insert into the inferior fascia of the urogenital diaphragm and the dorsal surface of the corpus spongiosum penis. Some of its most anterior fibers reach the dorsum of the penis. Each **ischiocavernosus muscle** arises from the ischial tuberosity and the inner aspect of the ischiopubic ramus; it inserts into the lateral aspect of the anterior part of the crus of the corpus cavernosum penis. Make an incision through the bulbospongiosus muscle along the midventral line of the corpus spongiosum penis and reflect the two parts of the muscle laterally. The ischiocavernosus muscle should also be reflected from the ventral surface of each crus (Fig. 15.4).

The **bulb of** the **penis** lies in the median plane. It is attached to the undersurface of the inferior fascial layer of the urogenital diaphragm. Anteriorly, it narrows to become continuous with the corpus spongiosum penis. Each **crus of** the **penis** is attached to the corresponding ischiopubic ramus and the inferior surface of the lateral parts of the urogenital diaphragm. The crura run forward and medially and unite in front of the lower part of the pubic symphysis with each other and the corpus spongiosum penis to form the **shaft of** the **penis.**

Free and elevate the crura from the ischiopubic rami and complete the separation of the three components of the penis. Then dissect between the bulb and the crura to expose the **inferior fascial layer (perineal membrane) of** the **urogenital diaphragm;** it is a tough, glistening sheet of connective tissue (Fig. 15.4). Attempt to separate the bulb from the diaphragm and observe that it is firmly attached superiorly to the diaphragm at a point in the midline about 1.5 cm in front of its posterior end. At this point, the urethra pierces the urogenital diaphragm to enter the bulb. Attempt to display the small **artery to** the **bulb,** which pierces the diaphragm on each side of the urethral orifice to enter the bulb. Draw the bulb forward to expose the lower surface of the urogenital diaphragm. Find the **dorsal nerve of** the **penis** and the **internal pudendal artery,** which here pierce the inferior fascial layer of the urogenital diaphragm under cover of the crura. Just as it emerges from the urogenital diaphragm, the internal pudendal artery terminates by dividing into the **deep artery of** the **penis,** which enters the crus, and the

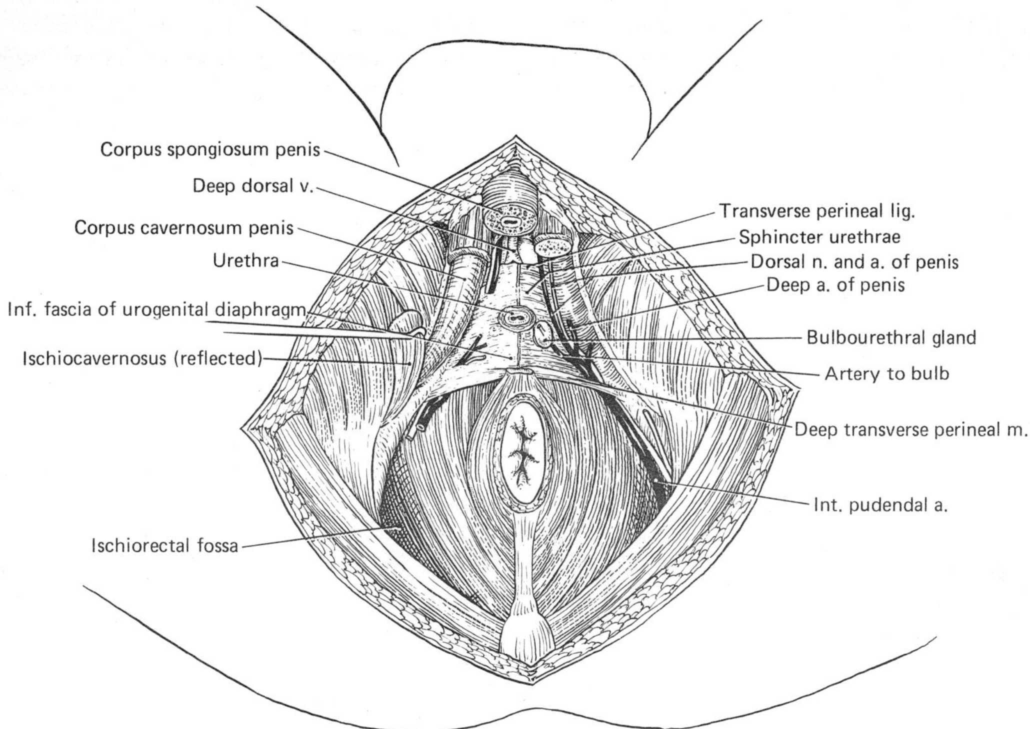

Figure 15.4 Male perineum; deep. The inferior fascia of the urogenital diaphragm and part of the crus of the penis have been removed on the left.

dorsal artery of the **penis,** which accompanies the dorsal nerve forward onto the dorsum of the penis (Fig. 15.4).

The inferior surface of the urogenital diaphragm is now exposed. Clean its sharp anterior border, the **transverse perineal ligament.** Observe that this ligament lies just behind the **arcuate pubic ligament,** which covers the lower border of the pubic symphysis, and that the **deep dorsal vein of** the **penis** enters the pelvic cavity by passing through the narrow interval between the transverse perineal and the arcuate pubic ligaments.

Now reflect the inferior layer of the fascia of the urogenital diaphragm to open the **deep pouch of** the **perineum.** This is the area enclosed by the two fascial layers of the urogenital diaphragm; it contains the diaphragm itself, nerves, arteries, and glands.

The **urogenital diaphragm** comprises the **sphincter urethrae** and the **deep transverse perineal muscles** (Fig. 15.4). The sphincter urethrae is a thin muscle that stretches transversely between the ischiopubic rami and encircles the membranous urethra. It is continuous posteriorly with the deep transverse perineal muscle, which also stretches between the ischiopubic rami.

The second or **membranous portion of** the **male urethra** is short and traverses the urogenital diaphragm from above downward. It is continuous with the third or spongy portion of the urethra. Attempt to find the small **bulbourethral glands;** they are embedded in the deep transverse perineal muscle a short distance behind the urethra. Their fine ducts pierce the inferior fascia of the diaphragm to enter the bulb and join the third part of the urethra.

The dorsal nerve of the penis and the internal pudendal artery were previously seen entering the urogenital diaphragm at the anterior end of the pudendal canal. They may now be traced forward along the lateral margin of the deep pouch to the point at which they were found to leave it by piercing the inferior fascia. Observe that while in the deep pouch the internal pudendal artery gives rise to the artery to the bulb, which pierces the inferior fascia independently to enter the bulb, as already noted.

The continuity of the pudendal nerve and the internal pudendal artery with their branches can now be effectively followed from the pelvis through the anal triangle to their termination in the urogenital triangle.

FEMALE UROGENITAL TRIANGLE

Beginning at the posterior part of the mons pubis, carefully dissect the terminal branches of the **posterior labial vessels** and **nerves** (Fig. 15.5). Trace them posteriorly though the superficial fascia of the urogenital triangle to the perineal nerve, which you localized in the anal triangle. As you do, notice that the fatty layer of fascia is continuous laterally over the ischiopubic rami with the same layer of fascia on the medial aspect of the thigh and posteriorly in the anal triangle.

Traced anteriorly, the **perineal nerve** divides into superficial and deep branches. The **superficial branches** are the two or three posterior labial nerves that you have just found. They supply cutaneous innervation to the skin of the urogenital triangle and to the posterior part of the labia.

The **deep branches** supply the muscles of the superficial perineal pouch, which you should now clean. Observe that these nerves are all accompanied by branches of the perineal artery.

The **superficial transverse perineal muscle** is a small paired muscle, variable in size and degree of development and, consequently, often difficult

Figure 15.5 Female perineum; superficial. Arteries and nerves have been omitted on the right.

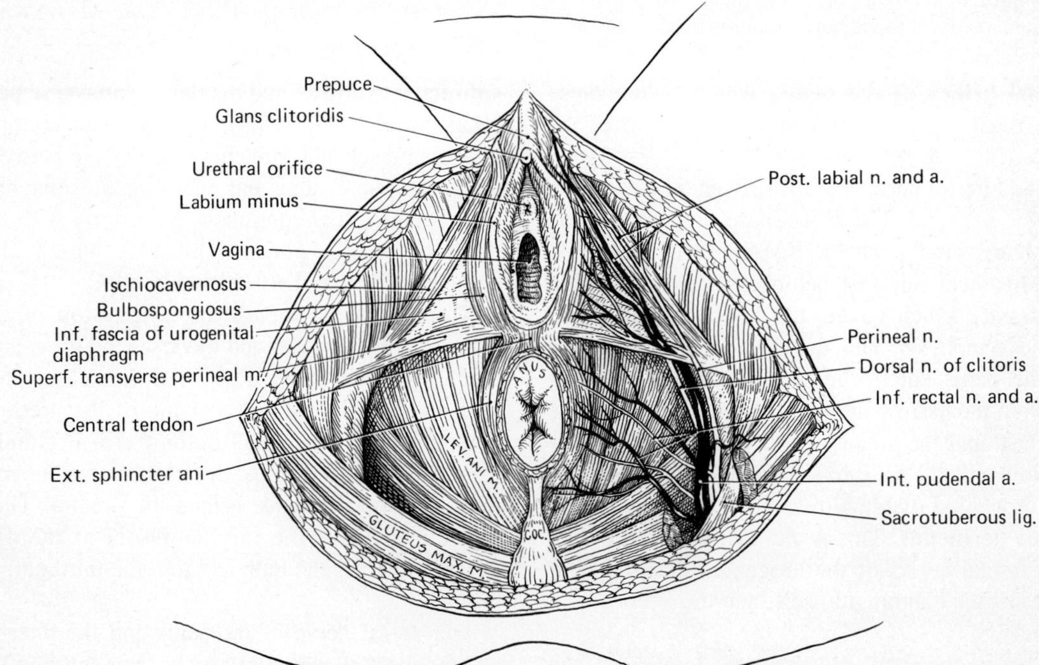

to demonstrate. It arises from the inner surface of the anterior part of the ischial tuberosity and inserts into the central tendon of the perineum, where it blends with the external sphincter ani and the bulbospongiosus muscles (Fig. 15.5).

The **ischiocavernosus muscle** is also present but is much smaller than the same muscle in the male. It arises from the ischiopubic ramus near the ischial tuberosity and covers the crus of the clitoris, upon which it inserts (Figs. 15.5 and 15.6). The **bulbospongiosus muscle** is homologous to the same muscle in the male, except that it is divided into two halves by the vagina; one half lies on each side of the vestibule, closely applied to the external surface of the corresponding bulb of the vestibule. Posteriorly, the muscle arises from the central tendon of the perineum; anteriorly, its two halves converge to attach to the sides of the clitoris (Fig. 15.5).

Examine the **clitoris.** The **body of** the **clitoris** (corpus clitoridis), which corresponds to the body or shaft of the penis excluding the urethra, is formed in front of the lower border of the pubic symphysis by the junction of the two **crura of** the **corpora cavernosa of** the **clitoris.** The crura, which correspond to the crura of the penis, diverge from each other posteriorly where they attach to the ventral aspect of the ischiopubic rami. Each crus is covered by the thin ischiocavernosus muscle and **deep muscular fascia.** From the symphysis, the body of the clitoris projects downward for a short distance to terminate at the **glans clitoridis,** the small, rounded tubercle of erectile tissue that was already seen at the anterior end of the urogenital fissure between the prepuce and the frenulum of the clitoris.

Carefully reflect the bulbospongiosus muscle to expose the **bulb of** the **vestibule.** It consists of two oblong halves, composed principally of erectile tissue, situated on each side of the vestibule. Anteriorly, the bulbs converge into a very thin **commissure** that connects to the glans. Remove the bulb from the inferior surface of the urogenital diaphragm to expose the **inferior fascial layer (perineal membrane) of** the **diaphragm** (Fig. 15.6). As the bulb is being removed, watch for the **artery to** the **bulb,** which pierces the inferior fascia to enter the bulb and the greater vestibular glands. Each **greater vestibular gland** lies under cover of the posterior end of the corresponding half of the bulb of the vestibule. From it a long duct passes into the wall of the vestibule to open lateral to the vaginal orifice.

Reflect the ischiocavernosus muscle and remove the crus of the clitoris from its attachment to the ischiopubic ramus. As the crus is reflected, secure the **dorsal nerve of** the **clitoris** and the **internal pudendal artery** (Fig. 15.6), which emerge through the inferior fascia of the urogenital diaphragm under cover of the crus. Observe that the internal pudendal artery here divides into its terminal branches, the **deep** and **dorsal arteries of** the **clitoris.** The former immediately enters the crus; the latter proceeds anteriorly with the dorsal nerve to reach the dorsum (anterior surface) of the body of the clitoris.

The inferior surface of the urogenital diaphragm is now exposed. Clean its sharp anterior border, the **transverse perineal ligament.** Observe that this ligament lies just behind the **arcuate pubic ligament,** which covers the lower border of the pubic symphysis.

Now reflect the inferior layer of fascia of the urogenital diaphragm to open the **deep pouch of** the **perineum.** This is the area enclosed by the two fascial layers of the urogenital diaphragm and contains the diaphragm itself, nerves, arteries, and glands.

The **urogenital diaphragm** comprises the **sphincter urethrae** and **deep transverse perineal muscles** (Fig. 15.6). The urogenital diaphragm is not as complete a partition as it is in the male, since it is pierced by the vaginal canal as well as the urethra. The sphincter urethrae is a thin muscle that stretches transversely between the ischiopubic rami and encircles the urethra. It is continuous posteriorly with the deep transverse perineal muscle, which also stretches between the ischiopubic rami.

The dorsal nerve of thc clitoris and the internal

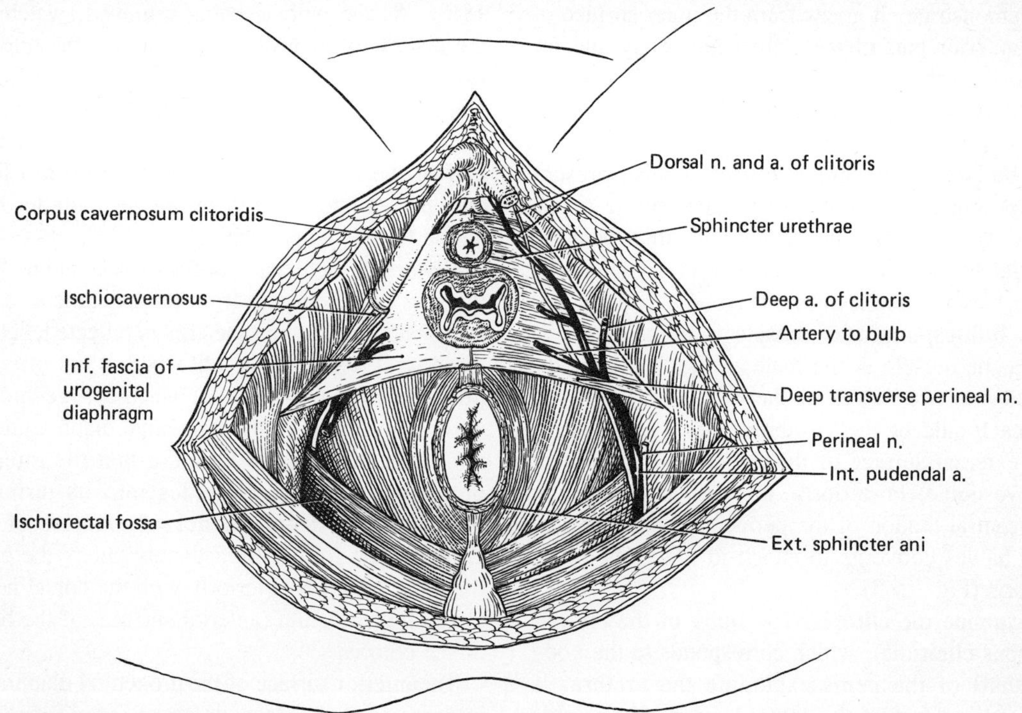

Figure 15.6 Female perineum; deep. The inferior fascia of the urogenital diaphragm and part of the crus of the clitoris have been removed on the left.

pudendal artery were previously seen entering the urogenital diaphragm at the anterior end of the pudendal canal. Now trace them forward along the lateral margin of the deep pouch to the point at which they were found to leave it by piercing the inferior fascia. Observe that while in the deep pouch the internal pudendal artery gives rise to the artery to the bulb, which pierces the inferior fascia independently to enter the bulb, as already noted.

The continuity of the pudendal nerve and the internal pudendal artery with their branches can now be effectively followed from the pelvis through the anal triangle to their terminations in the urogenital triangle.

Chapter 16

Pelvis Minor

The **pelvis** is the region enclosed by the **sacrum, coccyx,** and **coxal (hip) bones,** and their associated ligaments and muscles. It is subdivided into major and minor pelves. The **major pelvis** is the area bounded by the iliac fossae. The **minor** or **true pelvis** is the **most inferior** and **posterior portion** of the general **abdominopelvic cavity.** It is bounded anteriorly and laterally by the internal surfaces of the **coxal bones,** covered by the **obturator internus muscles** and **fasciae,** and posteriorly by the anterior surface of the **sacrum,** which is also covered by fascia. The minor pelvis communicates superiorly with the abdomen proper at the **pelvic brim** (pectineal line of pelvis, arcuate line, and sacral promontory). Inferiorly, the pelvis presents the **inferior pelvic aperture** (**outlet**); the **pelvic cavity** is separated from the **perineum** by the **pelvic diaphragm.** The diaphragm is composed of two paired muscles, the **levator ani** and the **coccygeus,** and is pierced by the anal canal and by genitourinary structures.

The peritoneum extends below the pelvic brim but does not reach as far as the pelvic diaphragm. Consequently, a considerable portion of the pelvic cavity is extraperitoneal. The coils of the small intestine and the sigmoid colon are the principal intraperitoneal structures within the pelvis; the rectum and bladder are only partially clothed with peritoneum. In the female, the uterus and ovaries project upward into the peritoneum and thus become intraperitoneal.

The surgical approach used in treatment of some of the pelvic viscera (e.g., prostatectomy) is through the anterior abdominal wall just superior to the pubic symphysis. By this route the peritoneum is not invaded; therefore, postoperative complications due to peritoneal infection are lessened.

Descriptions of the **pelvic fasciae** vary and are especially confusing due to inconsistent nomenclature. For now simply divide the fasciae into two parts, a **parietal pelvic fascia** and a **visceral**

pelvic fascia. The **parietal fascia** is an extension into the pelvis of the abdominal fascial layer (endoabdominal fascia) that is regionally designated as transversalis, quadratus, iliacus, and psoas fascia. In the pelvis, the fascia covering the internal surfaces of the obturator internus muscle (**obturator fascia**) and its extension across the front of the sacrum are part of the parietal pelvic fascia. Likewise, the **superior** and **inferior surfaces** of the **pelvic diaphragm** are covered by a layer of parietal pelvic fascia. The parietal fascia, from which the muscles of the pelvic diaphragm arise, not only forms the lateral wall of the cavity of the pelvis minor but extends into the perineum, where it helps form the lateral wall of the ischiorectal fossa.

The **visceral pelvic fascia** is on the same plane with the **extraperitoneal** (**subserous**) **fascia** that lies just external to the peritoneum. It is fatty, areolar connective tissue that varies in thickness and that forms fascial sheaths in which the pelvic viscera are completely enclosed. Blood vessels and nerves course through this layer to the viscera. In some cases, thickened portions of the visceral pelvic fascia are called ligaments because they are thought to support an associated organ (e.g., puboprostatic ligament).

For this dissection, you will first observe and study the disposition of the pelvic peritoneum. Then you will study the structures that occupy the extraperitoneal space. Third, the visceral pelvic fascia is described, and you will split the pelvis in half. Finally, you will examine the muscles that comprise the pelvic diaphragm and the pelvic wall.

Note that the following descriptions apply to normal, healthy, and moderately young persons. Diseased conditions of the female reproductive organs are common in older cadavers; the woman may have had a **hysterectomy** while living, in which case the uterus and sometimes the ovaries will have been removed.

Do not remove the peritoneum from the pelvis minor at this time. First identify the various structures that enter or leave the pelvis by crossing the pelvic brim external to the peritoneum.

MALE PELVIS

Begin by reviewing the structures that create the peritoneal folds on the inside of the anterior abdominal wall (see page 139). The **median umbilical ligament** (fetal urachus) runs upward toward the umbilicus from behind the pubic symphysis (Fig. 16.1). Somewhat lateral to this on each side, also running toward the umbilicus, find the **medial umbilical ligament,** a cordlike structure that represents the fetal umbilical artery. Still more laterally, after crossing lateral to the inferior epigastric artery (the **lateral umbilical fold**), the **ductus (vas) deferens** descends into the pelvis by crossing the external iliac artery and vein shortly before they pass behind the inguinal ligament. The **ureter** crosses the pelvic brim on each side at about the point where the common iliac arteries terminate. Here also the large **internal iliac artery** and **vein** descend into the pelvis. Identify the **middle sacral vessels** running downward anterior to the sacrum; slightly to their left, the **superior rectal vessels** cross in front of the left common iliac vessels to run downward into the pelvis minor. An **obturator artery** can occasionally be found running downward across the pelvic brim slightly anterior to the ductus deferens. In such cases, it is an abnormal branch of either the inferior epigastric or the external iliac artery. Most frequently, however, the obturator artery arises within the pelvic cavity as a branch of the internal iliac artery.

Next, study the disposition of the **peritoneum** within the pelvis (Fig. 16.2). Anteriorly, it covers the superior surface of the bladder. From the superior surface of the bladder, the peritoneum is reflected upward on each side onto the lateral wall of the pelvis. This portion of the peritoneum is sometimes called the **lateral false ligament of** the **bladder.** At the posterior border of the bladder, the peritoneum is reflected downward for a short distance over the posterior surface of the bladder and then upward onto the front of the rectum. Observe that here the rectum is covered only anteriorly by peritoneum. Slightly higher, it is covered anteriorly and on its sides. The **sigmoid colon,** which joins the rectum in front of the third

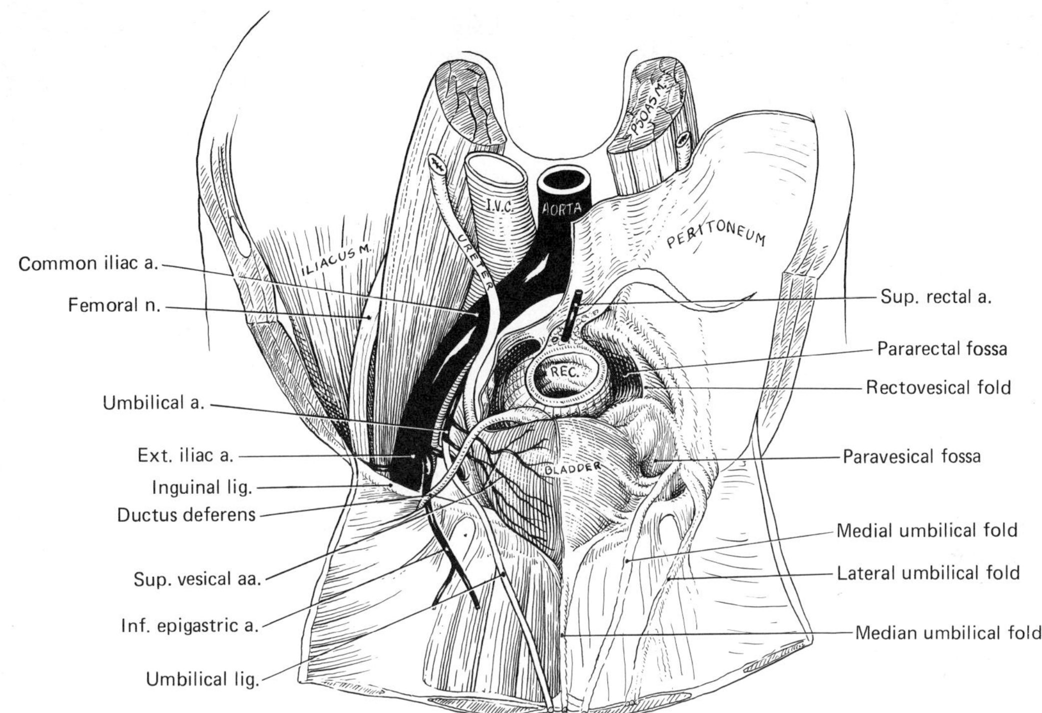

Figure 16.1 Male pelvis seen from above. The pelvic peritoneum has been removed on the right.

sacral vertebra, is completely intraperitoneal and is attached to the posterior left wall of the pelvis by the lower end of the **sigmoid mesocolon.**

The pelvic portion of the male peritoneal cavity is divided into **fossae** by **peritoneal folds** and **ridges** (Fig. 16.1). The **rectovesical** (**sacrogenital**) **folds** run horizontally from the posterior surface of the bladder backward and laterally toward the sacrum (Fig. 16.1). If the rectum and bladder are both contracted, these folds are usually visible with a sharp free margin within which, near the bladder, the seminal vesicles can be felt. Between the rectovesical fold and the rectum on either side is the **pararectal fossa.** The two pararectal fossae communicate with each other anterior to the rectum and posterior to the bladder at the **rectovesical peritoneal pouch.**

The peritoneum on the wall of the pelvis, anterior to the ureteral ridge and lateral to the upper surface of the bladder (i.e., the lateral false ligament of the bladder), forms the floor of the **paravesical peritoneal fossa,** which is especially evident when the bladder is distended. The ductus deferens can usually be seen through the peritoneum, crossing the paravesical fossa; when it reaches the rectovesical fold, it turns abruptly downward behind the bladder.

Remove and discard the peritoneum from the pelvic cavity except for the part that covers the superior surface of the bladder and the anterior surface of the rectum and the intervening rectovesical pouch.

Clean the **ductus deferens** (Fig. 16.1). It lies on the lateral pelvic wall external to the peritoneum and crosses, in turn, the superior vesical artery, the obturator nerve and vessels, and the ureter. From here it turns downward behind the bladder and enters the visceral pelvic fascia; its further course will be followed later.

Now clean the structures that occupy the extraperitoneal space by removing the fatty areolar tissue in which they are embedded. They are the

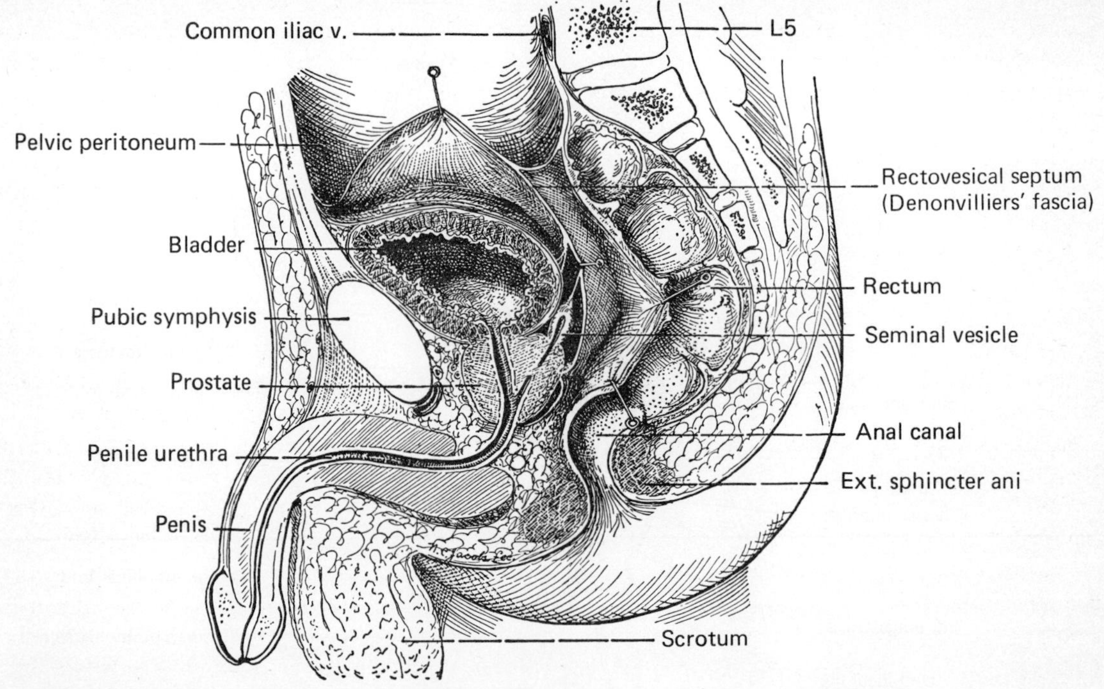

Figure 16.2 Sagittal section through the **male pelvis.** The rectum and its intrinsic fascia are retracted dorsally. The peritoneum over the bladder is lifted.

obturator vessels and nerve, the ureter, and the umbilical artery.

The **obturator nerve,** which you saw arising from the lumbar plexus, crosses the pelvic brim lateral to the common iliac vessels. It emerges from the medial side of the psoas major muscle behind the internal iliac artery and runs forward across the pelvic wall to enter the **obturator canal.** The **obturator artery** and **vein** enter the obturator canal just below the nerve. The parietal pelvic fascia is prolonged as a sheath for the obturator nerve and vessels through the obturator canal into the thigh.

Clean the pelvic portion of the **ureter.** It runs downward and forward in front of the internal iliac artery to the posterolateral angle of the bladder.

Distally, the **medial umbilical ligament** is a solid cord. Following it backward across the pelvic wall, observe that it becomes a patent artery, the **umbilical artery,** which springs from the **internal iliac artery,** of which it was, in the fetus, the original direct continuation. You will find two or three small vessels arising from it and passing to the bladder. They are the **superior vesical arteries** (Fig. 16.1).

Next, direct your attention to the **bladder.** It presents a **superior surface,** which is completely covered with peritoneum, a **posterior surface,** which is covered only on its upper part, and two **inferolateral surfaces,** which are devoid of peritoneum and abut the pelvic wall and pelvic diaphragm. The median umbilical ligament runs upward from the **apex of** the **bladder,** the point at which the superior and the two inferolateral surfaces meet. If you pull the apex upward and backward, the inferolateral surfaces will easily detach from the pelvic wall, exposing the **retropubic space,** which intervenes between the pelvic wall and the inferolateral surfaces of the bladder. This area is a potential rather than an actual space, since it is narrow and filled with fatty areolar tissue.

Its importance lies in the fact that an effusion of fluid into it, as from a rupture of the bladder, can spread laterally as far as the internal iliac arteries and upward into the extraperitoneal space at the sides of the pelvic and abdominal cavities.

As you turn the bladder upward and backward, you will see that its **neck** is firmly attached to the pelvic floor. The neck of the bladder is the region toward which the two inferolateral and the posterior surfaces converge. It lies immediately superior to the **prostate gland** (Fig. 16.2). After you remove the fatty areolar tissue from the retropubic space, you will see two white fascial bands running forward from the neck of the bladder to the inner surface of the body of the pubis, on each side of the pubic symphysis. They are the **anterior true ligaments of** the **bladder** or **puboprostatic ligaments** and represent thickenings of the visceral pelvic fascia. Clean the posterior surface of the bladder and observe its relationships. It lies above the prostate and is in direct contact with the anterior surfaces of the **seminal vesicles,** which separate its lower part from the **rectum.** The terminal portions of the **ductus deferentes** cross the posterior surface of the bladder along the medial borders of the seminal vesicles. The **ureter** joins the upper lateral angle of the bladder, where the posterior, superior, and inferolateral surfaces converge.

Before splitting the pelvis, attempt to define the line along which the pelvic diaphragm springs from the pelvic wall. Push the peritoneum of the pararectal fossae medially, open the retropubic space widely by displacing the bladder, and remove all the remaining fatty areolar tissue. The object of this dissection is to clean the upper surface of the lateral part of the pelvic diaphragm and the parietal pelvic fascia covering it.

Aided by reference to a bony pelvis, locate by touch the pelvic surface of the **ischial spine.** Find a tendinous fascial band running from the spine in a curve upward and forward to the lower border of the **obturator canal.** Anterior to the obturator canal, the same band turns downward and forward across the internal surface of the pubic bone as far as the anterior end of the **anterior true ligament of** the **bladder.** This band is the **arcus tendineus,** or tendinous arch, and is a thickened portion of the **obturator fascia.** It marks the line from the ischial spine to the obturator canal, along which the **pelvic diaphragm** (i.e., the levator ani and coccygeus muscles and the parietal pelvic fascia that covers them) arises from the obturator fascia; anterior to the obturator canal, the diaphragm arises directly from the internal surface of the pubic bone.

A helpful way to define the pelvic diaphragm and its attachment is to place one hand through the perineum into the ischiorectal fossa and the other hand into the pelvis from above. By gently pushing upward with the hand that is in the ischiorectal fossa, you can feel the thickness of the diaphragm, and at the same time the attachment along the tendinous arch is made more evident. Note that the obturator fascia is seen within the pelvis minor only posterior to the obturator canal. Here the fibers of the obturator internus muscle can usually be seen through the fascia, or if not, a portion of the fascia can be removed to expose them. It will also be apparent that the **pelvic diaphragm** does not stretch horizontally across the pelvis but runs downward and medially from each side, so that the diaphragm as a whole has roughly the shape of an inverted dome. That configuration explains the apparent contradiction that the inferior surface of the pelvic diaphragm forms the medial wall of the ischiorectal fossa.

Now split the pelvic viscera and skeleton into equal halves. Insert a probe, a director, or a catheter into the urethra and with a sharp knife bisect the corpus spongiosum penis by cutting to the instrument from both the dorsal and ventral surfaces. Cut through the midline of the pubic symphysis and extend the cut posteriorly through the pelvic viscera (bladder, prostate and rectum) to the sacrum. Sever one (right or left) pair of common iliac vessels at the level of the fourth lumbar vertebra. On the same side, divide the ureter near the renal pelvis and tie it to the testicular vessels, which you should also sever near their origins. Reflect the aorta and vena cava to one side and make a midline saw cut through the coccyx, sacrum, and lumbar vertebrae. Make a clean transverse cut (on the designated side) through the soft tissues above the iliac crest to the intervertebral disk between the third and fourth lumbar vertebrae. Remove the lower quadrant.

Dissect the peritoneum from the superior surface of the bladder and from the anterior surface of the rectum. Retract the peritoneum upward and note the **rectovesical fascial septum** (**rectogenital septum**) that extends from the pelvic peritoneum downward to the pelvic floor between the seminal vesicles and prostate anteriorly and the rectum posteriorly (Fig. 16.2). This condensation of visceral pelvic fascia is prolonged upward over the posterior surface of the prostate gland and, still higher, encloses the seminal vesicles.

Clean the **rectum** (inside and out) and observe that a considerable portion of it is entirely devoid of peritoneum, since it lies below the lowest part of the rectovesical peritoneal pouch. The rectum, which is about 12 cm long, curves along the ventral surface of the sacrum. The lowest part turns downward and backward (perineal flexure) at right angles to the upper part and passes through the pelvic diaphragm to join the **anal canal.** The **rectoanal junction** is at the pelvic diaphragm (Fig. 16.3). Externally, the rectum is rather nondescript. Internally, note the **transverse rectal folds** (three of them) that project inward toward the lumen in an alternating fashion.

A periodic rectal examination is essential in preventive and diagnostic medical care. A knowledge of the normal relationships of the pelvic viscera to the rectum is essential; only then can one identify pelvic abnormalities. What structures can be palpated through the rectum?

The **anal canal,** which is about 3 cm long, lies in the anal triangle of the perineum and ends at the **anus.** Attempt to demonstrate the **anal columns** that run longitudinally on the internal wall of the canal (Fig. 16.3). They represent folds of mucous membrane that overlie a **rectal venous plexus.** Distally, the vertical columns are joined together by the **anal valves,** semilunar-shaped folds of mucous membrane that enclose the **anal sinuses.** The scalloped line along the bases of the valves is called the **pectinate line.** Note that the mucous membrane is continuous with the skin of

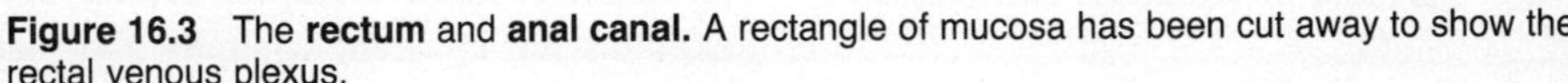

Figure 16.3 The **rectum** and **anal canal.** A rectangle of mucosa has been cut away to show the rectal venous plexus.

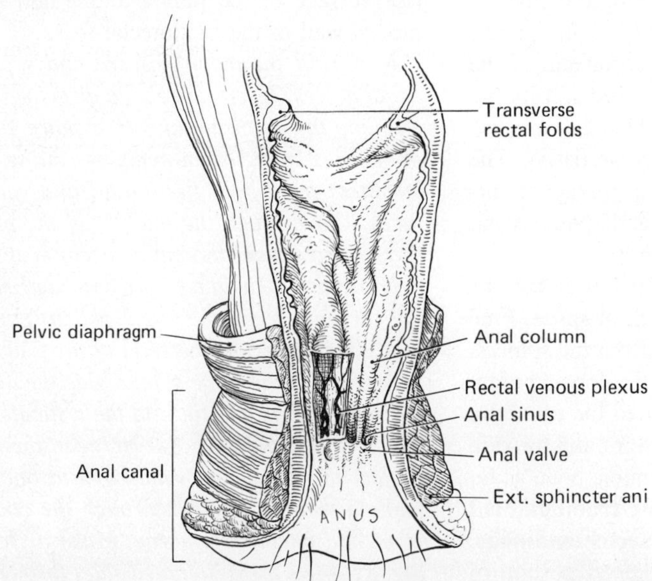

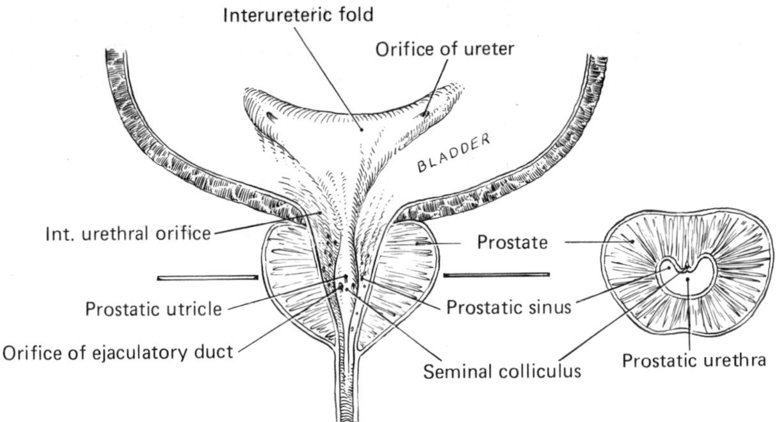

Figure 16.4 A frontal section through the **bladder** and **prostate** is shown on the left, and a cross section through the prostate and urethra at the level indicated is on the right.

the anus. The pectinate line marks the division of the anal canal with respect to blood supply (inferior mesenteric vs. internal iliac), venous drainage (portal vein vs. inferior vena cava), nerve supply (autonomic vs. somatic), and lymph drainage (internal iliac vs. inguinal).

Hemorrhoids (piles) are varicose masses of the rectal venous plexus. Internal hemorrhoids lie superior to the pectinate line, are covered by mucous membrane, and involve the superior rectal veins. External hemorrhoids lie below the pectinate line, involve the middle and inferior rectal veins, and are covered by skin. Anal infections are thought to be the primary cause of hemorrhoids. Poor venous return due to portal hypertension is also cited as a cause.

Trace the **superior rectal artery** downward along the posterior surface of the rectum. It divides into two main branches; one passes to each side of the rectum to anastomose with the right and left **middle rectal arteries,** which are branches of the internal iliac.

The **mucous membrane** lining the **bladder** is thrown into irregular folds over most of its surface when the bladder is empty. In the area known as the **vesical trigone,** however, the wall is always smooth. The vesical trigone is a triangular area corresponding to the lower portion of the posterior surface. It is bounded below by the **internal urethral orifice,** which is at the neck of the bladder leading downward into the first or prostatic portion of the urethra, and above on each side by the **ureteral orifice,** which appears slitlike (Fig. 16.4). Observe the **interureteric fold,** a transverse ridge extending between the two ureteral orifices. Pass a probe through one of these orifices into the ureter and observe that the ureter runs obliquely for some distance within the wall of the bladder before opening into its interior.

As the bladder wall stretches with filling or contracts when emptying, the ureteral orifices are compressed and closed, thus preventing reflux of urine.

Return to the posterior aspect of the bladder and attempt to demonstrate that each **seminal vesicle** is really a single, long, coiled tube that presents a lobulated appearance. At its lower medial angle, immediately above the prostate, this tube narrows to form the **excretory duct** of the seminal vesicle.

The **ductus deferens,** as it runs downward and medially along the medial border of the seminal vesicle, widens to form the **ampulla of** the **ductus deferens.** The ampulla terminates below by joining the **excretory duct of** the **seminal vesicle** to form the **ejaculatory duct.** The two ejaculatory ducts pass through the substance of the prostate gland to join the prostatic portion of the urethra.

Clean the **prostate.** Superiorly, it abuts the bladder. It rests upon the upper surface of the middle of the urogenital diaphragm, rather than, as you would expect, on the pelvic diaphragm. This is because the two levator ani muscles do not meet in the midline anteriorly, and the gap in the pelvic diaphragm between their free margins is closed below by the urogenital diaphragm. The prostate is enclosed in a strong **sheath** derived from the **visceral fascia.** Posteriorly, the fascia cannot easily be separated from the gland. Anteriorly and at the sides, the **prostatic plexus of veins** intervenes between the gland and its fascial covering. The deep dorsal vein of the penis drains into this plexus by passing beneath the pubic symphysis and above the anterior transverse perineal ligament of the urogenital diaphragm.

The prostate is traversed by the **first (prostatic) portion of** the **urethra.**

Enlargement of the prostate (median and lateral lobes) is common in older men. Compression of the urethra may cause difficulty in urinating, in which case the enlarged portion is removed.

If the entire course of the prostatic urethra is not exposed by the midline cut used to bisect the pelvic viscera, dissect that part of the prostate that still covers the prostatic urethra.

Observe the **urethral crest,** which is a median longitudinal ridge on the posterior wall of the prostatic urethra (Fig. 16.4). It is most prominent at about its middle, where it enlarges to form the **seminal colliculus.** At the summit of the colliculus, notice the orifice of a small blind pouch, the **prostatic utricle,** which runs backward for a varying distance into the substance of the prostate. Just below and to each side of the prostatic utricle are small terminal **orifices of** the **ejaculatory ducts.** The **ducts of** the **prostate gland** open by a number of minute orifices into troughs, the **prostatic sinuses,** on each side of the urethral crest; the orifices can often be made apparent by squeezing the prostate.

The **second** or **membranous portion of** the **urethra** traverses the urogenital diaphragm. It is short and narrower than the prostatic portion, and its wall presents no features of particular interest.

The **third** or **spongy portion of** the **urethra** is the longest of the three, traversing the whole length of the corpus spongiosum penis to terminate at the glans penis. The bulbourethral glands open into the spongy portion about 1.5 cm from its beginning. Its terminal portion, which is dilated in the glans, is the **fossa navicularis.**

Now pay particular attention to the internal iliac artery and its branches. The veins of the pelvis are numerous, often plexiform in character, and drain into the internal iliac vein. If they obscure the dissection, cut them away and discard them.

The **internal iliac artery,** as already seen, arises from the common iliac artery and runs down into the pelvis, crossing the pelvic brim opposite the sacroiliac articulation, where it lies medial to the external iliac vein and usually anterior to the internal iliac vein. It gives rise to **visceral** and **parietal branches.** The **visceral branches** are the umbilical, inferior vesical, and middle rectal; the **parietal branches** are the iliolumbar, lateral sacral, obturator, internal pudendal, and superior and inferior gluteal arteries. These branches are constant in their occurrence, but the manner in which they arise from the main trunk is subject to great variation. The **umbilical artery,** which you have already seen, may be regarded as the direct continuation of the main trunk. The superior gluteal, inferior gluteal, and internal pudendal arteries always arise in that order from above downward, but any two (frequently the inferior gluteal and internal pudendal) or all three may arise by a common stem. All other branches may arise directly from the internal iliac or indirectly by any combination of common stems. The iliolumbar and lateral sacral often arise in common with the superior gluteal. Identify the various branches and trace them as far as their course lies within the pelvis.

The **iliolumbar artery** runs upward and laterally to cross the pelvic brim external to the common iliac artery and vein, where it divides into iliac and lumbar branches. The iliac branch runs laterally behind the psoas major to enter the deep surface of the iliacus; the lumbar branch runs upward behind the psoas, supplying it and the quadratus lumborum.

The **lateral sacral artery** runs downward and medially over the anterior surface of the sacrum. There are frequently two lateral sacral arteries. The **superior gluteal artery** leaves the pelvis through the upper part of the greater sciatic foramen by passing between the lumbosacral trunk and the ventral ramus of the first sacral nerve. The **inferior gluteal** and **internal pudendal arteries** have a longer course in the pelvis, which they leave through the lower part of the greater sciatic foramen just above the spine of the ischium. The **obturator** has already been traced.

The inferior vesical and middle rectal arteries, which often arise in common, run medially through the fatty areolar tissue above the pelvic diaphragm. The **inferior vesical** supplies the lower part of the bladder and the prostate; the **middle rectal** reaches the side wall of the rectum, along which it sends branches to anastomose with the superior and inferior rectal arteries.

Reflect the pelvic viscera medially and clean the levator ani and coccygeus muscles of the pelvic diaphragm. Note the prominent **pelvic nerve plexus,** which represents the **inferior hypogastric plexuses** and subdivisions to the pelvic viscera. A major contribution to the nerve net is the **preganglionic parasympathetic fibers** (**pelvic splanchnic nerves**) derived from the second, third, and fourth sacral nerves. In addition, the pelvic plexus receives **preganglionic sympathetic fibers** from the superior hypogastric plexus through the **hypogastric nerves,** and from the lower lumbar segments of the spinal cord through the **lumbar** and **sacral splanchnic nerves,** which course via the lumbar and sacral sympathetic ganglia, respectively.

The parasympathetic components are particularly important in that they mediate the functions of urination, defecation, and erection. Besides their vasomotor effects, the sympathetics are thought to play a role in ejaculation.

The **levator ani** is a broad muscular sheet. Anterior to the obturator canal, it springs directly from the internal surface of the pubic bone; posterior to the obturator canal, it springs from the internal surface of the **obturator internus fascia** along a curved line (arcus tendineus) extending downward and backward to the spine of the ischium. Anteriorly, the muscle presents a free margin that passes backward and medially around the side of the prostate to join, behind the prostate and in front of the rectum, the muscle of the opposite side. More posteriorly, the levator ani inserts into the side of the rectum and, still more posteriorly, it passes behind the rectum to join the muscle of the opposite side. The most posterior fibers insert upon the coccyx. Its nerve supply is derived from the third and fourth sacral nerves; attempt to find them running forward on its superior surface.

The **coccygeus muscle** arises from the ischial spine and spreads out as it passes medially to insert on the coccyx and lower part of the sacrum. It is often more tendinous than muscular.

Observe that a portion of the parietal pelvic fascia covers the front of the sacrum above the coccygeus muscle. This is continuous on each side with the obturator fascia. The sacral nerves and the piriformis muscle lie external to it. The internal iliac artery and the beginning of its branches lie, as has been seen, internal to the parietal fascia. The parietal branches of the internal iliac pierce the parietal fascia as they leave the pelvis.

FEMALE PELVIS

Begin by reviewing the structures that create the peritoneal folds on the inside of the anterior abdominal wall (see page 139). The **median umbilical ligament** (fetal urachus) runs upward toward the umbilicus from behind the pubic symphysis (Fig. 16.5). Somewhat lateral to this on each side, also running toward the umbilicus, find the **medial umbilical ligament,** a cordlike structure that represents the fetal umbilical artery. Still more laterally, after crossing lateral to the inferior epigastric artery (the **lateral umbilical fold**), the **round**

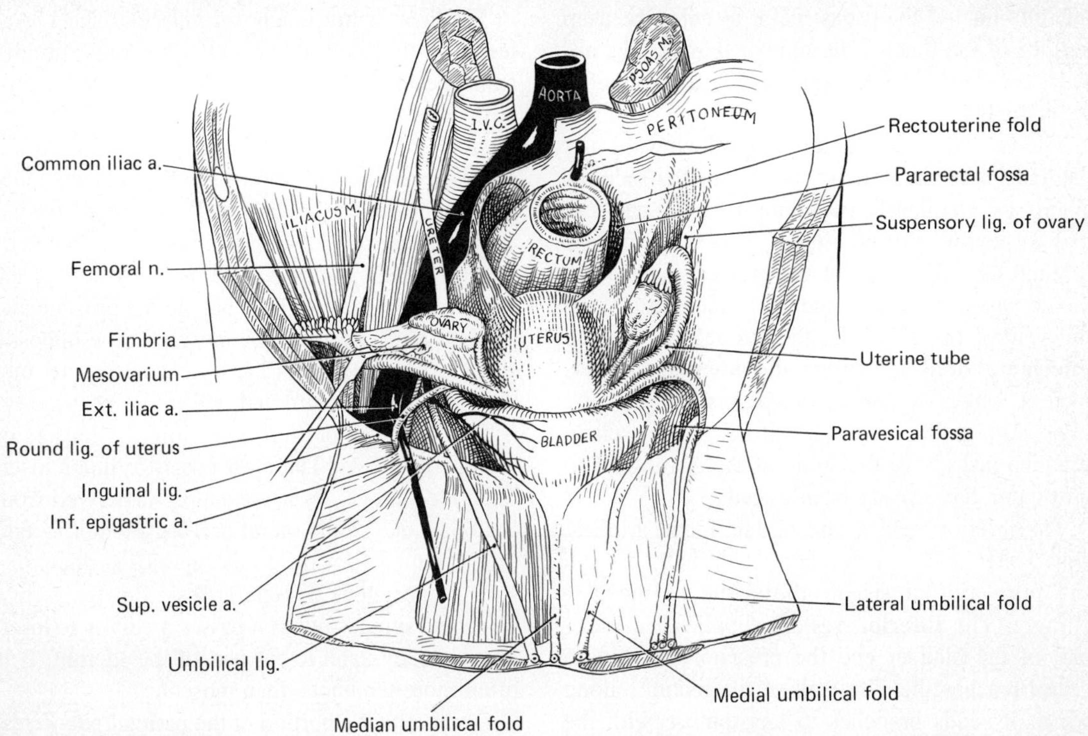

Figure 16.5 Female pelvis seen from above. The pelvic peritoneum has been removed on the right.

ligament of the **uterus** descends into the pelvis by crossing the external iliac artery and vein shortly before they pass behind the inguinal ligament. The **ureter** crosses the pelvic brim on each side at about the point where the common iliac arteries terminate. Here also the large **internal iliac artery** and **vein** descend into the pelvis. Identify the **middle sacral vessels** running downward anterior to the sacrum; slightly to their left the **superior rectal vessels** cross in front of the left common iliac vessels to run downward into the pelvis minor. An **obturator artery** can occasionally be found running downward across the pelvic brim slightly anterior to the round ligament. In such cases, it is an abnormal branch of either the inferior epigastric or the external iliac artery. Most frequently, however, the obturator artery arises within the pelvic cavity as a branch of the internal iliac artery. The **ovarian arteries** descend retroperitoneally to the pelvic brim. From here they turn medially, cross the external iliac vessels, and pass through peritoneal folds to the ovary.

Next, study the disposition of the **peritoneum** within the pelvis. Anteriorly, it covers the superior surface of the bladder. From the superior surface of the bladder, the peritoneum is reflected upward on each side onto the lateral wall of the pelvis. This portion of the peritoneum is sometimes called the **lateral false ligament of** the **bladder.** At the posterior border of the bladder, the peritoneum is reflected downward for a short distance over the posterior surface of the bladder and then upward onto the front of the **uterus,** thus forming the floor of a shallow fossa, the **vesicouterine pouch** (Fig. 16.6). Normally, the uterus is bent so that its anterior surface faces not only forward but also downward and overhangs the bladder. The **broad ligament** is the name given to the part of the peritoneum that clothes the uterus and that stretches on each side from the lateral border of the uterus to the lateral wall of the pelvis. Superiorly, it presents a free border in which the uterine tube is contained; at this border, the two layers of peritoneum that compose the broad ligament are continuous with each other. At its medial border, the broad ligament joins the lateral border of the uterus, and here its two layers of peritoneum are continuous with the peritoneum covering the anterior and posterior surfaces of the uterus. Along its lateral and inferior borders, the anterior and posterior peritoneal layers of the broad ligament are reflected anteriorly and posteriorly to become continuous with the peritoneum lining the pelvic wall and pelvic floor.

Projecting posteriorly from the lateral part of the broad ligament is a short peritoneal fold, the **mesovarium,** which supports the **ovary** (Fig. 16.5). The ovary is a small, oval body completely enclosed in peritoneum. The portion of the broad ligament that lies above the mesovarium and contains the uterine tube is known as the **mesosalpinx;** the portion below it is the **mesometrium.** As the ovarian vessels run downward and medially below the pelvic brim to reach the ovary, they cause a peritoneal fold in relation to the posterior surface of the lateral part of the broad ligament that is known as the **suspensory ligament of** the **ovary.** Notice another peritoneal fold projecting from the anterior surface of the broad ligament; the **round ligament of** the **uterus** is enclosed within it.

By carefully removing the posterior layer of the broad ligament, attempt to demonstrate the **epoophoron** and the **ligament of** the **ovary.** The former is a vestigial structure representing a part of the mesonephros of the embryo, which lies between the two layers of the peritoneum of the mesosalpinx. The ovarian ligament, also lying between the two layers of the peritoneum, is a band of smooth muscle and fibrous tissue that runs from the medial end of the ovary to the lateral border of the uterus.

The female pelvic peritoneal cavity is further subdivided into **fossae** by other **peritoneal folds.** The **rectouterine** (**sacrogenital**) **folds** pass backward and laterally from the lower part of the posterior surface of the uterus toward the sacrum and may be wholly or partially obliterated by distension of the bladder or rectum. Between the rectouterine folds and the rectum on each side is the **pararectal fossa.** The two pararectal fossae communicate with each other anterior to the rectum and posterior to the uterus, forming the **recto-uterine peritoneal pouch.** Since the peritoneum is carried downward below the lower border of the uterus onto the uppermost portion of the posterior surface of the vagina before being reflected backward and upward onto the front of the rectum, the lowest portion of the anterior wall of the recto-uterine pouch is formed by peritoneum on the vagina, not on the uterus (Fig. 16.6).

The peritoneum on the wall of the pelvis, anterior to the ureteral ridge and lateral to the upper surface of the bladder (i.e., the lateral false ligament of the bladder), forms the floor of the **paravesical peritoneal fossa,** which is especially evident when the bladder is distended.

At the upper lateral end of the broad ligament, the **uterine tube** usually turns downward and backward so that its **fimbriated end** spreads over the ovary (Fig. 16.5). The open end of this tube is the only place at which the peritoneal cavity is normally pierced. At the edges of this opening, the peritoneum becomes continuous with the mucous membrane lining the tube. Observe that the uterine tube joins the upper lateral angle of the uterus. Cut through the broad ligament on one side to expose the round ligament, which is attached to the uterus just below the uterine tube. Cut through the posterior layer of the broad ligament along the left lateral margin of the uterus to expose the **uterine artery.** It runs up along the lateral border of the uterus, to which it sends branches, accompanied by a plexus of veins. The uterine artery sends a few branches laterally through the broad ligament, toward the ovary, where they anastomose with the ovarian artery. The uterine artery may also send branches to the upper portion of the vagina.

Now clean the structures that occupy the extra-

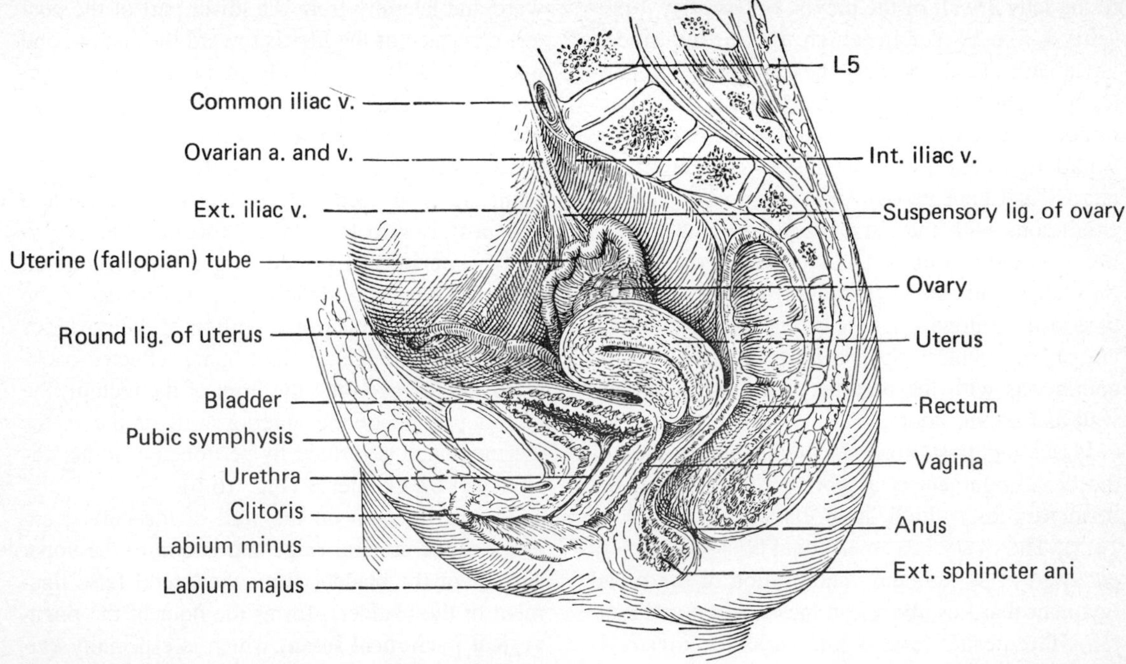

Figure 16.6 Midsagittal section through the **female pelvis.**

peritoneal space by removing the fatty areolar tissue in which they are embedded. They are the obturator vessels and nerve, the ureter, and the umbilical artery.

The **obturator nerve,** which you saw arising from the lumbar plexus, crosses the pelvic brim lateral to the common iliac vessels. It emerges from the medial side of the psoas major muscle behind the internal iliac artery and runs forward across the pelvic wall to enter the **obturator canal.** The **obturator artery** and **vein** enter the obturator canal just below the nerve. The parietal pelvic fascia is prolonged as a sheath for the obturator nerve and vessels through the obturator canal into the thigh.

Clean the pelvic portion of the **ureter.** It runs downward and forward in front of the internal iliac artery to the posterolateral angle of the bladder. The ureter crosses below the inferior border of the broad ligament to reach the upper lateral angle of the bladder. The uterine artery was seen running upward along the lateral border of the uterus; now follow it backward and laterally from the lower part of this border through the extraperitoneal space to the internal iliac artery. Note that the ureter passes inferior to the uterine artery.

Distally, the **medial umbilical ligament** is a solid cord. Following it backward across the pelvic wall, observe that it becomes a patent artery, the **umbilical artery,** springing from the **internal iliac artery,** of which it was, in the fetus, the original direct continuation. You will find two or three small vessels arising from it and passing to the bladder. They are the **superior vesical arteries** (Fig. 16.5).

Next, direct your attention to the **bladder.** It presents a **superior surface,** which is completely covered with peritoneum, a **posterior surface,** which is covered only on its upper part, and two **inferolateral surfaces,** which are devoid of peritoneum and abut the pelvic wall and pelvic diaphragm. The median umbilical ligament runs upward from the **apex of** the **bladder,** the point at which the superior and the two inferolateral surfaces meet. If you pull the apex upward and backward, the inferolateral surfaces will easily detach from the pelvic wall, exposing the **retropubic space,** which intervenes between the pelvic wall and the inferolateral surfaces of the bladder. This area is a potential rather than an actual space, since it is narrow and filled with fatty areolar tissue.

Its importance lies in the fact that an effusion of fluid into it, as from a rupture of the bladder, can spread laterally as far as the internal iliac arteries and upward into the extraperitoneal space at the sides of the pelvic and abdominal cavities.

As you turn the bladder upward and backward, you will see that its **neck** is firmly attached to the pelvic floor. The neck of the bladder is the region to which the two inferolateral and the posterior surfaces converge. It lies immediately superior to the urogenital diaphragm. After you remove the fatty areolar tissue from the retropubic space, you will see two white fascial bands running forward from the neck of the bladder to the inner surface of the body of the pubis, on each side of the pubic symphysis. They are the **anterior true ligaments of** the **bladder,** or **pubovesical ligaments,** and represent thickenings of the visceral pelvic fascia. Clean the posterior surface of the bladder and observe its relationships. It rests against the anterior wall of the **vagina,** except in its most superior part, where it is separated by peritoneum (vesicouterine pouch) from the lowest part of the anterior surface of the **uterus.** The **ureter** joins the upper lateral angle of the bladder, where the posterior, superior, and inferolateral surfaces converge.

Before splitting the pelvis, attempt to define the line along which the pelvic diaphragm springs from the pelvic wall. Push the peritoneum of the pararectal fossae medially, open the retropubic space widely by displacing the bladder, and remove all the remaining fatty areolar tissue. The object of this dissection is to clean the upper surface of the lateral part of the pelvic diaphragm and the parietal pelvic fascia covering it.

Aided by reference to a bony pelvis, locate by touch the pelvic surface of the **ischial spine.** Find a tendinous fascial band running from the spine in a curve upward and forward to the lower border of the **obturator canal.** Anterior to the obturator canal, the same band turns downward and forward across the internal surface of the pubic bone as far as the anterior end of the **anterior true ligament of** the **bladder.** This band is the **arcus tendineus,** or tendinous arch; it is a thickened portion of the **obturator fascia.** It marks the line from the ischial spine to the obturator canal, along which the **pelvic diaphragm** (i.e., the levator ani and coccygeus muscles and the parietal pelvic fascia that covers them) arises from the obturator fascia; anterior to the obturator canal, the diaphragm arises directly from the internal surface of the pubic bone.

A helpful way to define the pelvic diaphragm and its attachment is to place one hand through the perineum into the ischiorectal fossa and the other hand into the pelvis from above. By gently pushing upward with the hand that is in the ischiorectal fossa, you can feel the thickness of the diaphragm, and at the same time, the attachment along the tendinous arch is made more evident. Note that the obturator fascia is seen within the pelvis minor only posterior to the obturator canal. Here the fibers of the obturator internus muscle can usually be seen through the fascia, or if not, a portion of the fascia can be removed to expose them. It will also be apparent that the **pelvic diaphragm** does not stretch horizontally across the pelvis but runs downward and medially from each side, so that the diaphragm as a whole has roughly the shape of an inverted dome. That configuration explains the apparent contradiction that the inferior surface of the pelvic diaphragm forms the medial wall of the ischiorectal fossa.

Now split the pelvic viscera and skeleton into equal halves. Cut through the midline of the pubic symphysis and extend the cut posteriorly through the pelvic viscera (bladder, uterus, and rectum) to the sacrum. Sever one (right or left) pair of common iliac vessels at the level of the fourth lum-

bar vertebra. On the same side, divide the ureter near the renal pelvis and tie it to the ovarian vessels, which you should also sever near their origins. Reflect the aorta and vena cava to one side and make a midline saw cut through the coccyx, sacrum, and lumbar vertebrae. Make a clean transverse cut (on the designated side) through the soft tissues above the iliac crest to the intervertebral disk between the third and fourth lumbar vertebrae. Remove the lower quadrant.

Dissect the peritoneum from the superior surface of the uterus and from the anterior surface of the rectum. Retract the peritoneum upward and note the **rectovaginal fascial septum (rectogenital septum)**, which extends from the pelvic peritoneum downward to the pelvic floor between the vagina anteriorly and the rectum posteriorly (Fig. 16.6). This condensation of visceral pelvic fascia is prolonged upward over the posterior surface of the vagina and still higher onto the wall of the uterus.

Clean the **rectum** (inside and out) and observe that a considerable portion of it is entirely devoid of peritoneum, since it lies below the lowest part of the rectouterine peritoneal pouch. The rectum, which is about 12 cm long, curves along the ventral surface of the sacrum. The lowest part turns downward and backward (perineal flexure) at right angles to the upper part and passes through the pelvic diaphragm to join the **anal canal.** The **rectoanal junction** is at the pelvic diaphragm (Fig. 16.3). Externally, the rectum is rather nondescript. Internally, note the **transverse rectal folds** (three of them) that project inward toward the lumen in an alternating fashion.

A periodic rectal examination is essential in preventive and diagnostic medical care. A knowledge of the normal relationships of the pelvic viscera to the rectum is essential; only then can one identify pelvic abnormalities. What structures can be palpated through the rectum?

The **anal canal,** which is about 3 cm long, lies in the anal triangle of the perineum and ends at the **anus.** Attempt to demonstrate the **anal columns** that run longitudinally on the internal wall of the canal (Fig. 16.3). They represent folds of mucous membrane that overlie a **rectal venous plexus.** Distally, the vertical columns are joined together by the **anal valves,** semilunar-shaped folds of mucous membrane that enclose the **anal sinuses.** The scalloped line along the bases of the valves is called the **pectinate line.** Note that the mucous membrane is continuous with the skin of the anus. The pectinate line marks the division of the anal canal with respect to blood supply (inferior mesenteric vs. internal iliac), venous drainage (portal vein vs. inferior vena cava), nerve supply (autonomic vs. somatic), and lymph drainage (internal iliac vs. inguinal).

Hemorrhoids (piles) are varicose masses of the rectal venous plexus. Internal hemorrhoids lie superior to the pectinate line, are covered by mucous membrane, and involve the superior rectal veins. External hemorrhoids lie below the pectinate line, involve the middle and inferior rectal veins, and are covered by skin. Anal infections are thought to be the primary cause of hemorrhoids. Pregnancy and poor venous return due to portal hypertension are also cited as causes.

Trace the **superior rectal artery** downward along the posterior surface of the rectum. It divides into two main branches; one passes to each side of the rectum to anastomose with the right and left **middle rectal arteries,** which are branches of the internal iliac.

The **mucous membrane** lining the **bladder** is thrown into irregular folds over most of its surface when the bladder is empty. In the area known as the **vesical trigone,** however, the wall is always smooth. The vesical trigone is a triangular area corresponding to the lower portion of the posterior surface. It is bounded below by the **internal urethral orifice,** which is at the neck of the bladder leading downward into the urethra, and above on each side by the **ureteral orifice,** which appears slitlike (Fig. 16.4). Observe the **interureteric fold,** a transverse ridge extending between the two ureteral orifices. Pass a probe through one of these orifices into the ureter and observe that the ureter runs obliquely for some distance within the wall of the bladder before opening into its interior.

As the bladder wall stretches with filling or contracts when emptying, the ureteral orifices are compressed and closed, thus preventing reflux of urine.

The female **urethra** is a short, fibromuscular canal that lies immediately anterior to the vagina and ends below in the vestibule. It corresponds to the portion of the male prostatic urethra that lies above the opening of the prostatic utricle.

Now pay particular attention to the internal iliac artery and its branches. The veins of the pelvis are numerous, often plexiform in character, and drain into the internal iliac vein. If they obscure the dissection, cut them away and discard them.

The **internal iliac artery,** as already seen, arises from the common iliac artery and runs down into the pelvis, crossing the pelvic brim opposite the sacroiliac articulation, where it lies medial to the external iliac vein and usually anterior to the internal iliac vein. It gives rise to **visceral** and **parietal branches.** The **visceral branches** are the umbilical, inferior vesical, middle rectal, and uterine arteries; the **parietal branches** are the iliolumbar, lateral sacral, obturator, internal pudendal, and superior and inferior gluteal arteries. These branches are constant in their occurrence, but the manner in which they arise from the main trunk is subject to great variation. The **umbilical artery,** which you have already seen, may be regarded as the direct continuation of the main trunk. The superior gluteal, inferior gluteal, and internal pudendal arteries always arise in that order from above downward, but any two (frequently the inferior gluteal and internal pudendal) or all three may arise by a common stem. All other branches may arise directly from the internal iliac or indirectly by any combination of common stems. The iliolumbar and lateral sacral often arise in common with the superior gluteal. Identify the various branches and trace them as far as their course lies within the pelvis.

The **iliolumbar artery** runs upward and laterally to cross the pelvic brim external to the common iliac artery and vein, where it divides into iliac and lumbar branches. The iliac branch runs laterally behind the psoas major to enter the deep surface of the iliacus; the lumbar branch runs upward behind the psoas, supplying it and the quadratus lumborum.

The **lateral sacral artery** runs downward and medially over the anterior surface of the sacrum. There are frequently two lateral sacral arteries. The **superior gluteal artery** leaves the pelvis through the upper part of the greater sciatic foramen by passing between the lumbosacral trunk and the ventral ramus of the first sacral nerve. The **inferior gluteal** and **internal pudendal arteries** have a longer course in the pelvis, which they leave through the lower part of the greater sciatic foramen just above the spine of the ischium. The **obturator** has already been traced.

The inferior vesical and middle rectal arteries, which often arise in common, run medially through the fatty areolar tissue above the pelvic diaphragm. The **inferior vesical** supplies the lower part of the bladder (and occasionally the vagina); the **middle rectal** reaches the side wall of the rectum, along which it sends branches to anastomose with the superior and inferior rectals.

Draw the bladder forward and separate its posterior surface from the anterior surface of the **vagina,** to which it is loosely attached. At the same time, separate the posterior surface of the urethra from the vagina. Study the interior wall of the vagina. It is a wide canal whose anterior and posterior surfaces usually touch. Observe the **rugae vaginales,** transverse ridges found on both walls. Observe that the **cervix** of the uterus projects downward into the upper part of the vagina, into which it opens by a small circular or oval aperture, the **uterine ostium.** The portions of the vaginal canal that extend upward, anterior and posterior to the ostium, are known as the **anterior** and **posterior fornices of** the **vagina.**

The digital vaginal examination is important in identifying pelvic visceral abnormalities. Through the vagina, one can palpate the bladder, rectum, ureters, and cervix. With the other hand on the abdominal wall (bimanual palpation), the uterus and sometimes the ovaries can also be felt.

The **uterus** is a pear-shaped organ with thick, muscular walls. The uppermost, rounded portion of the uterus is called the **fundus.** The **body** is the segment that extends from the opening of the uterine tubes downward toward the cervix. The constricted portion between the body and the cervix is called the **isthmus.** The lining of the cervical canal is usually thrown into folds, while the lumen of the body has a smooth lining.

Reflect the pelvic viscera medially and clean the levator ani and coccygeus muscles of the pelvic diaphragm. Note the prominent **pelvic nerve plexus,** which represents the **inferior hypogastric plexuses** and subdivisions to the pelvic viscera. A major contribution to the nerve net is the **preganglionic parasympathetic fibers** (**pelvic splanchnic nerves**) derived from the second, third, and fourth sacral nerves. In addition, the pelvic plexus receives **preganglionic sympathetic fibers** from the superior hypogastric plexus through the **hypogastric nerves** and from the lower lumbar segments of the spinal cord through the **lumbar** and **sacral splanchnic nerves,** which course via the lumbar and sacral sympathetic ganglia, respectively.

The parasympathetic components are particularly important in that they mediate the functions of urination, defecation, and erection.

The **levator ani** is a broad muscular sheet. Anterior to the obturator canal, it springs directly from the internal surface of the pubic bone; posterior to the obturator canal, it springs from the internal surface of the **obturator internus fascia** along a curved line (arcus tendineus) extending downward and backward to the spine of the ischium. Anteriorly, the muscle presents a free margin that passes backward and medially around the side of the vagina and urethra to join, in front of the rectum, the muscle of the opposite side. More posteriorly, the levator ani inserts into the side of the rectum and, still more posteriorly, it passes behind the rectum to join the muscle of the opposite side. The most posterior fibers insert upon the coccyx. Its nerve supply is derived from the third and fourth sacral nerves; attempt to find them running forward on its superior surface.

The **coccygeus muscle** arises from the ischial spine and spreads out as it passes medially to insert on the coccyx and lower part of the sacrum. It is often more tendinous than muscular.

Observe that a portion of the parietal pelvic fascia covers the front of the sacrum above the coccygeus muscle. This is continuous on each side with the obturator fascia. The sacral nerves and the piriformis muscle lie external to it. The internal iliac artery and the beginning of its branches lie, as has been seen, internal to the parietal fascia. The parietal branches of the internal iliac pierce the parietal fascia as they leave the pelvis.

Chapter 17

Superior Extremity

SURFACE ANATOMY

The superior extremity consists of the shoulder (deltoid and scapular regions), arm (brachium), forearm (antebrachium), wrist (carpus), and hand (manus). Each region has an anterior (ventral) flexor surface and a posterior (dorsal) extensor surface.

Certain bony landmarks should be identified before the skin is reflected. The **humerus** is mostly covered by muscle except distally, where the **lateral** and **medial epicondyles** form the subcutaneous bony prominences on each side of the elbow. The broad bony prominence at the back of the elbow is the **olecranon process of** the **ulna.** Continuing into the forearm from the olecranon, the dorsal border of the **ulna** is subcutaneous throughout its length. It ends on the dorsomedial aspect of the wrist in the **styloid process of** the **ulna.** The **radius** is lateral and deeper, but its distal portion can usually be easily felt through the thin muscles and tendons that cover it. The bony projection at the lateral side of the wrist is the **styloid process of** the **radius.**

When the pectoral region was dissected, an incision was made in the skin on the anterior aspect of the arm a little below the shoulder. Make this incision circle the arm at this level (Fig. 17.1). Then make a median longitudinal incision through the skin on the anterior aspect of the arm and the forearm, extending from the upper transverse incision distally to the front of the wrist. Make two transverse incisions, one across the front of the wrist from the medial to the lateral border, and another in front of the elbow from the medial to the lateral epicondyle. This will mark out four skin flaps on the arm and forearm; reflect them medially and laterally. Then, starting at the upper

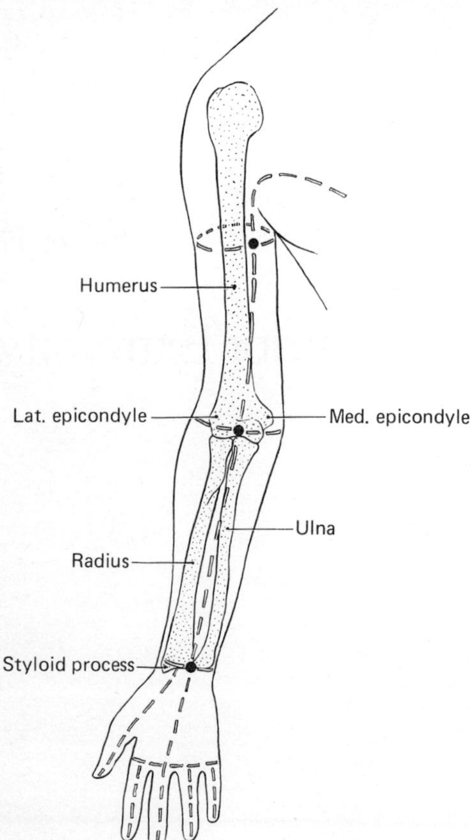

Figure 17.1 Surface landmarks and skin incisions on the superior extremity.

transverse incision on the back of the arm, reflect the skin off the back of the arm and forearm. The skin of the arm and forearm, reflected in a single piece, remains attached only at the back of the wrist, where it is still continuous with the skin of the hand.

Now reflect the skin from the hand by the following incisions: (1) a median longitudinal incision through the skin of the palm from the middle of the transverse incision already made across the wrist to the tip of the middle finger; (2) a transverse incision across the palm at the proximal ends of the fingers; (3) an oblique incision from the middle of the front of the wrist to the tip of the thumb; (4) longitudinal incisions, from incision 2, distally along the middle of the palmar surfaces of the index, ring, and little fingers to their tips. Starting with these incisions, reflect the skin from the hand and fingers, and remove it completely from the extremity.

CUTANEOUS VEINS AND NERVES

The **superficial veins** of the upper extremity are numerous and variable (Fig. 17.2). They often may be seen better in the living arm than in that of the cadaver. The two largest and most constant are the **cephalic vein** and the **basilic vein.** They begin at the lateral (radial) and medial (ulnar) sides, respectively, of a **venous arch** on the **dorsum of the hand.** Find the **cephalic vein** at the **lateral** side of the **wrist** and trace it upward through the superficial fascia along the **lateral** side of the anterior aspect of the **forearm.** Passing in front of the lateral side of the elbow, it ascends on the **lateral** aspect of the **arm.** The last part of its course is in the groove between the pectoralis major and deltoid muscles (the deltopectoral triangle) where the cephalic vein pierces the clavipectoral fascia to terminate in the **axillary vein.** The **basilic vein** ascends along the **medial** border of the **forearm** and crosses in front of the medial side of the elbow to reach the **medial** aspect of the **arm.** At the middle of the arm, it pierces the deep fascia to join the **deep veins** (venae comitantes), which accompany the **brachial artery.** The **median cubital vein** (extremely variable) is a large connecting channel usually present in front of the elbow running upward and medially from the **cephalic vein** to the **basilic vein.**

Due to their large size and superficial location, these veins are the most frequently used sites for withdrawing blood and for injecting various substances into the venous system.

Clean and study the **cutaneous nerves** of the arm, forearm, and hand (Fig. 17.3). First identify the nerves on the anterior aspect of the extremity

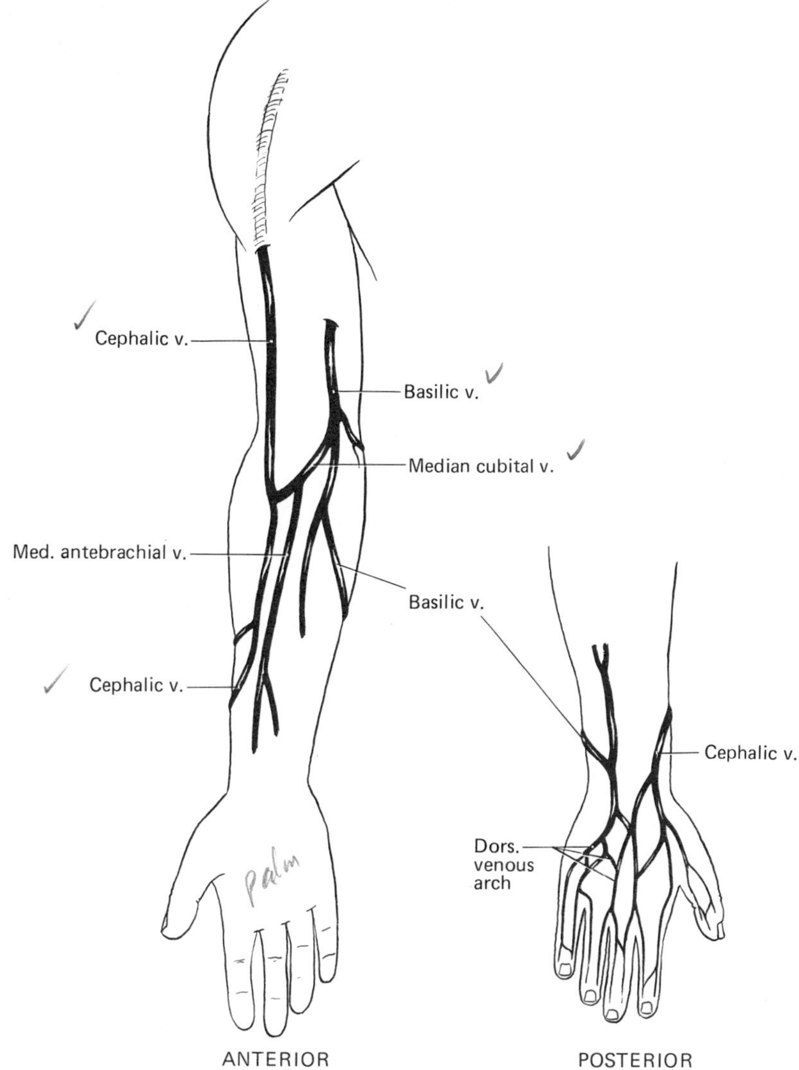

Figure 17.2 Primary **superficial veins** of the superior extremity.

at the points where they pierce the deep fascia; trace their distribution. Remove the superficial fascia as the nerves are cleaned.

A thorough knowledge of the cutaneous nerve distribution and of the spinal cord segments involved (dermatome pattern) is essential when the diagnostician tests for nervous system injury.

The origins of the **medial brachial** and **antebrachial cutaneous nerves** from the brachial plexus have been seen. The **medial brachial cutaneous nerve** pierces the deep fascia at about the middle of the medial aspect of the arm, just medial to the terminal part of the basilic vein. It descends on the medial side of the arm and, just above the

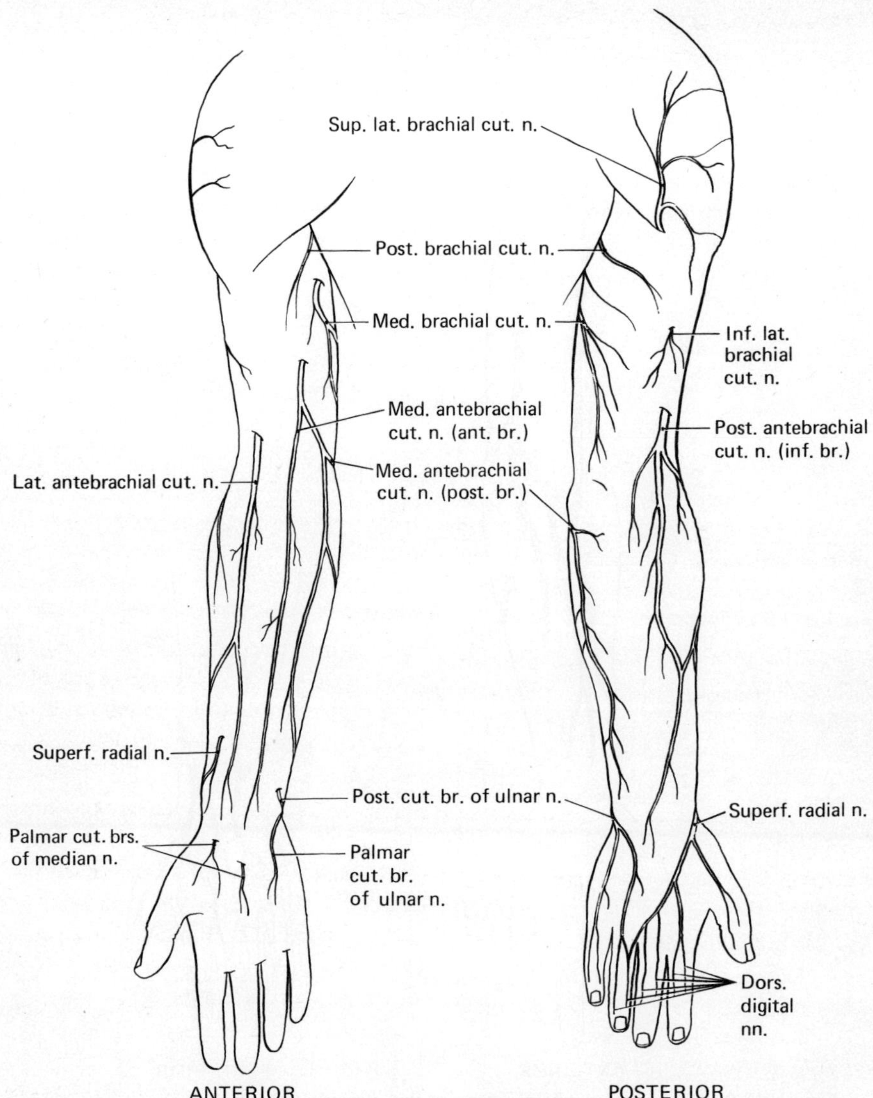

Figure 17.3 Cutaneous nerves of the superior extremity.

elbow, turns posteriorly to supply the skin over the olecranon. The **medial antebrachial cutaneous nerve** pierces the deep fascia slightly lower in the arm and lies just lateral to the basilic vein. It divides into **anterior** and **posterior branches:** both descend to supply the skin on the anteromedial and posteromedial aspects of the forearm as far as the wrist.

The **lateral antebrachial cutaneous nerve** is the direct continuation of the **musculocutaneous nerve.** It pierces the deep fascia on the anterolateral aspect of the arm a short distance above the elbow, close to the cephalic vein. It is distributed to the skin on the lateral and anterolateral aspects of the forearm as far down as the base of the thumb.

Turn to the posterior surface of the arm and identify the **posterior brachial cutaneous nerve,** which is given off in the axilla by the **radial nerve.** It pierces the deep fascia on the posteromedial aspect of the arm slightly inferior to the posterior border of the deltoid muscle and is distributed to the skin on the back of the arm below the deltoid. The **superior lateral brachial cutaneous nerve** is a branch of the **axillary nerve;** it pierces the deep fascia at about the middle of the posterior border of the deltoid and runs upward and laterally to supply the skin covering the lower half of that muscle.

The **posterior antebrachial cutaneous nerve** is a branch of the **radial nerve;** its two terminal branches usually pierce the deep fascia on the dorsolateral aspect of the arm separately. The **superior branch** (inferior lateral brachial cutaneous nerve) is relatively small; it appears about 5 cm above the lateral epicondyle and is distributed to the lower half of the lateral and anterolateral aspects of the arm. The **inferior branch** is large; it emerges slightly below the superior branch and descends posterior to the lateral epicondyle to supply the skin on the back of the forearm as far as the wrist.

Clean the **cutaneous nerves** on the **dorsum of** the **hand.** The **superficial radial nerve** emerges from under the lateral border of the brachioradialis muscle and winds dorsally around the lateral side of the distal forearm just proximal to the wrist. Reaching the lateral side of the dorsum of the wrist, it divides into branches that supply the skin on the lateral half of the dorsum of the hand, the dorsal surface of the thumb, and the dorsal surfaces of the index, middle, and lateral side of the ring fingers to the **distal interphalangeal joints.** The **posterior cutaneous branch of** the **ulnar nerve** is found winding dorsally around the medial border of the wrist to be distributed to the skin on the medial half of the dorsal surfaces of the hand, the little finger, and the medial side of the ring finger. The cutaneous nerves on the palmar surface of the hand and fingers will be studied as a dissection of those regions is done.

DELTOID REGION

Clean the **deltoid,** the large, thick, triangular muscle that forms the fleshy prominence of the shoulder. It arises from the anterior superior border of the lateral third of the **clavicle,** from the superior lateral surface of the **acromion,** and by an aponeurosis from the **spine of** the **scapula.** Its fibers converge laterally and inferiorly to form a strong tendon that is inserted into the **deltoid tuberosity of** the **humerus** between the brachialis and the lateral head of the triceps.

Cut the deltoid from its origin and reflect it downward and laterally toward its insertion. Do this carefully to avoid injuring the **axillary nerve** and the **posterior humeral circumflex artery,** which ramify on its deep surface (Fig. 17.4).

Now return to the axilla (Figs. 2.2 and 3.2). Review the **brachial plexus,** the **axillary artery,** and their branches. Remove any traces of axillary fat. Identify the insertion of the **pectoralis minor** on the upper medial border of the **coracoid process of** the **scapula.** Clean the **common tendon of** origin of the **coracobrachialis** and the **short head of** the **biceps brachii** at the tip of the **coracoid process** and follow them into the arm (Fig. 17.5). Observe that they separate from each other lateral to the coracoid process, the coracobrachialis lying medial to the biceps. The **long head of** the **biceps,** here narrow and tendinous, emerges from under the anterior border of the deltoid to join the short head on its lateral side. The proximal portions of these muscles rest deeply against the anterior aspect of the humerus and are embraced anteriorly by the tendon of insertion of the pectoralis major and posteriorly by the tendons of the latissimus dorsi and the teres major muscles.

SCAPULAR REGION

With the cadaver on its stomach, define and clean the infraspinatus, teres minor, and teres major muscles and the upper part of the long head of the triceps brachii, all of which were partially covered by the posterior part of the deltoid (Fig. 17.4).

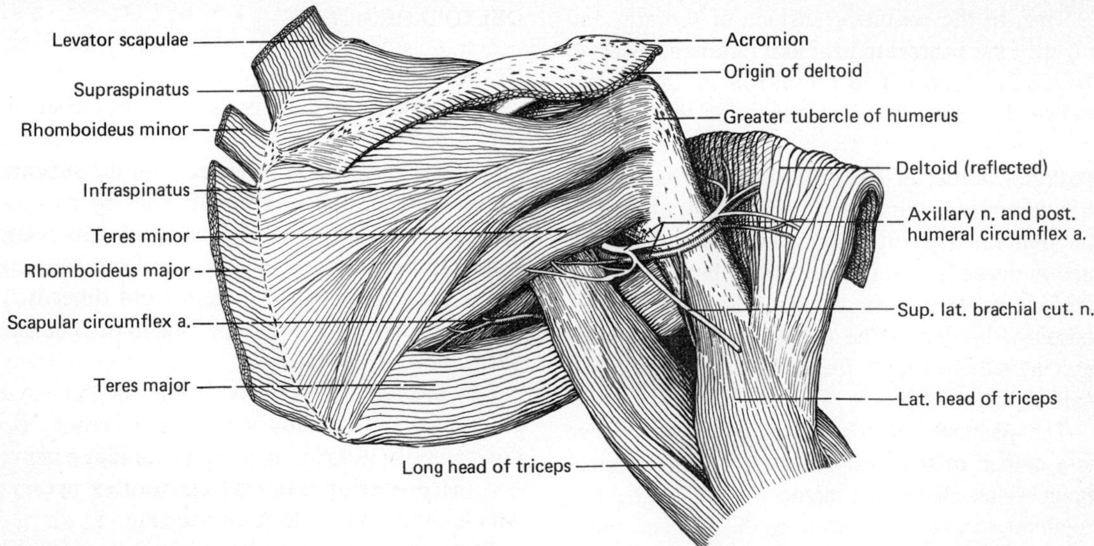

Figure 17.4 Posterior aspect of the **shoulder region** after reflection of the deltoid.

The **infraspinatus** occupies the **infraspinous fossa** of the scapula. It arises from the medial part of this fossa and, to some extent, from the layer of deep fascia that covers its outer surface. Its fibers converge laterally to form a strong, flat tendon that is closely attached to the posterior part of the capsule of the shoulder joint and is inserted on the **middle facet of** the **greater tubercle of** the **humerus.** The **teres minor** is a small muscle, often fused to the infraspinatus, below which it lies. It arises from the middle portion of the **axillary border of** the **infraspinous fossa;** its fibers extend laterally to form a tendon that crosses the lower posterior part of the capsule of the shoulder joint to insert on the **lowest facet of** the **greater tubercle of** the **humerus.** The origin of the **long head of** the **triceps** is covered posteriorly by the teres minor. Arising from the **infraglenoid tubercle** of the scapula, it descends in front of the teres minor and behind the teres major to reach the back of the arm. The **teres major** is a rounded, fleshy muscle that arises from the lower part of the **axillary border of** the **infraspinous fossa** and extends laterally, passing in front of the long head of the triceps, to reach the anterior aspect of the humerus. It inserts into the **crest of** the **lesser tubercle,** under cover of the coracobrachialis muscle and the tendon of insertion of the latissimus dorsi.

Clean the **coracoacromial ligament** (Fig. 17.5). This is a strong fibrous band that arches above the shoulder joint from the lateral border of the **coracoid process** to the tip of the **acromion;** it is wider at its coracoid than at its acromial attachment. Open the **subacromial bursa.** This large (synovial) bursa lies between the acromion and the coracoacromial ligament, and the muscles that cover the upper part of the shoulder joint. The subacromial bursa usually extends laterally between the deltoid muscle and the muscles attached to the capsule of the shoulder joint, where it is called the **subdeltoid bursa.**

Clean the **supraspinatus muscle** (Fig. 17.4). The supraspinatus occupies the **supraspinous fossa** and takes origin from its medial two-thirds. Extending laterally to pass below the acromion and the coracoacromial ligament, the muscle fibers join a strong, flat tendon, which is closely bound to the highest part of the capsule of the shoulder joint and inserts into the **highest facet on** the **greater tubercle of** the **humerus.**

The supraspinatus tendon is frequently torn in old people and in those involved in strenuous work. Moving the shoulder joint then becomes extremely painful, and the arm is nearly impossible to abduct without using compensating movements.

Draw the superior border of the supraspinatus backward to expose the superior border of the scapula. Clean the **superior transverse ligament** of the scapula. This strong, fibrous band converts the **scapular notch** in the superior border of the scapula into a foramen. Observe that the **suprascapular nerve,** whose origin from the upper trunk of the brachial plexus has already been seen, passes **through** this foramen to enter the supraspinous fossa. The **suprascapular artery** passes **above** the ligament to enter the supraspinous fossa close to the nerve (Fig. 17.5).

Divide the supraspinatus slightly lateral to the scapular notch by an incision at right angles to the direction of its fibers. Reflect the medial segment of the muscle backward and medially and follow the course of the suprascapular nerve. Observe that it runs inferiorly through the supraspinous fossa close to the bone, giving twigs of supply to the supraspinatus, and then passes through the **great scapular notch** to enter the infraspinous fossa. Attempt to define the **inferior transverse ligament.** This fibrous band, not as well defined as the superior ligament, converts the medial part of the great scapular notch into a foramen through which both the **suprascapular nerve** and the **suprascapular artery** pass.

Divide the infraspinatus about 4 cm medial to its insertion and reflect the medial segment backward and medially from the bony surface of the infraspinous fossa. Observe that the **suprascapular nerve** terminates in twigs that supply the **infraspinatus.** The **suprascapular artery** is also distributed to the **supraspinatus** and **infraspinatus muscles.** It clearly enters into anastomoses near the axillary border of the scapula with terminal branches of the **scapular circumflex artery.** The teres minor should also be dissected free from the adjacent structures and transected to expose the origin of the **long head of** the **triceps.** Observe that at its origin the long head lies between the teres minor and the lower part of the subscapularis.

The **axillary nerve** has already been seen to arise as a branch of the **posterior cord of** the **brachial plexus** within the axilla, which it leaves by passing between the adjacent borders of the subscapularis and teres major muscles in company with the **posterior humeral circumflex branch of** the **axillary artery.** The nerve and artery will now be found reaching the back of the shoulder region by passing through a small **quadrangular space** bounded by the lower border of the **teres minor,** the upper border of the **teres major,** the lateral margin of the **long head of** the **triceps,** and the medial aspect of the **surgical neck of** the **humerus.** Note that the teres minor lies immediately behind the lower part of the subscapularis. Clean the entire course of the axillary nerve and the posterior humeral circumflex artery (Fig. 17.4).

The **axillary nerve,** soon after it reaches the back of the shoulder, separates into a superior and an inferior division. The **superior division** is distributed entirely to the **deltoid muscle,** entering the deep surface of the muscle. The **inferior division** gives rise to a branch that supplies the **teres minor** and a few twigs to the deltoid. It ends as the **superior lateral brachial cutaneous nerve,** which winds around the posterior border of the deltoid to reach the skin covering the muscle. The largest branches of the **posterior humeral circumflex artery** accompany the branches of the superior division of the axillary nerve into the **deltoid.** A small branch winds anteriorly around the lateral side of the neck of the humerus to anastomose with the **anterior humeral circumflex artery.**

The origin of the **scapular circumflex artery** as a branch of the subscapular artery in the axilla has already been seen. It leaves the axilla by passing between the adjacent borders of the subscapularis and the teres major. It may now be seen passing through the **triangular space** bounded by the teres minor, the teres major, and the long head of the triceps (Fig. 17.4). It is distributed to the muscles near the axillary border of the scapula.

SUBSCAPULAR REGION

Turn to the anterior aspect of the shoulder region and clean the **subscapularis** (Fig. 17.5). This wide, thick muscle takes origin from the entire **subscapular fossa.** Stretching laterally across the front of the shoulder joint, the muscle narrows toward its insertion on the **lesser tubercle of** the **humerus.** Its tendon of insertion passes below the coracoid process and behind the common origin of the coracobrachialis and the short head of the biceps. The subscapularis is supplied by the **upper subscapular nerve** and by twigs from the **lower subscapular nerve.** The latter nerve is distributed principally to the **teres major.** Draw the upper border of the subscapularis forward and downward and open the **subscapular bursa.** This large synovial bursa lies between the deep surface of the **subscapularis** and the inner surface of the **scapula** near the glenoid border; it communicates laterally with the synovial cavity of the shoulder joint.

Clean the anterior surface of the teres major and the tendon of insertion of the latissimus dorsi, if this has not already been done, and examine the manner of insertion of these muscles. Observe that the tendon of the **latissimus dorsi** winds upward over the anterior surface of the teres major to insert into the **floor of** the **intertubercular sulcus,** while the **teres major** inserts into the **crest of** the **lesser tubercle.** Both insertions lie deep to the coracobrachialis and the biceps. The tendon of insertion of the **pectoralis major** should also be cleaned. It crosses in front of the coracobrachialis and the biceps to insert into the **crest of** the **greater tubercle** under cover of the anterior border of the deltoid (Fig. 17.5).

FLEXOR REGION OF THE ARM

Clean the **coracobrachialis** to its insertion. Be careful not to damage the brachial artery or the median nerve crossing its surface. The coracobrachialis is a bandlike muscle extending almost straight downward from its origin to insert into the **medial surface of** the **humerus** above the middle of the shaft. It is partially overlapped on its lateral side by the biceps. Observe that the **musculocutaneous nerve,** which arises from the lateral cord of the brachial plexus, enters the medial border of the muscle and passes obliquely downward through its substance to emerge under cover of the biceps. The coracobrachialis is supplied by a branch of the musculocutaneous nerve, which arises proximal to the point where the main trunk enters the muscle.

Clean the **biceps brachii muscle.** The origin of its **short head** has already been seen. The **long head** arises within the capsule of the shoulder joint from the **supraglenoid tubercle of** the **scapula.** Its round tendon emerges from the capsule and descends in the **intertubercular sulcus** to join the short head. The tendon is held in the sulcus by the **transverse humeral ligament,** which passes from the lesser to the greater tubercle of the humerus (Fig. 17.5). The fusiform belly of the biceps narrows to a strong tendon that enters the cubital fossa, where its insertion on the **tuberosity of** the **radius** will be seen more satisfactorily later. While cleaning the distal part of the biceps, note the **bicipital aponeurosis.** This thickened, fibrous band passes from the distal part of the medial border of the biceps medially and distally to join the deep fascia on the proximal part of the medial side of the forearm. Draw the biceps forward and secure its nerve supply from the **musculocutaneous nerve** (Fig. 17.5).

Emerging from the coracobrachialis, the **musculocutaneous nerve** descends laterally between the **biceps** and the **brachialis muscles,** both of which it supplies. A short distance above the elbow, it emerges from behind the lateral border of the biceps and pierces the deep fascia as the **lateral antebrachial cutaneous nerve** (Fig. 17.5). The brachialis is the thick, fleshy muscle that lies posterior to the biceps in the lower part of the arm. Its attachments will be seen later in the dissection. Note that it is a large muscle and forms one of the

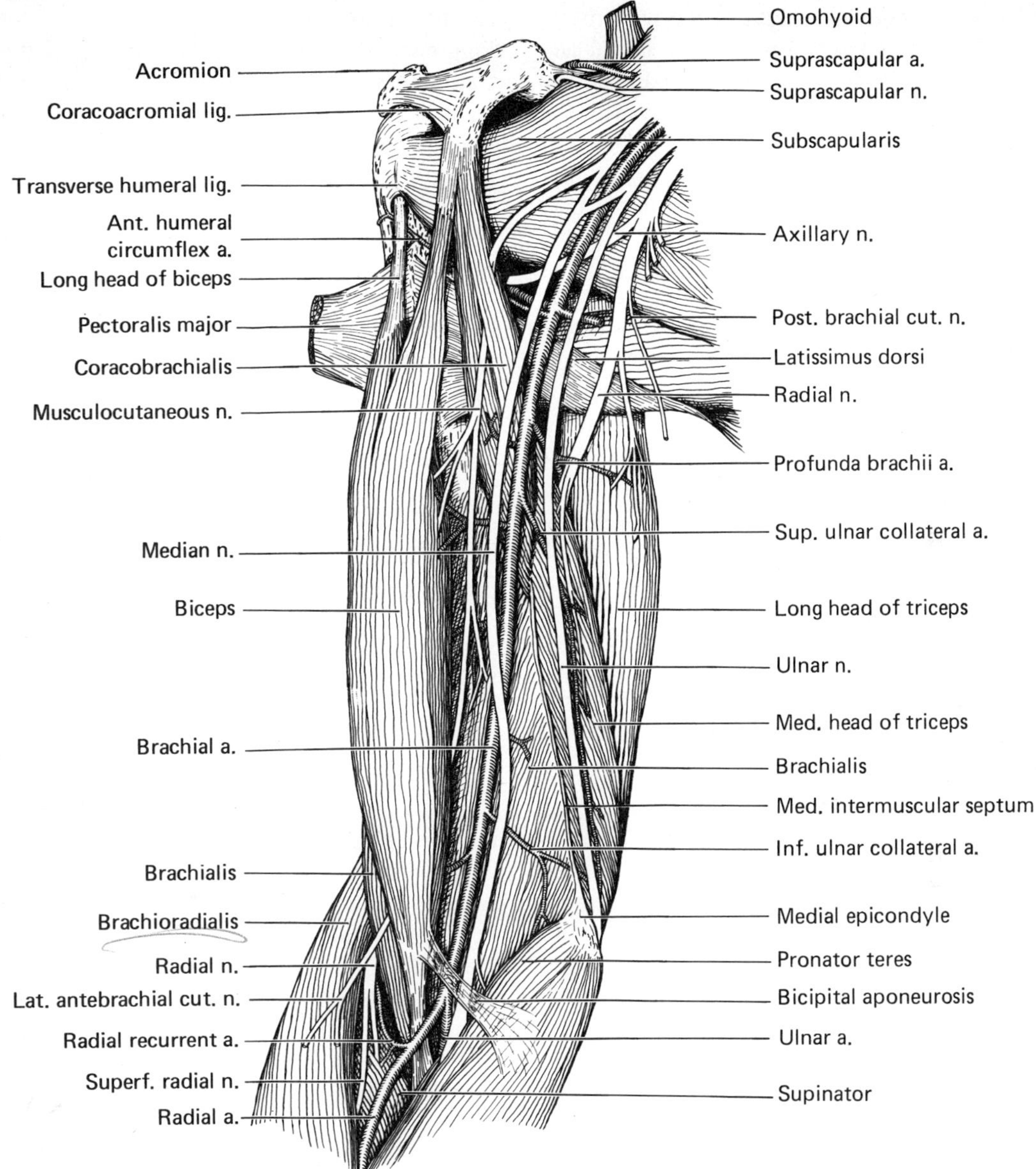

Figure 17.5 The **anteromedial** aspect of the **arm** with the biceps slightly displaced anterolaterally.

main constituents of the anterior (flexor) compartment of the arm.

The **arm,** below the level of the insertions of the deltoid and the coracobrachialis, is divided into **two compartments,** an **anterior** (flexor) and a **posterior** (extensor). The compartments are separated from each other by the humerus and the **lateral** and **medial intermuscular septa.** The septa are strong, aponeurotic, fascial bands that stretch laterally and medially from the lateral and medial **supracondylar ridges** of the humerus to the deep brachial fascia covering the lateral and medial surfaces of the arm. They extend inferiorly to the epicondyles and blend superiorly with the fasciae covering the deltoid and the coracobrachialis muscles. The **anterior compartment** contains the brachialis, the lower part of the biceps, and the origins of the brachioradialis and extensor carpi radialis longus muscles. It is traversed by the brachial artery and the median and musculocutaneous nerves. The **posterior compartment** and its contents will be dissected later.

The **brachial artery** begins at the lower border of the teres major as a continuation of the **axillary artery** and descends on the anteromedial aspect of the arm to terminate anterior to the elbow joint by dividing into the **radial** and **ulnar arteries** (Fig. 17.5). It is superficial throughout its course, with the exception that it is crossed superficially at about the middle of the arm by the median nerve and it may be overlapped anteriorly by the biceps.

The brachial artery pulse can be felt in the arm, and pressure can be applied to the artery to stem severe bleeding lower in the extremity.

At its termination, it is deep to the bicipital aponeurosis. The medial antebrachial cutaneous nerve also crosses its proximal portion. Deeply, it rests successively from above downward on the triceps, the coracobrachialis, and the brachialis muscles. Proximally, the ulnar nerve lies on its medial side but soon passes posteriorly away from the artery. The median nerve lies at first lateral to the brachial artery but crosses it at about the middle of the arm to come to lie on its medial side. The **median nerve,** like the **ulnar nerve,** has **no muscular branches in** the **arm,** though it is not uncommon to find a twig of communication between it and the musculocutaneous nerve.

In addition to numerous muscular branches, the **brachial artery** gives rise to the profunda brachii and the superior and inferior ulnar collateral arteries (Fig. 17.5). The **profunda brachii** is a large branch that arises from the medial side of the beginning of the brachial artery. Running distally and posteriorly, it passes between the medial and long heads of the triceps, in company with the **radial nerve,** to reach the back of the arm, where its further course will be seen later. The **superior ulnar collateral** usually arises at about the level of the insertion of the coracobrachialis. Running downward and posteriorly, it pierces the medial intermuscular septum to join the ulnar nerve, which it accompanies distally on the outer surface of the medial head of the triceps and behind the medial epicondyle. The **inferior ulnar collateral** arises from the brachial about 5 cm above its bifurcation and runs medially across the brachialis to divide into an anterior and a posterior branch. The posterior branch pierces the medial intermuscular septum to reach the back of the medial epicondyle; the anterior branch descends in front of the medial epicondyle, where its termination is at present hidden by the muscles arising there.

CUBITAL FOSSA

Now define the boundaries of the **cubital fossa,** the triangular space on the anterior aspect of the elbow (Fig. 17.6). The **base** of the triangle is formed by an imaginary transverse line between the two epicondyles. Its **medial boundary** is the lateral border of the **pronator teres muscle;** its **lateral boundary** is the medial border of the **brachioradialis muscle.** Its **apex,** which is directed distally, is the point where these two muscles meet. The **pronator teres** is the most lateral of the superficial group of muscles of the forearm that take origin by a **common tendon** from the **medial epicondyle of** the **humerus.** Its fibers pass distally and laterally across the front of the forearm to insert on the middle third of the **lateral surface of** the **radius;** its insertion is covered by the brachioradialis. The brachioradialis is ordinarily grouped with the extensor muscles that spread over the posterior surface of the forearm and hand. It acts, however, principally as a flexor of the elbow and does not reach the hand at all. It may, therefore, be cleaned and studied now.

The **brachioradialis** arises from the upper two-

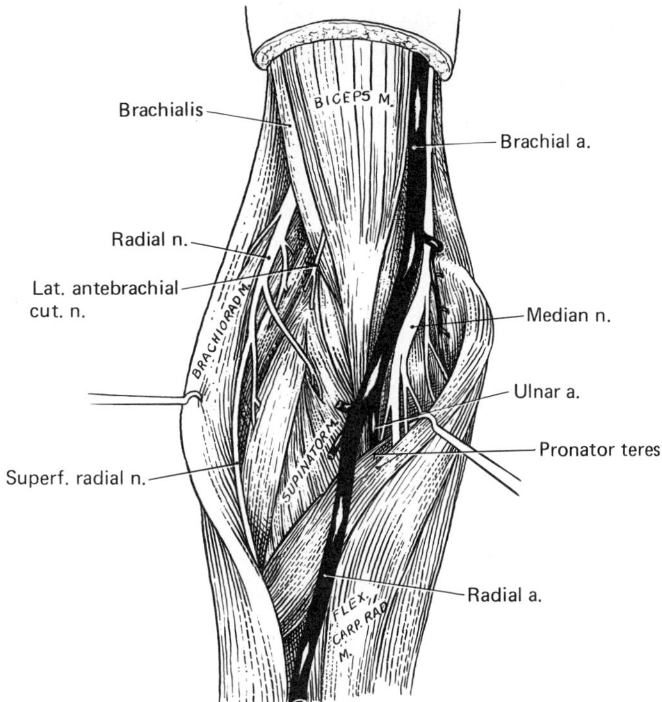

Figure 17.6 The **cubital fossa.**

thirds of the lateral **supracondylar ridge of** the **humerus** and from the anterior surface of the **lateral intermuscular septum.** Its upper portion lies, therefore, in the anterior compartment of the arm, where it overlaps the lateral part of the brachialis. It extends distally along the lateral side of the anterior surface of the forearm and gives rise to a strong, flat tendon that inserts into the base of the **styloid process of** the **radius.** The origin of the extensor carpi radialis longus muscle is also in the anterior compartment, from the lateral supracondylar ridge immediately distal to the origin of the brachioradialis.

The **floor of** the **cubital fossa** is formed proximally by the **brachialis muscle** and distally by the **supinator muscle.** Its **roof** is formed by **skin** and **fascia,** and it is crossed by the **bicipital aponeurosis.**

When a needle is inserted into the median cubital vein, the bicipital aponeurosis serves as a firm base against which the vein is pressed and also as protection for the deeper median nerve and brachial artery.

Clean the radial and ulnar arteries. The **radial artery** passes distally and somewhat laterally from its origin, crossing anterior to the tendon of the biceps and the supinator muscle. It leaves the cubital fossa at the apex, where it lies anterior to the pronator teres overlapped anteriorly by the brachioradialis. Near its origin it gives rise to the **radial recurrent artery.** This vessel runs laterally on the supinator and then turns proximally to ascend anterior to the lateral epicondyle between the brachialis and the brachioradialis.

The **ulnar artery** runs distally and medially to leave the cubital fossa by passing deep to the pronator teres. In the fossa it gives rise to the anterior and posterior ulnar recurrent arteries, which may arise separately or by a common stem. The **anterior ulnar recurrent** ascends between the pronator teres and the brachialis to anastomose with the anterior branch of the inferior ulnar collateral. The **posterior ulnar recurrent** passes medially, deep to the pronator teres. The further courses and anastomoses of the recurrent arteries can be seen to better advantage during the dissection of the joints.

The anastomosing recurrent and collateral arteries form an important collateral circulation around the elbow joint.

Follow the median nerve as it passes distally through the cubital fossa lying medial to the brachial artery, and medial and anterior to the ulnar artery (Fig. 17.6). It leaves the fossa by passing through the pronator teres, thus splitting the muscle into superficial and deep heads with respect to the median nerve. Look for the **deep head of** the **pronator,** small and sometimes absent, which arises from the medial border of the **coronoid process of** the **ulna** and joins the large superficial head. If present, it will intervene between the ulnar artery and the median nerve. In the fossa, the median nerve supplies the pronator teres.

Clean the insertion of the **biceps** on the **tuberosity of** the **radius;** it is overlapped by the pronator teres. Spread the proximal parts of the brachioradialis and the extensor carpi radialis longus laterally from the brachialis to expose the terminal part of the radial nerve. The **radial nerve** enters the anterior compartment of the arm by piercing the lateral intermuscular septum close to the lateral supracondylar ridge of the humerus. It is accompanied by the **radial collateral artery,** a branch of the **profunda brachii artery,** which anastomoses with the radial recurrent. After giving branches to the brachioradialis and the extensor carpi radialis longus and brevis, and one or two small twigs to the brachialis, the nerve ends by dividing into the **superficial** and **deep radial nerves.** The **superficial radial nerve** is a cutaneous branch; it passes distally in the forearm under cover of the brachioradialis (Fig. 17.6). Some distance above the wrist, it emerges from behind the lateral border of that muscle and winds dorsally around the lateral side of the wrist to reach the dorsum of the hand. The **deep radial nerve** passes from view at present by entering the substance of the supinator.

Displace the brachioradialis and the pronator teres as far laterally and medially, respectively, as can conveniently be done. Clean the **brachialis.** This muscle arises from the entire **anterior surface** of the distal half of the **humerus,** from the entire anterior surface of the **medial intermuscular septum,** and from the anterior surface of the **lateral intermuscular septum** proximal to the origin of the brachioradialis. Its distal portion lies anterior to the capsule of the elbow joint, to which it is closely bound, and narrows to a strong tendon that is inserted on the **tuberosity of** the **ulna.** Its nerve supply is derived chiefly from the **musculocutaneous nerve,** but it receives additional small twigs from the **radial.**

FLEXOR REGION OF THE FOREARM

The **anterior** and **medial portions of** the **forearm** are occupied by **muscles** that primarily **flex** the **wrist** and **fingers** and **pronate** the **hand.** These muscles are arranged in **three layers.** The muscles of the **superficial layer** arise by a **common tendon** from the **medial epicondyle of** the **humerus** and from the **deep fascia,** which invests their proximal portions (Fig. 17.7). They spread distally and laterally over the anterior aspect of the forearm, becoming distinct from one another about 8 cm distal to the medial epicondyle.

Near its insertion the **pronator teres** is crossed by the radial artery and overlapped by the brachioradialis. The **flexor carpi radialis** narrows to a round tendon that descends along the medial side of the radial artery

(the arterial pulse is most commonly taken here)

and enters the palm superficially. Its insertion on the **bases of** the **second** and **third metacarpals** will be seen later.

The **flexor carpi ulnaris** arises by the common tendon and also has a second head of origin from the medial border of the **olecranon** and from an aponeurosis attached to the proximal two-thirds of the dorsal border of the **ulna.** It inserts into the

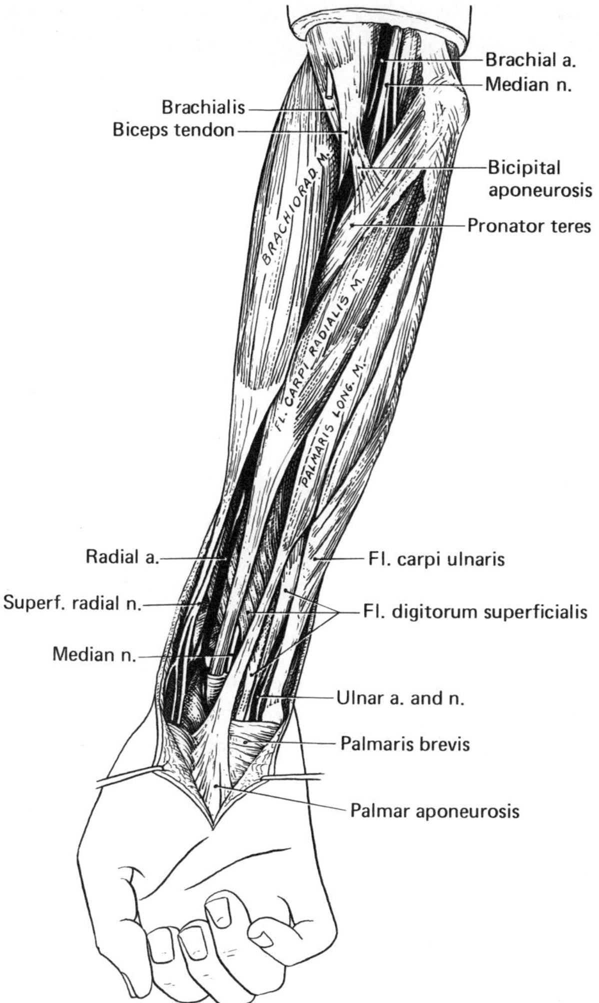

Figure 17.7 Superficial muscles of the **anterior** aspect of the **forearm.**

pisiform bone. Observe that the **ulnar nerve** passes posterior to the medial epicondyle and enters the forearm by passing deep to a fibrous arch that unites the two heads of the flexor carpi ulnaris.

In this superficial location, the ulnar nerve is often accidentally bumped, sending tingling sensations down the extremity. Severe injury to the nerve most frequently occurs here as well, resulting in a functional deformity, "claw hand," which is characterized by extended metacarpophalangeal and flexed interphalangeal joints. Why?

A nerve that passes through a muscle may become damaged ("trapped") within the muscle by encroaching fibroses or calcifications. Other muscles supplied by the nerve distal to the injury, therefore, become paralyzed. Examples in the superior extremity are the ulnar, median, and radial nerves in association with the flexor carpi ulnaris, pronator teres, and supinator muscles, respectively.

The tendon of the **palmaris longus** crosses the middle of the front of the wrist to insert into the **palmar aponeurosis** (Fig. 17.7). In the distal part of the forearm it lies immediately **anterior to** the

median nerve. In about 12 percent of the population, this muscle is absent; in such cases the median nerve is hazardously superficial.

The median nerve is subject to serious damage in the distal forearm and wrist. Loss of sensation in the fingertips and of opposition of the thumb makes this a severely incapacitating impairment.

Clean the **palmar aponeurosis.** This is a dense thickening of the **deep fascia of** the **palm** that radiates from the tendon of the palmaris longus toward the bases of the fingers, where it divides into four slips. On its deep surface, the aponeurosis joins the **fibrous sheaths,** which hold the **flexor tendons** in place against the palmar surfaces of the phalanges. As the aponeurosis is cleaned, look for the **palmaris brevis muscle** in the superficial fascia over the hypothenar area.

Reflect the palmar aponeurosis with the attached tendon of the palmaris longus and the palmaris brevis, as shown in Fig. 17.8. Do this carefully to avoid injuring the **superficial palmar arterial arch** and the terminal branches of the **median nerve,** which lie immediately subjacent to the aponeurosis. The aponeurosis should be cut at the bases of the fingers where its four divergent slips join the fibrous sheaths of the flexor tendons.

Bisect the pronator teres about 2.5 cm from its insertion; free and elevate the tendons of the flexor carpi radialis, the palmaris longus, and the flexor carpi ulnaris. While doing this, secure and clean the nerves that enter their deep surfaces. The **pronator teres** is supplied by the **median nerve** in the cubital fossa. The **flexor carpi radialis** and the **palmaris longus** receive branches of the **median nerve** arising under cover of the pronator teres. The **flexor carpi ulnaris** is supplied by two or three twigs from the **ulnar nerve** in the upper part of the forearm.

The **second layer** of the anterior aspect of the forearm is represented by a single large muscle, the **flexor digitorum superficialis** (Fig. 17.8). It arises in part from the common tendon off the **medial epicondyle of** the **humerus** and, more extensively, from the medial borders of the **ulnar tuberosity** and the **coronoid process of** the **ulna,** from the **oblique line on** the anterior surface of the **radius,** and from a **fibrous arch** that bridges the gap **between** its **ulnar** and **radial origins.** Observe that the median nerve and the ulnar artery pass into the forearm deep to this fibrous arch. As the wrist is approached, the muscle divides into **four tendons;** those for the **middle** and **ring fingers** are **anterior to** those for the **index** and **little fingers.**

At the wrist, the investing antebrachial fascia is thickened to form the **palmar carpal ligament,** a fibrous band anchored to the styloid processes of the radius and ulna. Anteriorly, the ligament is attached to the **flexor retinaculum,** which will be found deep to the palmar carpal ligament (Fig. 17.8). It is a strong, dense, fibrous band that stretches across the wrist from the **scaphoid** and **trapezium** laterally, to the **pisiform** and **hook of** the **hamate** medially. Together with the anterior surfaces of the carpal bones, the retinaculum completes an osteofibrous canal, the **carpal tunnel,** through which the flexor tendons of the digits and the median nerve enter the palm. The tendon of the flexor carpi radialis pierces the lateral side of the retinaculum in its own compartment as it crosses the wrist. Note that the ulnar nerve and artery enter the palm superficial to the flexor retinaculum but deep to the palmar carpal ligament. As the four flexor tendons enter the palm, they pass deep to the flexor retinaculum and are enclosed in one common **synovial sheath,** which also surrounds the four tendons of the flexor digitorum profundus muscle.

Because of its compactness and rigid walls, the carpal tunnel is unable to accommodate any swelling, pus infiltration, or pathological growth without compressing the structures, especially the median nerve, that traverse it. The condition known as the "carpal tunnel syndrome" is usually characterized by numbness of the fingers supplied by the median nerve, and in severe cases, by muscular paralysis marked by loss of thumb opposition.

Before dissecting the deep layer of muscles, study the course of the radial and ulnar arteries

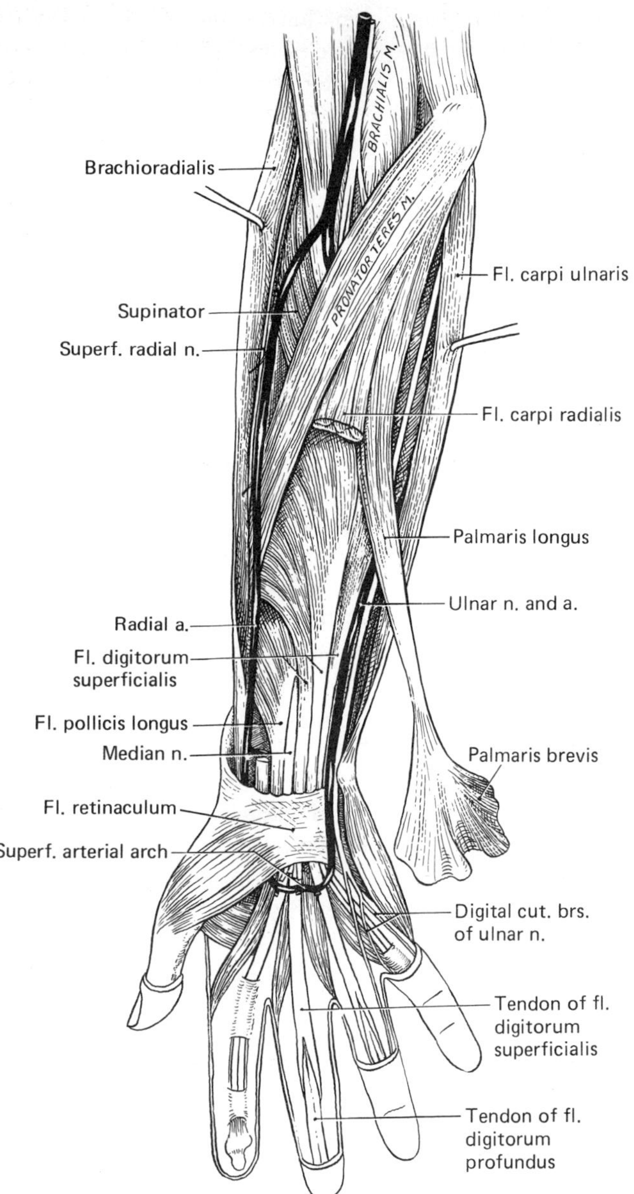

Figure 17.8 Deep muscles of the **anterior** aspect of the **forearm** and of the palm.

and the median and ulnar nerves in the forearm. The **radial artery** is **superficial** throughout its course **in** the **forearm,** with the exception that distal to the apex of the cubital fossa, it is overlapped for a variable distance by the brachioradialis. Deeply, it rests successively against the tendon of the biceps, the supinator, the insertion of the pronator teres, the radial head of the flexor digitorum superficialis, the flexor pollicis longus, the pronator quadratus, and the anterior surface of the radius. Just proximal to the wrist, it turns laterally and dorsally toward the dorsum of the wrist, where it will be traced later.

In addition to the radial recurrent artery, the **radial artery** gives rise in the forearm to numerous small muscular branches and to a palmar carpal branch and a superficial palmar branch. The **palmar carpal branch** is small and passes medially across the distal end of the radius, deep to the flexor tendons, to anastomose with the **palmar carpal branch of** the **ulnar artery.** The **superficial palmar branch** arises just as the radial artery turns dorsally at the wrist and runs forward over or through the intrinsic muscles of the thumb to take part in the formation of the **superficial palmar arterial arch.**

Detach the radial head of the flexor digitorum superficialis from the radius and displace it medially. Then clean the **ulnar artery,** which, in the **proximal** half of the **forearm,** is **covered by** the four muscles of the **superficial layer** and by the **flexor digitorum superficialis.** It is also crossed, under cover of the pronator teres, by the median nerve, which passes from its medial to its lateral side. In the **distal** half of the **forearm,** the **ulnar artery** is more **superficial,** being overlapped only by the tendon of the flexor carpi ulnaris. Deeply, it rests first upon the brachialis and then, for the remainder of its course in the forearm, upon the flexor digitorum profundus; at the wrist, it crosses the medial end of the flexor retinaculum superficially to enter the palm (Fig. 17.8).

In the forearm, the ulnar artery gives rise to many muscular branches as well as to distinct named branches. The origins of the **ulnar recurrent arteries** have been seen. Trace the **posterior ulnar recurrent** as it ascends between the flexors digitorum superficialis and profundus to pass posterior to the medial epicondyle. It anastomoses with the **superior ulnar collateral** and the posterior branch of the **inferior ulnar collateral.**

The **common interosseous artery** arises from the **ulnar** near the point where that vessel is crossed by the median nerve. It passes posteriorly and distally between the borders of the flexor pollicis longus and the flexor digitorum profundus muscles and divides almost immediately into the posterior and the anterior interosseous arteries. The **posterior interosseous** passes straight posteriorly between the proximal ends of the radius and the ulna and above the proximal border of the interosseous membrane to reach the posterior aspect of the forearm. The **anterior interosseous** passes distally anterior to the interosseous membrane and is covered by the overlapping borders of the flexor pollicis longus and the flexor digitorum profundus. Near its origin it gives rise to the **median artery,** which accompanies the **median nerve.** Usually small and unimportant, the median artery is occasionally enlarged and may accompany the nerve into the hand to take part in the formation of the superficial palmar arch.

The dorsal carpal branch of the ulnar artery arises near the proximal border of the flexor retinaculum and winds dorsally and medially to reach the dorsal surface of the wrist. The **palmar carpal branch** arises at about the same level and passes laterally deep to the flexor tendons to anastomose with the **palmar carpal branch** of the radial.

Passing **between** the two **heads of** the **flexor carpi ulnaris,** the **ulnar nerve** courses through the forearm, covered only by that muscle. Proximally, the ulnar nerve is separated from the ulnar artery by the flexor digitorum superficialis, but distally it closely accompanies the artery, lying on its medial side. Proximally in the forearm, the ulnar nerve gives branches that supply the **flexor carpi ulnaris** and the **medial portion of** the **flexor digitorum profundus;** there are no other muscular branches in the forearm. In the distal part of the forearm, it gives rise to the **dorsal cutaneous branch,** whose distribution to the skin on the dorsum of the hand has already been traced; and to a small **palmar cutaneous branch,** which passes anterior to the ulnar artery to reach the medial half of the **palm.** Near the distal border of the flexor retinaculum, the ulnar nerve terminates by dividing into a **deep** and a **superficial branch.**

The **median nerve** runs almost vertically through the forearm into the hand, passing deep to the flexor retinaculum with the flexor tendons. In the upper two-thirds of the forearm, it lies between the flexors digitorum superficialis and profundus; in the distal third, it is covered superficially only by the tendon of the palmaris longus. In the cubital fossa, or just distal to it under cover of the pronator teres, it gives rise to branches that supply the **pronator teres,** the **flexor carpi radialis,** the **palmaris longus,** and the **flexor digitorum superficialis.** More distally, it gives rise to a branch known as the **anterior interosseous nerve;** this nerve accompanies the anterior interosseous artery along the anterior surface of the interosseous membrane and is distributed to the deep muscles of the forearm. Immediately before the flexor retinaculum, the median nerve gives off a small **palmar cutaneous branch,** which crosses the retinaculum superficially to supply the skin of the lateral half of the palm (i.e., the thenar eminence).

Carefully feed a probe along the course of the median nerve through the carpal tunnel; note that it is compact and unyielding. Bisect the flexor retinaculum. All the long flexor tendons to the fingers and their synovial sheaths should be elevated to facilitate the dissection of the deeper structures in the distal forearm and in the hand. The digital fibrous sheaths over the flexor tendons may be opened to facilitate the elevation of the flexor tendons and straightening of the fingers (Fig. 17.8).

Now clean the deepest layer of the anterior muscles, which includes the flexor digitorum profundus, the flexor pollicis longus, and the pronator quadratus. The **flexor digitorum profundus** has a wide, fleshy origin from the **proximal two-thirds** of the anterior and medial surfaces of the **ulna** and the adjacent **interosseous membrane;** it also arises from the deep surface of the aponeurosis of the flexor carpi ulnaris on the dorsal border of the ulna. The muscle gives rise to **four tendons** that pass into the hand side by side, deep to the flexor retinaculum and the tendons of the flexor digitorum superficialis.

The **flexor pollicis longus** arises from the **middle half** of the anterior surface of the **radius** and from the adjacent portion of the **interosseous membrane;** its origin is limited proximolaterally by the line of origin of the radial head of the flexor digitorum superficialis. Its tendon passes deep to the flexor retinaculum, lying lateral to the tendons of the flexor digitorum profundus.

Spread the flexors digitorum profundus and pollicis longus apart to expose the pronator quadratus and the anterior interosseous artery and nerve. The **pronator quadratus** is a flat, quadrangular muscle arising from the medial side of the **distal fourth of** the anterior surface of the **ulna.** Its fibers pass transversely to insert on the anterior surface of the **radius.**

The **anterior interosseous artery** supplies branches to the deep flexors. It terminates at the proximal border of the pronator quadratus by dividing into **posterior** and **anterior branches.** The larger **posterior branch** pierces the interosseous membrane to reach the back of the forearm. The **anterior branch** descends deep to the pronator quadratus to anastomose with the **palmar carpal branches of** the **radial** and **ulnar arteries.** The **anterior interosseous nerve** accompanies the artery. It is distributed to the **lateral part of** the **flexor digitorum profundus,** the **flexor pollicis longus,** and the **pronator quadratus;** and it also sends a twig that accompanies the anterior branch of the artery to the wrist joint.

PALM OF THE HAND

Clean the **superficial palmar arterial arch** and the superficial branch of the ulnar nerve (Fig. 17.9). The superficial palmar arch is formed principally by the continuation of the **ulnar artery** into the palm but is usually completed laterally by the **superficial palmar branch of** the **radial artery.** The superficial arch crosses the palm at about the middle of the metacarpal bones. The superficial palmar branch of the radial artery may cross the base of the thenar eminence superficially to join the arch, or it may pass deep to the abductor pollicis brevis. The branches of the superficial palmar arch are somewhat variable but usually include a **proper palmar digital artery** for the ulnar

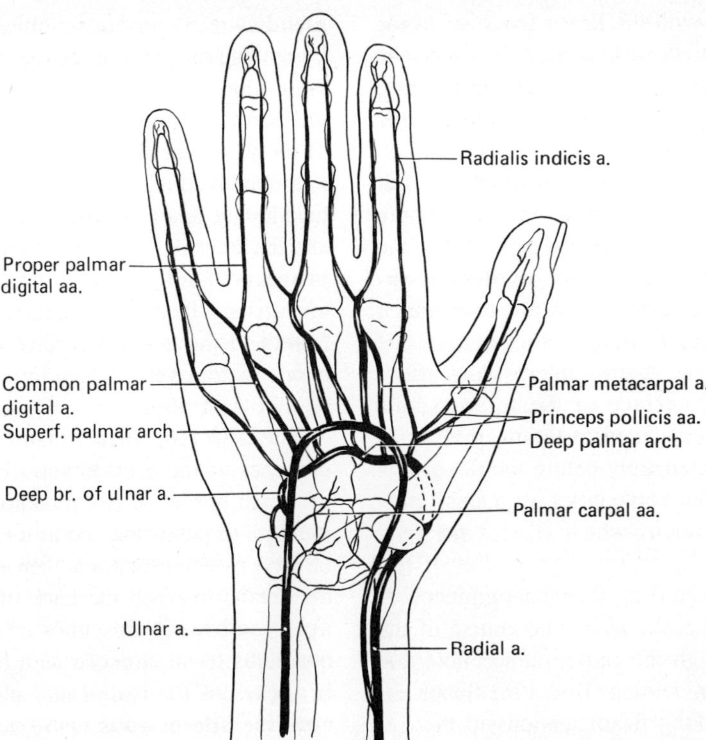

Figure 17.9 Diagrammatic presentation of the **palmar arterial system.**

side of the little finger and three **common palmar digital arteries,** which pass distally superficial to the three medial intermetacarpal spaces. At the bases of the interdigital clefts, each common artery divides into two **proper palmar digital arteries,** which supply the medial side of the index finger, both sides of the middle and ring fingers, and the radial side of the little finger.

As it reaches the distal border of the flexor retinaculum, the ulnar artery gives off a **deep branch,** which accompanies the deep branch of the ulnar nerve into the palm by passing between the short muscles of the little finger.

The **superficial branch of** the **ulnar nerve** terminates in the palm by dividing into three **palmar digital branches** distributed to the skin of both sides of the little finger and the medial side of the ring finger.

Attempt to locate the **two synovial sheaths** that envelop the flexor tendons as they pass through the carpal tunnel. One (the **radial bursa**) encloses the **tendon of** the **flexor pollicis longus;** it extends from several centimeters above the proximal border of the flexor retinaculum almost to the insertion of the tendon. The second (the **ulnar bursa**) encloses the **four tendons of** the **flexor digitorum superficialis** and the **four tendons of** the **flexor digitorum profundus.** It begins about 2.5 cm proximal to the flexor retinaculum and extends about 2.5 cm beyond the distal border of the retinaculum. The most **medial part,** however, is prolonged distally to enclose the two **flexor tendons for** the **little finger** as far as the base of the distal phalanx. **Three** individual **synovial sheaths** enclose the **tendons** for the **index, middle,** and **ring fingers;** each extends from the level of the metacarpophalangeal joint to the base of the distal phalanx.

The **digital fibrous sheaths** are bands of dense connective tissue that attach to the margins of the phalanges and that bridge their palmar aspects, thus forming, in each finger, an **osteofibrous canal.** Through them the flexor tendons, invested by synovial sheaths, pass to their respective insertions. The very strong **annular portions** of the fibrous sheaths lie opposite the bodies of the first and second phalanges of each finger (Fig. 17.10). The **cruciform portions** lie opposite the joints and therefore are thin and flexible.

Trace the **median nerve** in the palm. As it emerges from under the flexor retinaculum, the median nerve terminates by dividing into three **common palmar digital nerves.** The first passes distally and laterally to supply the short abductor, the short flexor, the opponens of the thumb, and the first lumbrical muscle. Then it divides into three **proper palmar digital nerves,** which supply the skin on both sides of the thumb and the lateral side of the index finger. The second and third common palmar digital branches each divide into two proper palmar digitals for the medial side of the index finger, both sides of the middle finger, and the lateral side of the ring finger. These median digital branches also innervate the dorsal aspects of the distal phalanges. The second common palmar digital usually supplies the second lumbrical muscle.

Observe that as the **long flexor tendons** diverge toward the bases of the fingers, those of the **flexor superficialis** lie **superficial to** those of the **flexor profundus.** Study the manner of insertion of the two tendons by opening the fibrous sheaths longitudinally along the fingers. This will aid in straightening the fingers and will facilitate the deeper dissection of the hand. Observe that in front of the body of the proximal phalanx, the **tendon of** the **flexor superficialis** is **pierced by** the **tendon of** the **flexor profundus.** The **superficialis tendon** inserts on the **base of** the **middle phalanx,** while the **tendon of** the **profundus** in-

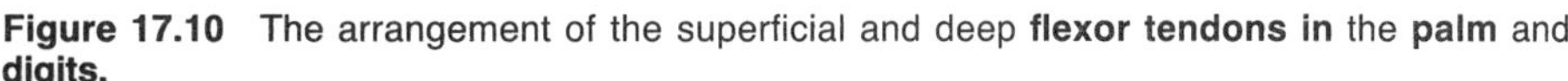

Figure 17.10 The arrangement of the superficial and deep **flexor tendons in** the **palm** and **digits.**

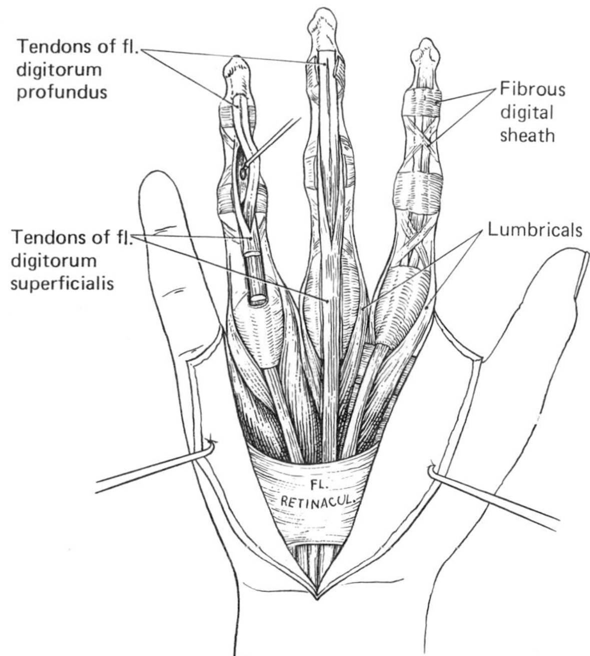

serts on the **base of** the **distal phalanx** (Figs. 7.8 and 7.10). Note the delicate **vincula longa** and **brevia,** which extend from the tendons to the phalanges.

Elevate the tendons of the flexor digitorum superficialis and clean the four **lumbrical muscles.** These small muscles arise in the distal part of the palm from the **tendons of** the **flexor digitorum profundus.** The **first** arises from the lateral side of the tendon for the index finger and the **second** from the lateral side of the tendon for the middle finger; the **third** and **fourth** originate from the adjacent sides of the tendons between which they lie. Each passes to the lateral side of the corresponding finger and, at the metacarpophalangeal joint, inserts into the **expansion extensor tendon** on the dorsum of that finger.

With the flexor tendons and lumbrical muscles elevated, note a **potential space** (an interfascial plane) between these tendons and muscles and the deeper palmar interossei, the adductor pollicis, and the metacarpal bones. This space is divided into two by a fibrous **oblique septum** extending from the palmar aponeurosis to the shaft of the middle metacarpal bone. A medial compartment (the **midpalmar space**) is beneath the tendons to the middle, ring, and little fingers and their accompanying lumbrical muscles. A lateral compartment (the **thenar space**) is found between the deep surface of the tendon to the index finger, with its accompanying lumbrical muscle, and the superficial surface of the adductor pollicis muscle.

These interfascial spaces are clinically noteworthy because they serve as an unobstructed route for the spread of infection from the digits into the palm via the synovial bursae. By the same token, the opposing fasciae confine the infection, thereby preventing it from invading the entire hand.

Clean the short muscles of the little finger, which form the **hypothenar eminence** on the medial side of the palm. The **abductor digiti minimi** is the most medial; it arises from the **pisiform bone** and inserts into the medial side of the **base of** the **proximal phalanx** of the little finger. The **flexor digiti minimi brevis** arises from the **hook of** the **hamate** and the medial end of the **flexor retinaculum** and inserts with the **abductor.** The **opponens digiti minimi** is covered superficially by the short flexor, with which it is often partially blended. It arises from the **hook of** the **hamate** and the adjacent border of the **flexor retinaculum** and inserts into the whole length of the medial palmar surface of the **fifth metacarpal.** All three of these muscles are supplied by twigs from the **deep branch of** the **ulnar nerve.** Observe that as they sink into the palm, the deep branches of the ulnar nerve and artery pass between the origins of the abductor and the flexor brevis.

Clean the short muscles of the thumb, which form the **thenar eminence,** or ball of the thumb. Of these, the **abductor pollicis brevis** is the most superficial. It arises from the **trapezium** and the lateral end of the **flexor retinaculum** and inserts into the lateral side of the base of the **proximal phalanx** of the thumb. When clean, it should be detached from its origin and reflected toward its insertion to expose the deeper muscles. The **opponens pollicis** is a thick, fleshy muscle arising from the **trapezium** and the adjacent part of the **flexor retinaculum.** It inserts into the lateral side of the entire palmar surface of the **first metacarpal.** The **flexor pollicis brevis** is divided into deep and superficial heads by the tendon of the flexor pollicis longus. The **superficial head** lies along the medial side of the opponens pollicis and covers the tendon of the flexor longus. It arises from the **trapezium** and the **flexor retinaculum** and inserts into the base of the **proximal phalanx,** just medial to the insertion of the abductor brevis. Divide the superficial head close to its origin and turn it laterally to its insertion. Trace the tendon of the **long flexor** to its insertion on the base of the **distal phalanx** of the thumb. The small **deep head of** the **flexor pollicis brevis** is now visible; it arises from the **trapezoid bone** and runs laterally and distally deep to the tendon of the flexor longus to insert with the **superficial head.**

The **adductor pollicis** arises by two heads, which are distinguished from each other by the deep palmar arch passing medially into the palm between them. The **oblique head** arises from the **capitate** and the bases of the **second** and **third metacarpals;** the **transverse head** arises from the palmar aspect of the shaft of the **third metacarpal.** The two heads converge to form a tendon that inserts into the medial side of the base of the **proximal phalanx of** the **thumb.**

To render the **deep palmar arterial arch** accessible for study, retract the tendons of the flexor digitorum superficialis, flexor digitorum profundus, and flexor pollicis longus upward. The lateral end of the deep palmar arch is covered by the oblique head of the adductor pollicis. This muscle and the deep head of the short flexor should be divided close to their origins and turned laterally. The **deep palmar arch** begins at the base of the first interosseous space, where the radial artery enters the palm. The arch is formed principally by the **radial artery** but is usually completed medially by the **deep branch of** the **ulnar artery,** which enters the palm under cover of the flexor digiti minimi brevis (Fig. 17.9). If that muscle is now detached from its origin and reflected, the full course of the deep palmar arch will be exposed. It crosses the palm at the bases of the metacarpal bones, resting deeply against the proximal portions of the interosseous muscles. Its two largest branches arise from its lateral end, at the base of the first interosseous space. The **princeps pollicis artery** passes along the metacarpal of the thumb, under cover of the oblique head of the adductor, and at the base of the proximal phalanx divides into two branches, which are distributed to the two sides of the palmar aspect of the thumb. The second branch, the **radialis indicis artery,** passes distally under cover of the transverse head of the adductor and along the lateral side of the index finger. In addition to these branches, the deep palmar arch gives rise to three **palmar metacarpal branches,** which descend in the three medial interosseous spaces. At the base of the proximal phalanx, each palmar metacarpal divides into two perforating branches; one passes dorsally to join the dorsal metacarpal artery, and the other anastomoses with the common palmar branch of the superficial arch.

The **deep branch of** the **ulnar nerve** accompanies the medial part of the deep palmar arch. It is distributed to the three **short muscles of** the **little finger,** the **third** and **fourth lumbricals,** the **adductor pollicis,** and all of the **interosseous muscles.**

The **interossei** are small muscles that occupy the interosseous spaces. They are arranged in two groups consisting of **three palmar** and **four dorsal interossei.** Detach the transverse head of the adductor pollicis from its origin and reflect it laterally. Then study the interossei. The **first palmar interosseous muscle** arises from the medial palmar surface of the second metacarpal and inserts into the medial side of the base of the proximal phalanx of the index finger. The **second** and **third palmar interossei** arise from the lateral palmar surfaces of the fourth and fifth metacarpals, respectively, and insert into the lateral sides of the bases of the proximal phalanges of the ring and little fingers. The **dorsal interossei** lie on a slightly deeper plane; one dorsal interosseus muscle is found in each space, each arising from the adjacent sides of two metacarpals. The **first** and **second** insert into the lateral sides of the bases of the proximal phalanges of the index and middle fingers, respectively. The **third** and **fourth** insert into the medial sides of the bases of the proximal phalanges of the middle and ring fingers. In addition to these insertions, the tendons of the interossei also attach to the **extensor expansions of** the **fingers.**

EXTENSOR REGION OF THE ARM

Turn to the back of the arm and clean the **triceps brachii.** The distal part of this muscle occupies the entire posterior compartment of the arm. The triceps arises by three heads. The **long head** originates from the **infraglenoid tubercle of** the **scapula.** The medial and lateral heads arise from the posterior aspect of the humerus, separated by the **radial sulcus (groove)** for the radial nerve.

The **lateral head** arises from the posterior surface of the **humerus** superior and lateral to the sulcus. The origin of the medial head is lower and much more extensive, and partly covered by both the long and the lateral heads. The **medial head** arises from the entire posterior surface of the **humerus** below and medial to the radial groove, from the entire posterior surface of the **medial intermuscular septum,** and from the lower part of the posterior surface of the **lateral intermuscular septum.** The **common tendon** of insertion of the triceps forms a strong aponeurotic band on the posterior surface of the distal part of the muscle; it inserts into the **olecranon.** Observe that the **ulnar nerve** lies on the external surface of the **medial head,** close to the medial intermuscular septum, as it descends through the arm to pass behind the medial epicondyle. It is joined at the middle of the arm by the **superior ulnar collateral artery,** which pierces the medial intermuscular septum at about this point. Separate the three heads of the triceps as completely as possible to expose the **radial sulcus.** Clean the radial nerve and the profunda brachii artery.

Follow the **radial nerve** from its origin in the axilla from the **posterior cord of** the **brachial plexus.** It crosses the subscapularis, the teres major, the tendon of the latissimus dorsi, and the long head of the triceps, and enters the **radial sulcus of** the **humerus** by passing between the long and medial heads of the triceps (Fig. 17.11). Three branches arise from the radial nerve **before** it enters the sulcus. The first is the **posterior brachial cutaneous nerve,** whose distribution to the skin on the back of the arm has already been traced. The second supplies the **long head of** the **triceps.** The third is distributed to the **medial head;** it is sometimes known as the **ulnar collateral nerve** because it descends on the external surface of the medial head close to the ulnar nerve for some distance before finally entering the substance of the muscle (Fig. 17.5).

As the **radial nerve** passes laterally and distally in the sulcus, it gives rise to a branch to the **lateral head** and a second branch to the **medial head** and to the **posterior antebrachial cutaneous nerve.** The latter nerve passes through the substance of the triceps to reach the posterior lateral surface of the arm, from which point it has been traced (Fig. 17.11). At the distal end of the sulcus, the radial nerve pierces the lateral intermuscular septum to enter the anterior compartment of the arm.

The radial nerve is subject to injury in the arm either from the jagged edges of a fractured humerus or from prolonged pressure applied against the nerve, as can happen when a drunk falls asleep with his arm slung over the back of a barstool or park bench (''Saturday night palsy''). The resultant functional loss, commonly called ''wrist drop,'' is characterized by an inability to extend the wrist. Why?

The **profunda brachii artery** is a branch of the **brachial artery.** It accompanies the **radial nerve** in the radial sulcus and is distributed principally to the **triceps.** One branch ascends deep to the deltoid to anastomose with the **posterior humeral circumflex.** Another branch, the **middle collateral artery,** descends to anastomose with the **interosseous recurrent artery.** The continuation of the profunda, known as the **radial collateral artery,** accompanies the nerve into the anterior compartment of the arm to anastomose with the **radial recurrent artery.**

EXTENSOR REGION OF THE FOREARM AND HAND

Remove any superficial fascia remaining on the posterior aspect of the forearm and dorsum of the hand. Observe that the **deep antebrachial fascia** on the posterior aspect of the forearm is denser than that on the anterior aspect. Proximally, it forms an aponeurotic sheet from the deep surface of which the superficial extensor muscles take partial origin. At the wrist, the fascia is strengthened by a strong transverse fibrous band known as the **extensor retinaculum** (dorsal carpal ligament). Laterally, the extensor retinaculum is attached to the **lateral border of** the distal end of the **radius;** medially, it is bound to the **styloid process of** the

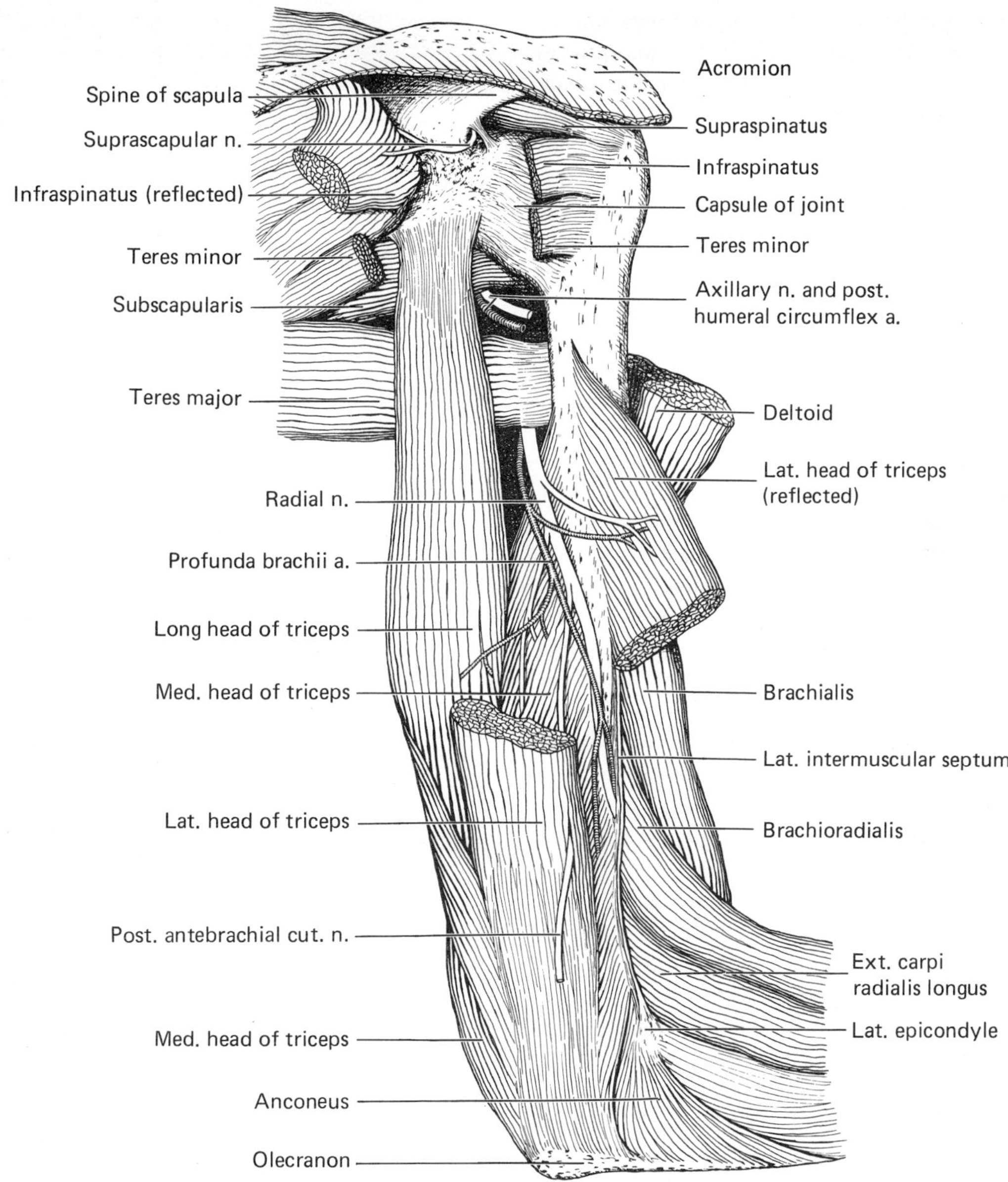

Figure 17.11 The **posterolateral** aspect of the **arm.**

ulna and the **triquetrum** and **pisiform bones.** In addition to its lateral and medial attachments, the extensor retinaculum is firmly attached to a series of bony ridges on the **posterior aspect of** the distal ends of the **radius** and **ulna.** There are thus formed, deep to the ligament, **six osteofibrous compartments** or **canals** through which the **extensor tendons** pass to the dorsum of the hand. Identify the compartments and the tendons that traverse them (Fig. 17.13).

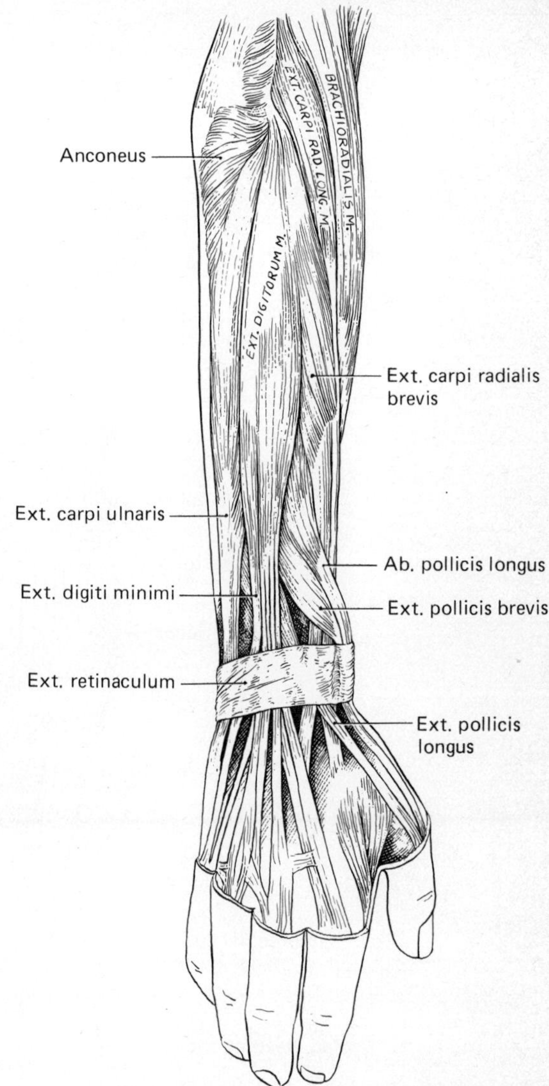

Figure 17.12 Superficial muscles of the **posterior** aspect of the **forearm** and hand.

Most laterally, the **first compartment** is in relation to the lateral surface of the styloid process of the radius; through it pass the tendons of the **abductor pollicis longus** and the **extensor pollicis brevis.** Just medial to this is a broad **second** compartment for the tendons of the **extensor carpi radialis longus** and the **extensor carpi radialis brevis.** The **third** compartment is a narrow one for the slender tendon of the **extensor pollicis longus.** Medial to this is a wider **fourth** compartment through which pass the four (sometimes only three) tendons of the **extensor digitorum** and the tendon of the **extensor indicis.** The **fifth** compartment lies over the groove between the radius and the ulna and transmits the tendon of the **extensor digiti minimi.** The **sixth** compartment is in relation to the dorsal surface of the ulna, just lateral to the styloid process, and transmits the tendon of the **extensor carpi ulnaris.**

Explore with a blunt probe the limits of the **synovial sheaths** that surround the tendons as they pass deep to the extensor retinaculum. Each tendon has its own synovial sheath, except for a single sheath enclosing the tendons of the extensor digitorum and the tendon of the extensor indicis. The synovial sheaths begin proximal to the extensor retinaculum and extend distally to about the middle of the dorsum of the hand.

Clean the **anconeus muscle.** It arises from the back of the **lateral epicondyle of** the **humerus** and spreads distally and medially to insert on the **lateral border of** the **olecranon.** It is more or less continuous superiorly with the medial head of the triceps; its nerve supply is derived from a branch of the **radial nerve,** which supplies the medial head of the triceps.

Retaining the extensor retinaculum, clean the **superficial layer of muscles** on the posterior aspect of the forearm (Fig. 17.12). The **extensor carpi radialis longus** is the most lateral and is partially overlapped near its origin by the brachioradialis. It arises from the distal portion of the lateral **supracondylar ridge of** the **humerus.** The **remaining muscles** of the superficial layer arise by a **common tendon** from the **lateral epicondyle** and from the **deep fascia** that covers them; they spread distally and medially over the dorsal aspect of the forearm.

The **extensor carpi radialis longus** and **brevis** descend along the lateral side of the forearm, the tendon of the former partially covering that of the latter. Just proximal to the extensor retinaculum,

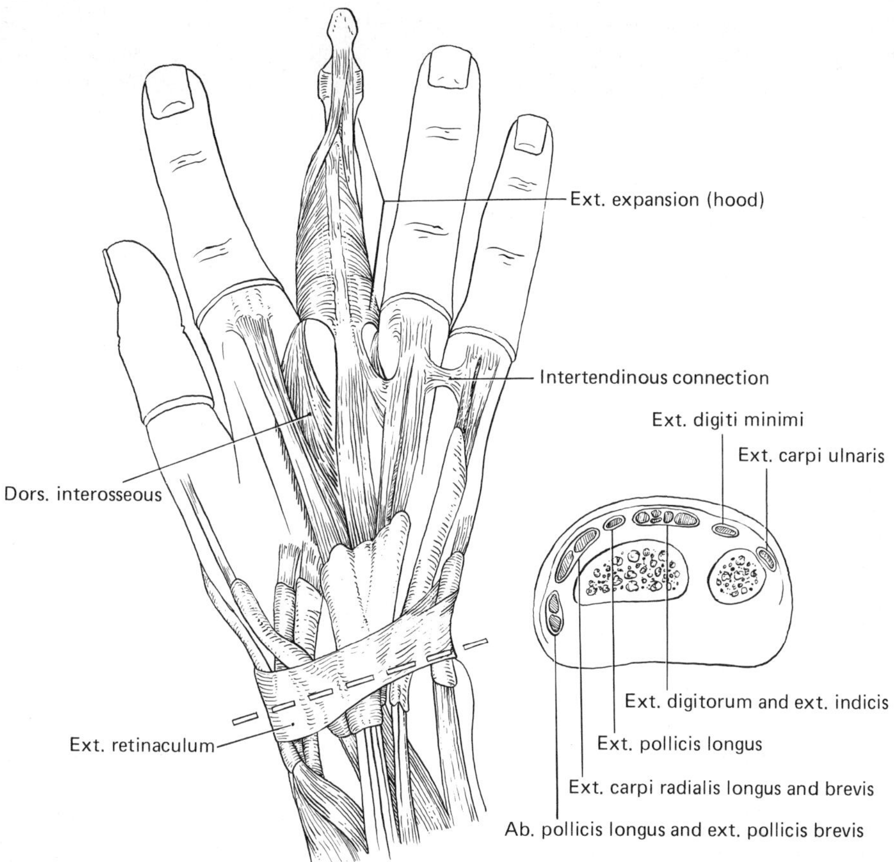

Figure 17.13 The arrangement of the **extensor tendons at** the **wrist** and **on** the **hand.**

they are crossed superficially by two deeper muscles, the abductor pollicis longus and the extensor pollicis brevis. The tendons of the two radial extensors pass deep to the extensor retinaculum as previously noted. Just distal to the retinaculum, they are crossed superficially by the tendon of the extensor pollicis longus. The **extensor carpi radialis longus** inserts into the dorsal aspect of the **base of** the **second metacarpal;** the **extensor carpi radialis brevis** into the adjacent portions of the **bases of** the **second** and **third metacarpals.** The two radial extensors are supplied by branches arising from the **radial nerve** just proximal to its termination or from the **deep radial nerve** before it enters the supinator muscle.

The **extensor digitorum** gives rise, some distance above the wrist, to **four tendons** that pass side by side deep to the extensor retinaculum and radiate toward the fingers. Opposite the dorsal aspect of the metacarpophalangeal joint, each tendon spreads into a fibrous **extensor expansion,** the central portion of which is attached to the **base of** the **proximal phalanx** (Fig. 17.13). This expanded tendon is sometimes called the **extensor hood.** On the dorsum of the proximal phalanx, each expansion divides into **three slips.** The **middle slip** inserts into the base of the **middle phalanx,** and the two **collateral slips** pass distally to insert together into the base of the **distal phalanx.** At about the middle of the proximal phalanx, each extensor tendon receives on its lateral side the tendon of **insertion of** a **lumbrical muscle.** Note further that, while the main insertion of the interossei is directly into the bases of the proximal phalanges, each **interosseous muscle** also inserts into the corresponding **extensor expansion.** The **adjacent tendons** of the extensor digitorum are usually united by oblique **intertendinous connections** on the dorsum of the hand (Fig. 17.13)

The tendon of the **extensor digiti minimi** passes deep to the extensor retinaculum in its own compartment and, at the back of the fifth metacarpophalangeal joint, joins the **fourth tendon of** the **extensor digitorum.**

The **extensor carpi ulnaris** has an accessory origin from the proximal part of the dorsal border of the **ulna.** Its tendon passes deep to the most medial part of the extensor retinaculum and inserts on the base of the **fifth metacarpal.**

Free and elevate the tendons of the extensor digitorum, the extensor digiti minimi and the extensor carpi ulnaris. Detach the ulnar head of the extensor carpi ulnaris and retract the superficial group laterally to expose the deep muscles. While doing this, clean and preserve the nerve twigs that enter the deep surfaces of the muscles in the proximal part of the forearm. In the interval between the superficial and the deep extensors are the **posterior interosseous artery** and **nerve** and their branches. These should be cleaned as the deep muscles are cleaned.

The **supinator** is partly covered by the anconeus, which may be removed. The supinator arises in part from the common tendon on the **lateral epicondyle** but has a more extensive **ulnar origin** from the area just below the radial notch (**supinator fossa** and **crest**). Its fibers form a muscular sheet that wraps laterally around the proximal part of the **radius** to insert on the anterior surface of that bone from the tuberosity to the insertion of the pronator teres. The **deep radial nerve** enters the supinator in the cubital fossa, supplies the muscle, and emerges from its distal part at the back of the forearm. As it emerges from the supinator, the deep radial nerve supplies the extensor digitorum, the extensor digiti minimi, and the extensor carpi ulnaris. The continuation of the nerve is known as the **posterior interosseous nerve.**

The **abductor pollicis longus** arises from the posterior surface of the middle third of both the **radius** and the **ulna** and the intervening portion of the **interosseous membrane.** Its tendon runs distally and laterally, in company with the tendon of the extensor pollicis brevis, to cross the tendons of the radial extensors of the wrist superficially and to pass through the most lateral of the extensor retinacular compartments. It inserts on the lateral side of the **base of** the **first metacarpal.**

The **extensor pollicis brevis** arises from the posterior surface of the middle third of the **radius** (distal to the abductor pollicis) and the adjacent part of the **interosseous membrane.** It inserts on the **base of** the **proximal phalanx of** the **thumb.**

The **extensor pollicis longus** arises from the posterior surface of the middle third of the **ulna** (distal to the abductor pollicis) and the adjacent portion of the **interosseous membrane.** Its tendon passes deep to the extensor retinaculum in a compartment of its own and inserts into the **base of** the **distal phalanx of** the **thumb.**

The **extensor indicis** takes origin from a small area on the posterior surface of the **ulna** and the **interosseous membrane,** just distal to the origin of the extensor pollicis longus. Its tendon crosses the wrist in the same compartment with the tendons of the extensor digitorum. Both here and on the dorsum of the hand, it is covered by the first tendon of the latter muscle, which it joins at the back of the **second metacarpophalangeal joint.**

The **posterior interosseous artery** was seen to arise in the anterior part of the forearm and to pass posteriorly above the interosseous membrane. It appears at the back of the forearm between the adjacent borders of the supinator and the abductor pollicis longus and descends between the deep and superficial muscles, to all of which it gives branches. Near the lower border of the supinator, it gives rise to the **interosseous recurrent artery,** which ascends, under cover of the anconeus, to anastomose behind the lateral epicondyle with

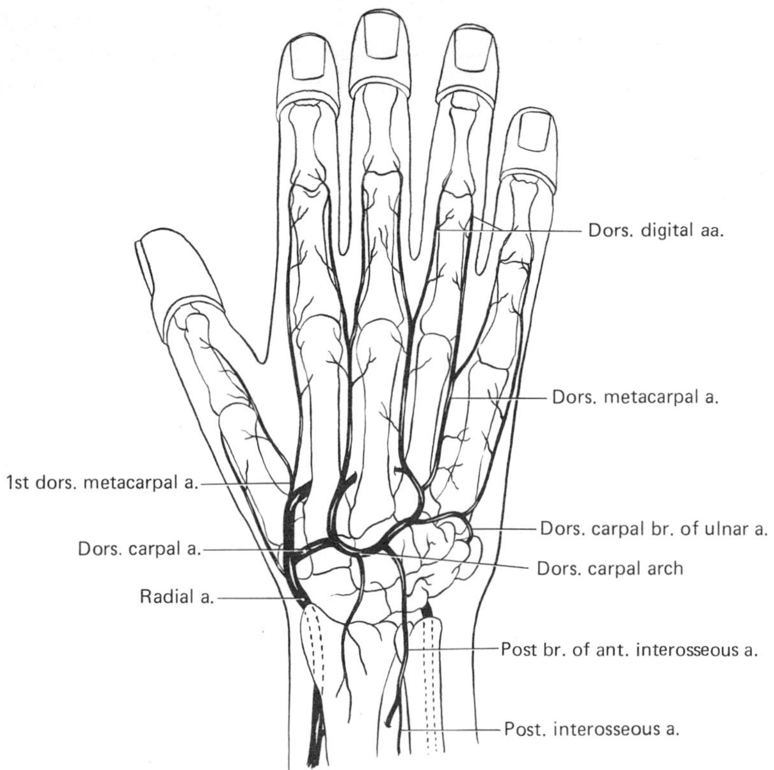

Figure 17.14 Diagrammatic presentation of the **arterial system on** the **dorsum of** the **hand.**

the **middle collateral branch of** the **profunda brachii.**

The **posterior interosseous nerve** descends between the deep and the superficial muscles, supplying branches to the four deep extensor muscles. A slender continuation of the nerve descends on the dorsal surface of the interosseous membrane, deep to the extensor pollicis longus and extensor indicis and, passing deep to the tendons of the extensor digitorum, is distributed to the **carpal joints.** To expose this nerve and the posterior branch of the anterior interosseous artery, divide the extensor retinaculum over the tendons of the extensor digitorum. The **posterior branch of** the **anterior interosseous artery** pierces the interosseous membrane some distance proximal to the wrist and descends in company with the posterior interosseous nerve to the back of the wrist.

As it winds laterally and dorsally around the wrist, the **radial artery** passes deep to the tendons of the abductor pollicis longus and the extensors pollicis longus and brevis. At the base of the first interosseous space, it turns into the palm as the **deep palmar arch.** At this point, the radial artery gives two branches, the **dorsal carpal artery** and the **first dorsal metacarpal artery.** The **dorsal carpal branch** runs medially across the back of the wrist to anastomose with the **dorsal carpal branch of** the **ulnar artery** and with terminal twigs of the **posterior branch of** the **anterior interosseous** to form the **dorsal carpal arch** (Fig. 17.14). From it arise the second, third, and fourth dorsal metacarpal arteries. The **dorsal metacarpals** descend in the interosseous spaces; each divides into two small **dorsal digital branches** for the adjacent sides of two fingers.

JOINTS

Dissect the joints of only one extremity (Figs. 17.15 and 17.16); the other should be saved for reviewing the entire dissected limb and for relating the various structures to the joints. While dissecting the muscles and other structures away from the joints, take the opportunity to follow the course of the anastomotic, **collateral vessels** and the **nerves to** the **joints,** which could not be dissected adequately in the preceding dissection of the superior extremity.

Acromioclavicular Joint

The clavicle is joined to the scapula by means of a synovial (diarthrodial) joint between the **lateral end of** the **clavicle** and the **acromion process** and by a ligamentous union between the inferior surface of the flattened lateral part of the clavicle and the **coracoid process.** These should now be studied. Push the clavicle upward from in front and clean the two portions of the **coracoclavicular ligament.** The **conoid ligament** is the **more medial;** it is a strong fibrous cord that passes upward and laterally from the medial side of the root of the **coracoid process** to the **conoid tubercle** on the inferior surface **of** the **clavicle.** The **trapezoid ligament** is a flat fibrous band; it is attached below to a rough ridge on the medial border of the **coracoid process** and above to an oblique line on the **inferior surface of** the **clavicle,** which runs forward and laterally from the conoid tubercle. The **acromioclavicular joint** is surrounded by a fibrous capsule attached to the margins of the opposing articular surfaces of the two bones. Open this capsule and observe the articular surfaces of the two bones. Divide the conoid and trapezoid ligaments and disarticulate the clavicle.

Shoulder Joint

The **shoulder joint** is a ball and socket synovial joint. To clean its **articular capsule,** divide the coracoacromial ligament along its line of attachment to the coracoid. Then saw through the acromion at its junction with the scapular spine and remove the acromion and the coracoacromial ligament. The **fibrous capsule** of the shoulder joint is attached medially to the **margin of** the **glenoid fossa** and laterally to the **anatomical neck of** the **humerus.** It is almost entirely surrounded by the muscles that pass from the scapula to the tubercles of the humerus. The **supraspinatus, infraspinatus,** and **teres minor** have already been divided; reflect the lateral segments of these muscles laterally and posteriorly toward their insertions and observe that they are firmly bound to the articular capsule. Anteriorly, the capsule is covered by the **subscapularis.** Divide this muscle about 5 cm medial to the lesser tubercle and reflect its lateral segment laterally, thus exposing the opening in the fibrous capsule by which the **articular synovial cavity communicates with** the **subscapular bursa.**

Fusion of the tendons of the supraspinatus, infraspinatus, teres minor, and subscapularis muscles to the shoulder joint capsule in addition to their bony attachments forms a musculotendinous (rotator) cuff that strengthens the capsule and helps maintain the head of the humerus in the shallow glenoid cavity. Although the shoulder joint is the most movable joint in the body, it is also the most frequently dislocated (inferiorly where the capsule is not buttressed by tendons and ligaments).

Clean the **coracohumeral ligament,** a strong band stretching from the lateral border of the coracoid downward and laterally to the upper part of the **greater tubercle.** Only at its medial end is it distinctly separable from the fibrous capsule. The **transverse ligament of** the **humerus** is a fibrous band, closely connected with the capsule, that extends **between** the **two tubercles** roofing over the proximal portion of the intertubercular sulcus. The **glenohumeral ligaments** are thickenings in the anterior part of the capsule, which may best be seen from the inside (Fig. 17.15). Divide the posterior part of the capsule vertically and turn the head of the humerus laterally and anteriorly, so that the internal surface of the anterior part of the capsule may be seen. The **superior glenohumeral ligament** stretches from the **glenoid border** at the

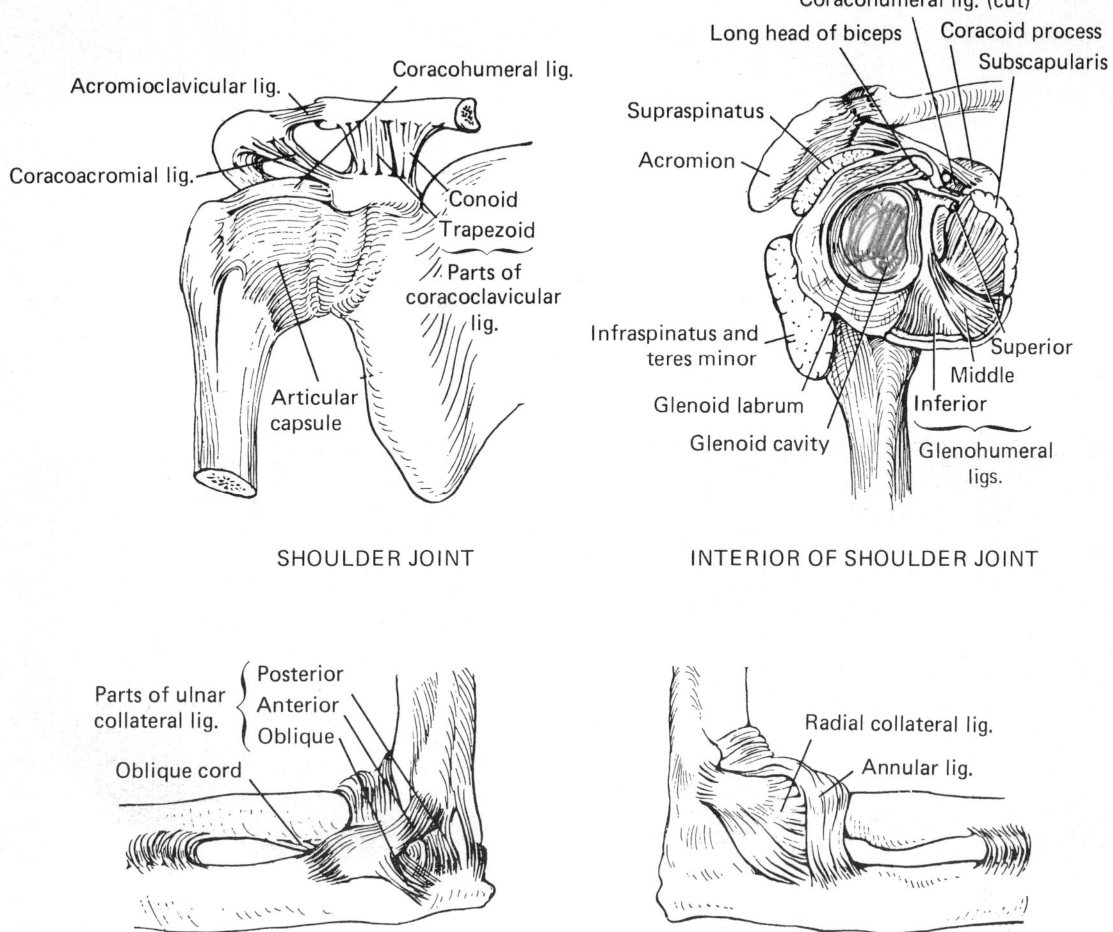

Figure 17.15 Joints of the superior extremity.

root of the coracoid downward and laterally to the summit of the **lesser tubercle.** The **middle** and **inferior glenohumeral ligaments** are less distinct thickenings in the lower anterior part of the capsule. The **opening into** the **subscapular bursa** lies between the superior and the middle glenohumeral ligaments.

Observe that the tendon of the **long head of** the **biceps** arises from the **supraglenoid tubercle of** the **scapula** and passes through the articular cavity to reach the **intertubercular sulcus.** Divide this tendon and the anterior part of the capsule and separate the humerus from the scapula. Observe the **glenoid labrum.** This narrow fibrocartilaginous ring surmounts the edge of the bony glenoid cavity and slightly deepens it.

Elbow Joint

Clean the **capsule of** the **elbow joint.** Anteriorly, the distal part of the **brachialis** is closely applied to the capsule; posteriorly, it is covered by the **triceps** and the **anconeus.** These muscles must be removed in cleaning the capsule. The origins of the superficial flexors and extensors should also be cut away from the medial and lateral epicondyles. Now is a good time to review the attachments of the supinator muscle. At the **elbow joint** (hinge type), the distal end of the **humerus** meets the proximal articular surfaces of the **radius** and the **ulna.** Enclosed in the same capsule, however, and with a common articular cavity, is the proximal **radioulnar joint** (pivot type). The **fibrous capsule** is attached above to the **humerus** and below to the margins of the **articular surfaces of** the **ulna** and the neck of the **radius.** All the **ligaments of** the **elbow joint** are merely thickenings of the fibrous capsule. The strongest of these are the radial and the ulnar collateral ligaments. The **ulnar collateral ligament** spreads distally from the **medial epicondyle** to attach to a ridge on the medial borders of the **coronoid** and **olecranon processes of** the **ulna.** The **radial collateral ligament** arises from the **lateral epicondyle.** Its fibers pass distally, and most of them end by joining the lateral part of the **anular ligament;** some fibers, however, reach as far as the neck of the radius. The **anular ligament** is a strong fibrous band whose two ends are attached to the anterior and posterior margins of the **radial notch of** the **ulna.** It encircles the **head of** the **radius** and holds it in place as it rotates against the radial notch in the actions of **pronation** and **supination.** The anular ligament may be seen to better advantage if the joint capsule is opened by a transverse incision across its anterior portion. Observe that the bony articular surfaces are covered by a layer of **cartilage** and that the **articular cavity** is elsewhere lined by the **synovial membrane.**

Wrist Joint

Clean the fibrous capsules of the distal radioulnar joint and the wrist joint. At the **distal radioulnar joint** (pivot type), the **ulna** articulates with the **ulnar notch on** the **radius** and with the proximal surface of the **radial articular disk.** Its external ligaments are the **palmar** and **dorsal radioulnar ligaments,** which connect the distal ends of the

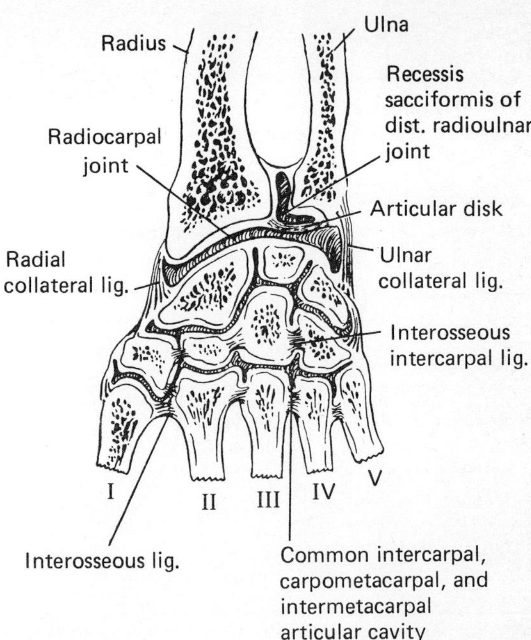

VERTICAL SECTION THROUGH WRIST JOINTS

Figure 17.16 Joints of the wrist and fingers.

two bones (Fig. 17.16). At the **wrist joint,** the distal surfaces of the **radius** and **radial articular disk** articulate with the proximal surfaces of the **scaphoid** and **lunate.** Its external ligaments are the radial and ulnar collateral ligaments of the wrist and the palmar and dorsal radiocarpal ligaments. The **ulnar collateral (medial) ligament** is a fibrous cord that descends from the **ulnar styloid process** to the **pisiform** and **triquetrum bones.** The **radial collateral (lateral) ligament** consists of fibers that radiate from the tip of the **styloid process of** the **radius** to the **scaphoid** and **trapezium bones.** The **dorsal** and **palmar radiocarpal ligaments** are thickened parts of the capsule that spread distally from the lateral part of the distal end of the **radius** to the dorsal and palmar surfaces of the **carpal bones.** Open the joint by a transverse incision across the anterior part of the capsule and study the articular surfaces. The **articular disk** is a **plate of fibrocartilage** attached laterally to the medial border of the **radial ar-**

ticular surface and medially to the **styloid process of** the **ulna.** It articulates distally with the **triquetrum bone** and separates the cavity of the wrist joint from that of the distal radioulnar joint.

Carpal and Metacarpal Joints

The carpal bones are joined by dorsal, palmar, and interosseous ligaments. **Four separate articular cavities,** in addition to that of the wrist joint, are found in connection with the carpal bones. These may be investigated by dividing the ligaments that bind the dorsal surfaces of the bones and spreading the bones apart to expose the articular surfaces. The **first,** a single large cavity, includes the articulations of the **scaphoid, lunate,** and **triquetrum** with each other and with the four **bones of** the **distal row.** It is further prolonged along both sides of the trapezoid to include the articulations between the **second** and **third metacarpals** and between the **capitate** and **trapezoid.** A **second** articular cavity is found at the junction of the **trapezium** and the **first metacarpal.** A **third** cavity is for the articulation of the **fourth** and **fifth metacarpals** with the **hamate.** The **fourth** is a small cavity between the **pisiform** and the **triquetrum.**

Chapter 18

Inferior Extremity

SURFACE ANATOMY

The sequence of this dissection is based on the assumption that you have already dissected the abdomen and pelvis and that you have separated one-half of the pelvis from the vertebral column. If you dissect the extremity while the abdomen is still intact, it is advisable to make a slight rearrangement to avoid the necessity of turning the body too frequently. You can accomplish this by dissecting the anterior part of the thigh, leg, and foot while the body is in the supine position. Then turn the body over and dissect the gluteal region, posterior part of the thigh, popliteal fossa, and flexor surfaces of the leg and foot.

Before you reflect the skin from the inferior extremity, direct your attention to its surface anatomy. Anteriorly, the **thigh** is marked off from the **anterior abdominal wall** by a depressed line running from the anterior superior iliac spine to the pubic tubercle that corresponds to the **inguinal ligament.** The **gluteal region** or buttock, the prominence of which is caused principally by the **gluteus maximus muscle,** forms the upper lateral and posterior portion of the inferior extremity. It is bounded above by the **iliac crest,** which generally can be palpated, and inferiorly, it is demarcated from the posterior thigh region by the gluteal skin crease. Medially, the thigh is separated from the perineum by the border of the **ischiopubic ramus.** The head and shaft of the **femur** are for the most part deeply placed and covered by thick layers of muscle, which give the thigh its rounded contour. The lateral surface of the **greater trochanter,** however, is subcutaneous. It lies about 7 cm below the anterior superior iliac spine and usually projects farther laterally than the most lateral portion of the iliac crest. At the front of the knee, the anterior surface of the **patella** (kneecap) is subcutaneous. At the lateral side of the knee, the **lateral condyle of** the **femur** can be palpated; immediately below it is the **lateral condyle of** the **tibia** and the **head of** the **fibula.** At the medial side of the knee, locate the **medial condyle of** the **femur** and the **medial condyle of** the **tibia.**

Identify some surface landmarks of the **leg** and **foot.** Observe that the broad, flat, medial surface of the **tibia** is subcutaneous throughout its length and is continuous below with the **medial malleolus,** which is also subcutaneous. The shaft of the fibula is, for the most part, covered by muscles. The **head of** the **fibula,** however, can be palpated just below the posterior part of the lateral condyle of the tibia. It becomes very prominent when the knee is flexed. At the lateral side of the ankle, the **lateral malleolus of** the **fibula** is subcutaneous. All the individual tarsal bones cannot be recognized. However, the **tuberosity of** the **calcaneus,** which forms the prominence of the heel, and the **tendon of** the **calcaneus** (Achilles tendon), which attaches to it posteriorly, can be easily recognized. Identify the **tuberosity of** the **navicular bone** on the medial border of the foot, slightly below and in front of the medial malleolus. Somewhat farther anteriorly, on the lateral margin of the foot, you may be able to feel the **tuberosity of** the **fifth metatarsal,** which forms a prominent bony projection.

Now reflect the skin from the entire extremity. Make a longitudinal incision through the skin downward along the medial aspect of the thigh from the lower border of the pubic symphysis to the medial condyle of the tibia as shown in Fig. 18.1. From the lower end of this incision, make a transverse incision across the front of the leg, about 2.5 cm below the patella, to the head of the fibula. Starting at the upper end of the longitudinal incision, reflect the skin laterally from the entire anterior aspect of the thigh; then continue the reflection posteriorly and downward from the buttock and the posterior aspect of the thigh. The incisions made over the sacrum and coccyx during the dissection of the back will aid

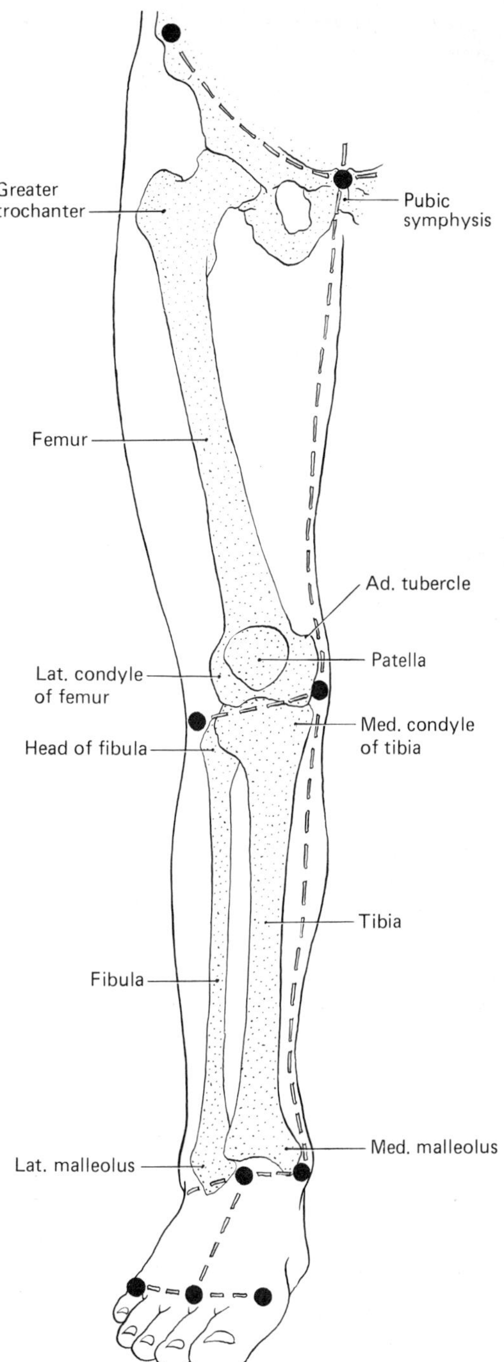

Figure 18.1 Surface projections and skin incisions on the inferior extremity.

you in reflecting the skin laterally over the gluteal region.

Now remove the large skin flap reflected from the thigh by cutting it along the line where it remains attached to the upper posterior part of the leg. Then make a longitudinal incision through the skin of the leg along the medial surface of the tibia as far as the lower tip of the medial malleolus. From the lower end of this incision, make another one that completely encircles the posterior part of the foot; it must go transversely across the front of the ankle downward and backward below the lateral malleolus, then across the lower back part of the heel, and upward and forward below the medial malleolus to the starting point. Reflect and remove this large skin flap from the entire circumference of the leg.

Then make a transverse incision across the dorsum of the foot at the bases of the toes and a longitudinal incision running backward along the dorsum from the middle of this transverse incision to the front of the ankle. This will mark out two flaps of skin on the dorsum of the foot, which you should reflect to the lateral and medial borders of the foot, respectively. Make a transverse incision through the skin across the sole of the foot at the bases of the toes. From the middle of this incision, carry a longitudinal incision backward to the heel. Then reflect the two skin flaps thus marked out to each side. The skin should also be reflected from the plantar aspect of the toes. Do this by making a longitudinal incision along the middle of each toe. Observe that the plantar skin is very thick and closely bound to the superficial fascia by means of fibrous strands, which extend from the plantar aponeurosis through the superficial fascia to the skin.

CUTANEOUS VEINS AND NERVES

The **superficial fascia of** the **thigh** is typical and usually moderately thick. There are numerous **superficial veins** within it (Fig 18.2). The largest and most constant of them is the **great saphenous vein,** which you should now clean. It begins from the medial side of the **dorsal venous arch of** the **foot** and passes anterior to the medial malleolus. From there it ascends on the **medial side of** the **leg** and courses behind the medial side of the knee. The great saphenous vein then continues upward along the **medial side of** the **thigh,** inclining somewhat anteriorly, and joins the **femoral vein** about 2.5 cm below the inguinal ligament by passing through the **saphenous hiatus.** This is an oval opening in the deep fascia (fascia lata) of the thigh that lies immediately in front of the femoral vein, below the middle part of the inguinal ligament. The hiatus is filled with loose connective tissue called the **cribriform fascia.** Look for an **accessory saphenous vein** that ascends on the medial side of the thigh to drain into the great saphenous vein near the hiatus. You will encounter numerous unnamed veins as well.

The **small (lesser) saphenous vein** begins from the lateral side of the dorsal venous arch, ascends posterior to the lateral malleolus along the lateral aspect of the leg, and terminates posteriorly in the popliteal vein (Fig. 18.2).

The superficial veins connect with the deeper veins by **perforating** or **communicating veins** (Fig. 18.2). Elevate the superficial veins near the ankle, and note some of the perforating veins.

The valves in this venous system are arranged to allow unidirectional blood flow toward the deep veins. Muscular massage, therefore, becomes an important factor in returning the long column of blood to the heart. An increase in the venous pressure here, such as could occur during pregnancy, by proximal venous obstruction, or simply by long hours of standing, will cause varicose veins, particularly if the valves are incompetent.

Observe the **superficial inguinal lymph nodes.** There are from 10 to 20 of them, and they are often of considerable size. They lie in the superficial fascia along the inguinal ligament and in the region of the saphenous hiatus. In many cases, the fine **lymphatic vessels** that communicate with them can be seen. In addition to receiving the lymph drainage from the lower extremity, these nodes also receive afferent channels from the ab-

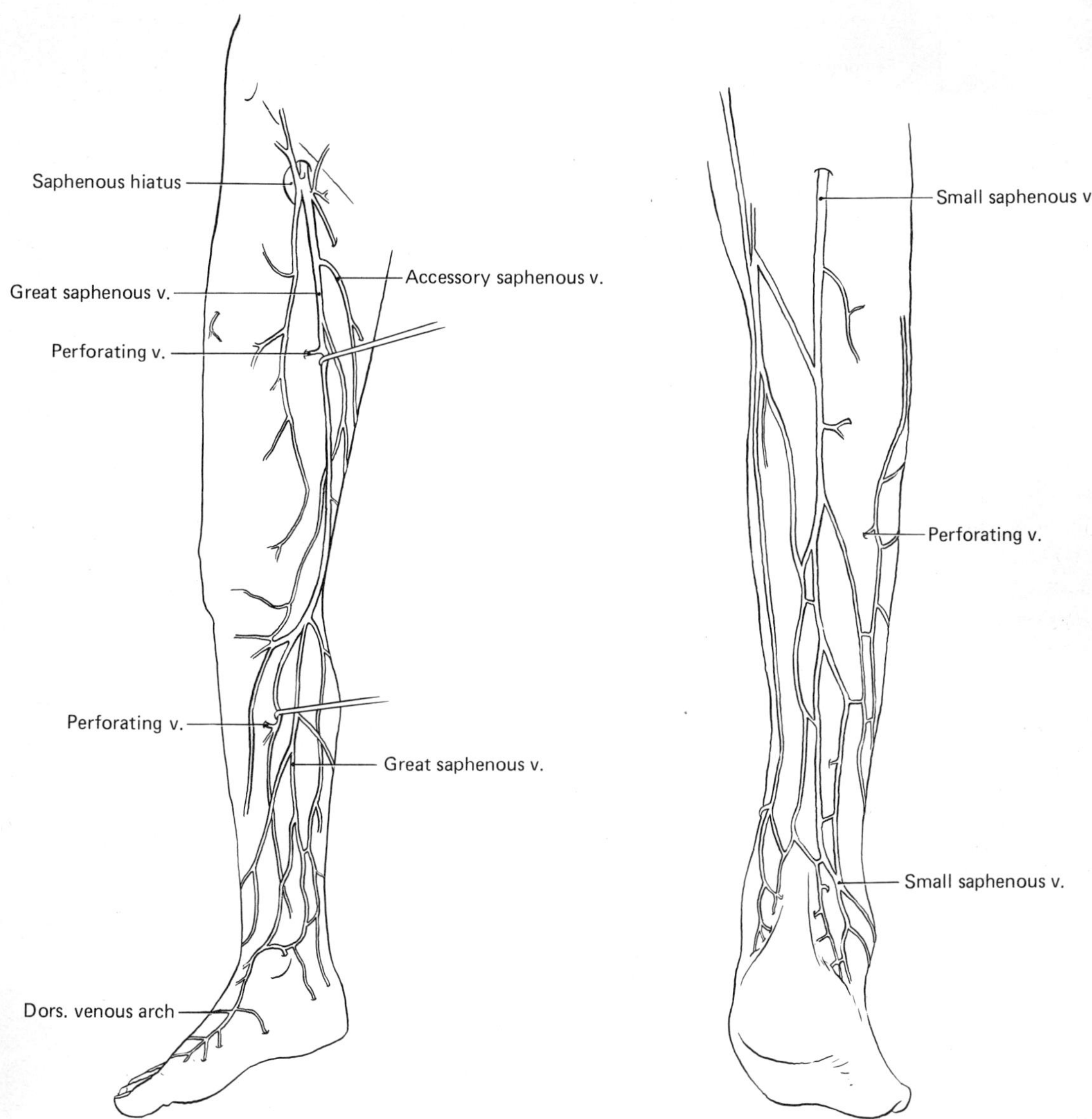

Figure 18.2 Primary **superficial veins** of the anteromedial aspect of the lower extremity (*left*) and of the posterior aspect of the leg (*right*).

dominal wall below the level of the umbilicus, the penis and scrotum (vulva in the female), the perineum, and the gluteal region. The superficial inguinal lymph nodes drain into the external iliac nodes.

Direct your attention next to the **cutaneous nerves of** the **thigh.** The main trunks and branches pierce the fascia lata at variable distances below the inguinal ligament or the iliac crest and descend along the deep surface of the superficial fascia. Remove the superficial fascia as you display them.

The **lateral femoral cutaneous nerve,** a **branch**

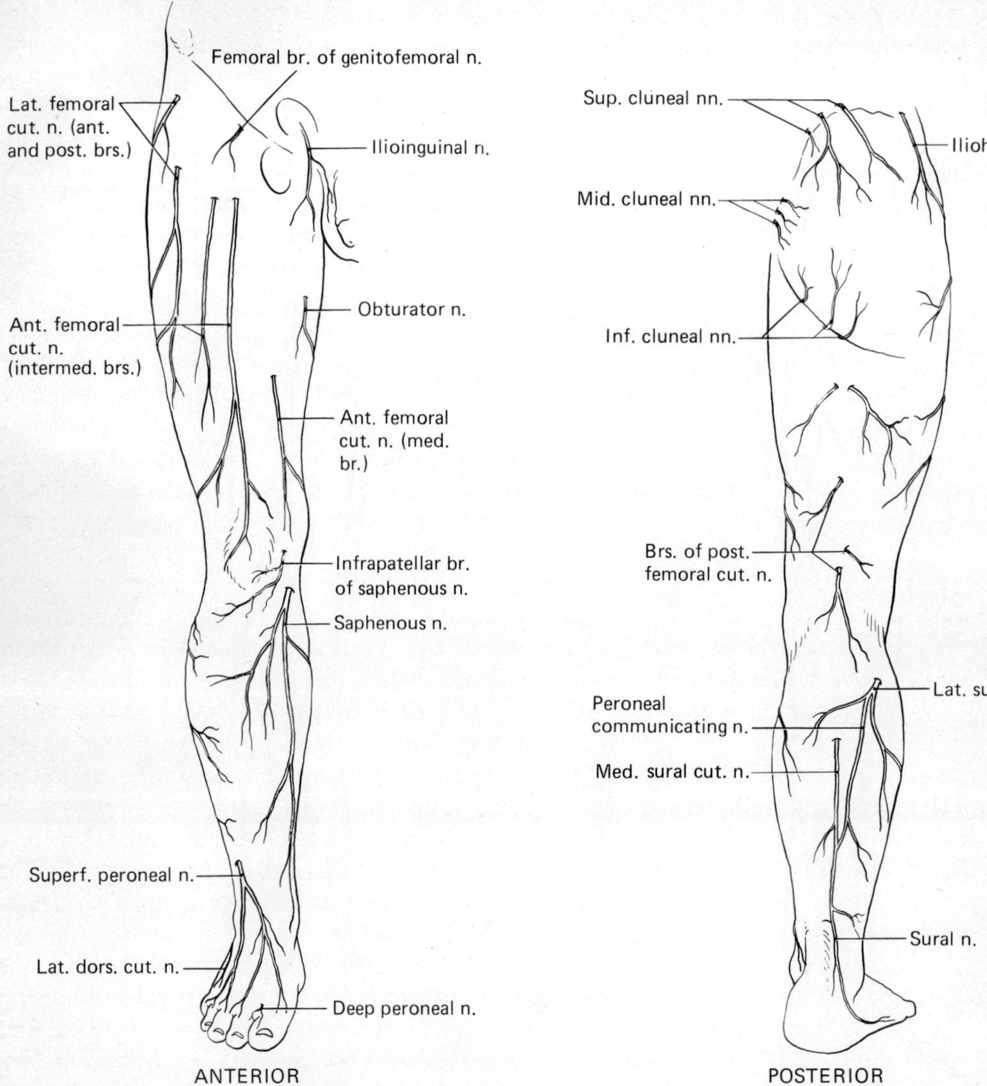

Figure 18.3 Cutaneous nerves of the inferior extremity.

of the lumbar plexus, enters the thigh by passing behind the lateral end of the inguinal ligament. Below the inguinal ligament, it divides into anterior and posterior branches that pierce the fascia lata separately (Fig. 18.3). The **posterior branch** supplies the skin on the upper lateral part of the thigh and buttock. The **anterior branch** becomes superficial somewhat lower and more anteriorly and supplies the skin on the lower anterolateral part of the thigh.

The **femoral branch** is one of the terminal branches of the **genitofemoral nerve.** It emerges through the saphenous hiatus or may pierce the fascia lata near the opening. It supplies the skin below the inguinal ligament on the upper anterior aspect of the thigh over the femoral triangle.

The **anterior cutaneous branches of** the **femoral nerve** are divided into intermediate and medial branches. Their origin from the femoral nerve will be seen when the femoral triangle is dissected. Find the terminal branches piercing the fascia lata and trace them downward on the thigh. The branches of the **intermediate cutaneous nerve** pierce the fascia lata close together, at the middle of the anterior aspect of the thigh about a third of the distance between the inguinal ligament and the knee. The branches of the **medial cutaneous nerve** usually appear close to the great saphenous vein, piercing the fascia lata at any point along the course of the vein in the thigh.

The **infrapatellar branch of** the **saphenous nerve** is a cutaneous nerve that becomes superficial at the medial side of the knee, from where it takes a curved course downward and forward below the patella.

The **cutaneous nerves of** the **gluteal region** include the lateral cutaneous **branch of** the **iliohypogastric nerve** and a group of small nerves known as the **cluneal nerves.** They are small and usually difficult to demonstrate, but you should attempt to identify them as you remove the superficial fascia. The **lateral cutaneous branch of** the **iliohypogastric nerve** runs downward over the iliac crest at about the junction of its anterior and middle thirds and is distributed to the skin over the upper anterolateral buttock. The **superior cluneal nerves** are the lateral branches of the **dorsal rami of** the first three **lumbar nerves.** They cross the iliac crest in series behind the lateral cutaneous branch of the iliohypogastric nerve and are distributed to the skin of the gluteal region. The **middle cluneal nerves** are small nerves derived from the lateral branches of the **dorsal rami of** the first three **sacral nerves.** They pierce the gluteus maximus in a line running from the posterior superior iliac spine to the tip of the coccyx and supply the skin over the medial part of the gluteus maximus. The **inferior cluneal nerves** are branches of the **posterior femoral cutaneous nerve;** they curve upward around the lower border of the gluteus maximus to supply the skin on the lower part of the gluteal region. Their identification is easier when the gluteus maximus is cleaned.

Continue with the **cutaneous nerves of** the posterior aspect of the **leg.** Although some variation occurs in their distribution, you will find most of them by following the descripton given here. The **medial** and **lateral sural cutaneous nerves** arise in or near the popliteal fossa. The **lateral sural cutaneous nerve** is distributed to the skin on the upper lateral and anterolateral part of the leg. The **medial sural cutaneous nerve** accompanies the **small saphenous vein** down the back of the calf. The **peroneal communicating nerve,** which is usually a branch of the lateral sural cutaneous nerve, passes downward and backward across the calf and joins the medial sural cutaneous nerve to form the **sural nerve.** The sural nerve supplies the lower lateral part of the leg and turns forward, below the lateral malleolus, to supply the lateral margin of the foot, where it is known as the **lateral dorsal cutaneous nerve;** it may be traced as far forward as the lateral side of the little toe.

The **saphenous nerve** becomes superficial inferomedial to the knee. It descends in company with the **great saphenous vein** and supplies the skin on the medial and anteromedial part of the leg as far down as the medial malleolus; branches of the saphenous nerve can often be followed for a considerable distance along the medial margin of the foot.

The **superficial peroneal nerve** is one of the terminal branches of the **common peroneal nerve.** Piercing the deep fascia on the anterolateral aspect of the leg about halfway between the knee and the ankle, it divides almost at once into a medial and a lateral branch. The **medial branch** passes downward in front of the ankle and divides into **medial** and **lateral trunks.** The **medial trunk** passes forward to the skin along the medial side of the great toe. The **lateral trunk** reaches the cleft between the second and third toes and divides into two dorsal digital branches that supply the skin on the adjacent sides of these toes. The **lateral branch** of the superficial peroneal also gives rise to **two trunks,** from which **dorsal digital nerves** arise to supply the adjacent sides of the third and fourth, and fourth and fifth toes.

The skin on the adjacent sides of the great and second toes is supplied by two dorsal digital branches of the terminal part of the **deep peroneal nerve.** Find it emerging in the cleft between these toes.

The cutaneous innervation to the sole of the foot will be examined later.

THIGH

At this point, the **superficial fascia** should have been removed from the anterior and lateral aspects of the thigh to expose the **deep fascia.** If it has not been removed, do it now. Retain the **medial** and **intermediate rami of** the **anterior cutaneous nerves** so that their origin from the femoral nerve can later be recognized. The deep fascia that invests the thigh is known as the **fascia lata.** Superiorly, it is attached to the inguinal ligament and the iliac crest. Toward the medial aspect of the thigh, the fascia lata is relatively thin and does not differ appreciably from the deep fascia that is ordinarily found investing muscles. Along the lateral aspect of the thigh, however, it is resolved into a very dense aponeurotic band known as the **iliotibial tract,** which you should now investigate. Superiorly, it is attached to the **anterior part of** the **iliac crest** through the fascia covering the gluteus medius muscle. Inferiorly, it extends over the lateral side of the knee joint to attach to the **lateral condyle of** the **tibia.** The iliotibial tract receives the insertions of the **tensor fasciae latae muscle** and most of the fibers of the **gluteus maximus.** Clean the external surfaces of these two muscles and study their relationship to the fascia lata.

The **tensor fasciae latae** is a flat quadrilateral muscle that arises from the **anterior portion of** the **external lip of** the **iliac crest** and the **anterior superior iliac spine.** Its fibers run downward and somewhat laterally to join the **iliotibial tract** about one-third of the distance down the thigh.

The **gluteus maximus** is a large, thick quadrangular muscle, made up of very coarse muscle fiber bundles. It arises from the most **posterior part of** the **iliac crest** and the **dorsum of** the **ilium** behind the **posterior gluteal line,** from the lateral part of the posterior surface of the **sacrum** and **coccyx,** and from the **sacrotuberous ligament.** Its fibers pass downward and laterally across the buttock, the greater portion of them inserting into the **iliotibial tract** of the fascia lata. The remainder insert into the **gluteal tuberosity** of the femur.

Carefully define the two borders of the **gluteus maximus.** Stretching across a roughly triangular area bounded by the superior border of the gluteus maximus, the posterior border of the tensor fasciae latae, and the iliac crest, the fascia lata covers the external surface of the gluteus medius (Fig. 18.4). This portion of the fascia lata is usually covered by a thick layer of superficial fascia, all of which should be removed.

As you clean the inferior border of the gluteus maximus, look for the **inferior cluneal branches of** the **posterior femoral cutaneous nerve;** they curve upward around this border. The trunk of the posterior femoral cutaneous nerve will emerge from under the middle of the lower border of the gluteus maximus to run downward on the posterior aspect of the thigh.

As described above, the **iliotibial tract** is a greatly thickened portion of the fascia lata and is continuous with the thinner portion of the deep fascia surrounding the rest of the thigh. The fascia covering the anterior thigh muscles must be removed, but you should retain the iliotibial tract. To do this, make a longitudinal incision through the fascia lata, running downward from the lower end of the anterior border of the tensor fasciae latae to the lateral condyle of the tibia. The thick portion of the fascia lata behind the incision is the iliotibial tract. As you clean the anterior thigh muscles, remove the continuation of the fascia lata across the thigh anterior to the incision. Be sure to retain the relative positions of the muscles.

Extensor Region of the Thigh

Clean the **sartorius,** a long, narrow straplike muscle that crosses the anterior aspect of the thigh obliquely. Arising from the **anterior superior iliac spine,** its fibers run downward to the medial

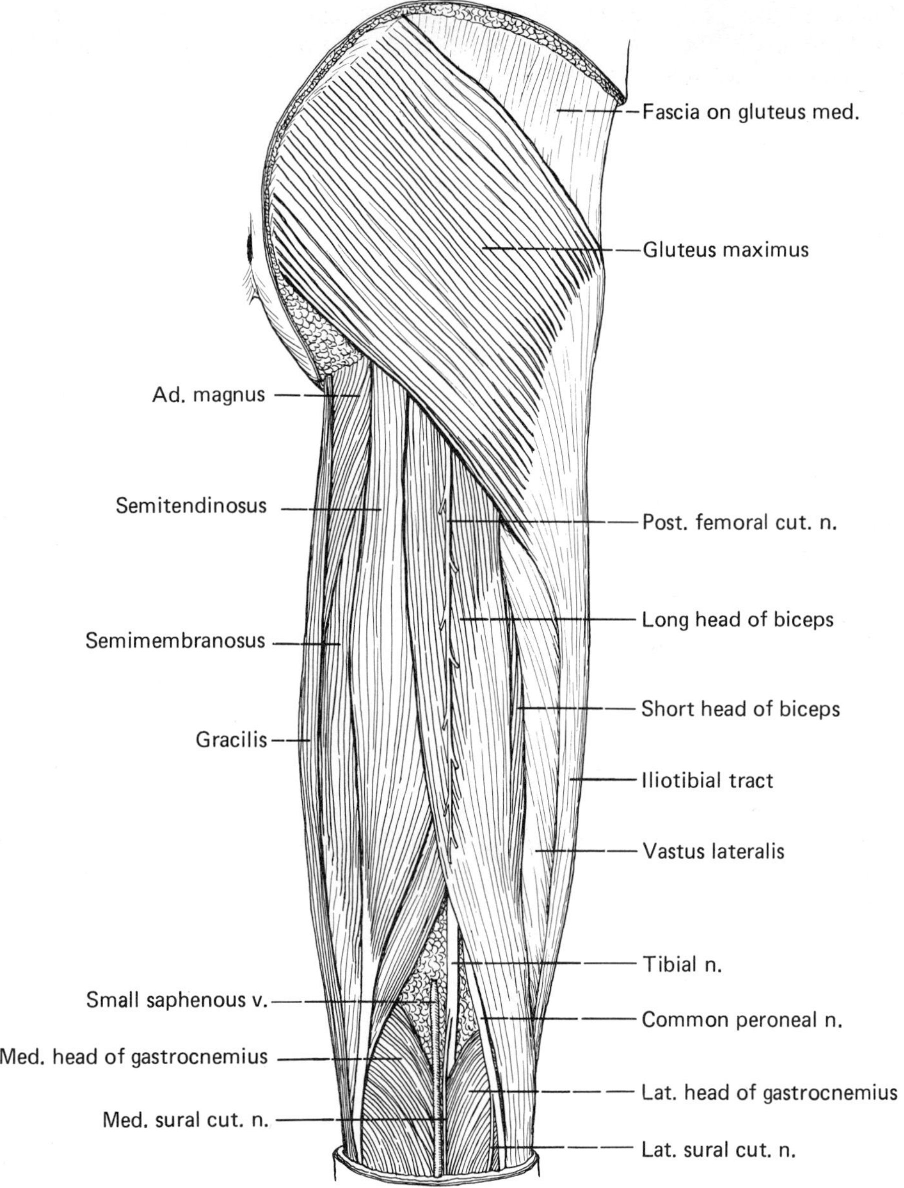

Figure 18.4 The **posterior** aspect of the **thigh.**

side of the knee; from here, the muscle continues downward as a flat tendon that inserts into the upper part of the **medial surface of** the **tibia.** The insertion will be seen later.

The portion of the thigh below and lateral to the sartorius is occupied by four muscles that make up the **quadriceps femoris;** they are the **rectus femoris,** the **vastus medialis, vastus intermedius,** and **vastus lateralis** (Fig. 18.5).

The uppermost portion of the **rectus femoris** is overlapped by the sartorius medially and the tensor fasciae latae laterally. It arises from the **coxal**

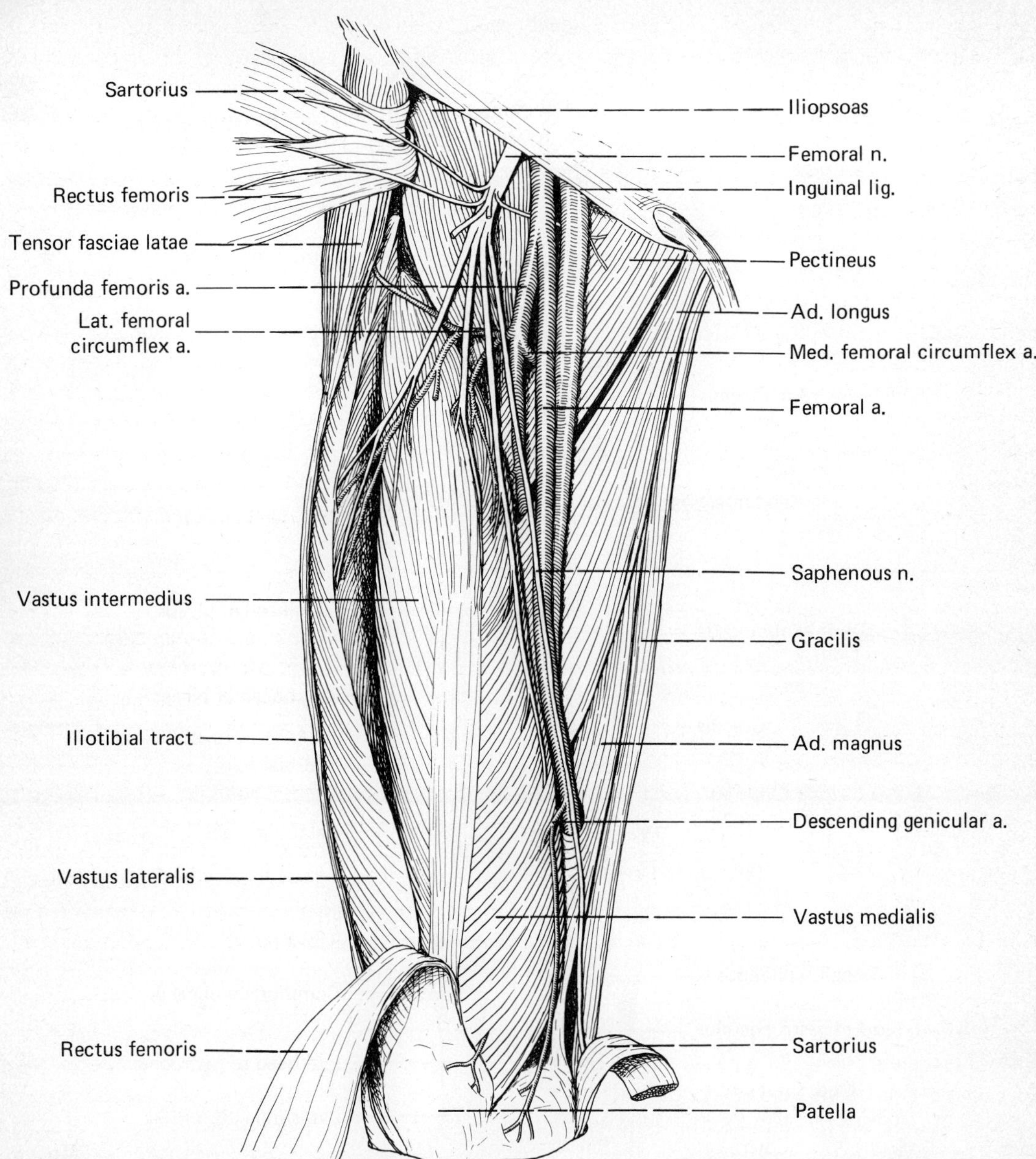

Figure 18.5 The **anterior** aspect of the **thigh.**

(hip) bone by two separate short tendons, which may be seen better later. The **straight tendon** arises from the **anterior inferior iliac spine,** and the **reflected tendon** from the upper surface of the **rim of** the **acetabulum.** The two tendons unite to form an aponeurotic expansion, whose anterior surface can now be seen in the interval between the upper part of the sartorius and the tensor fasciae latae. Observe that muscle fibers spread downward from this aponeurosis to form a thick, spindle-shaped muscle that inserts by a strong, flat tendon into the **upper border of** the **patella.**

Lateral to the rectus femoris, clean the exposed portion of the **vastus lateralis.** Draw the iliotibial tract laterally and observe that it lies immediately external to the broad lateral surface of the vastus lateralis. Pass your hand posteriorly in the interval between the tract and the vastus lateralis, and observe that a short fascial septum extends inward from the deep surface of the posterolateral portion of the fascia lata to the lateral lip of the linea aspera and the lateral supracondylar ridge. This is the **lateral intermuscular septum** of the thigh, which **separates** the anterior **extensor group** of muscles **from** the posterior **flexor** or hamstring **muscles.**

Turn next to the medial aspect of the thigh and clean the external surface of the **gracilis.** It arises by a flat tendon from the margin of the **inferior ramus of** the **pubis.** Its upper portion is flat and relatively broad, and as it descends on the medial aspect of the thigh, it becomes narrower and thicker, finally giving rise to a rounded tendon that descends behind the medial condyle of the femur. Its insertion on the **medial surface of** the **tibia** will be seen later. In the lower half of the thigh, the gracilis lies immediately posterior to the sartorius. The interval on the upper anterior part of the thigh, between the medial border of the sartorius and the anterior border of the gracilis, from which the deep fascia has not yet been removed, is occupied by the **adductor muscles.**

Before you dissect the adductor muscles, define the **femoral triangle.** It is bounded **above** by the **inguinal ligament, laterally** by the medial border of the upper part of the **sartorius,** and **medially** by the medial border of the **adductor longus.** Its **roof** is formed by the **fascia lata,** which here is relatively thin. The **floor** of the triangle is formed by the anterior surfaces of the **adductor longus, pectineus,** and **iliopsoas muscles.** The contents of the femoral triangle include the upper portions of the **femoral vessels** and the terminal branches of the **femoral nerve.** Remove the fascial roof of the femoral triangle, define the medial border of the adductor longus, and study the femoral vessels and the femoral sheath.

The **adductor longus** arises by a narrow, flat tendon from the **superior ramus of** the **pubis** near the pubic tubercle. The muscle widens as it passes downward and laterally toward its insertion on the middle third of the medial lip of the **linea aspera.** Its medial border, particularly near the origin, is usually adjacent to the anterior border of the gracilis (Fig. 18.5).

The **femoral artery** begins behind the inguinal ligament as a direct continuation of the **external iliac artery.** It descends in the femoral triangle, which it leaves a short distance above the apex of the triangle, by passing deep to the sartorius. At its **beginning,** the **femoral artery** is **lateral to** the **femoral vein; lower** down, it lies **anterior to** the **vein.** In the uppermost part of the femoral triangle, both the artery and the vein are enclosed within the femoral sheath; study it.

The **femoral sheath** is a funnel-shaped fascial sheath that represents a prolongation behind the inguinal ligament into the thigh of portions of the **transversalis fascia** and the **iliac fascia.** Its **anterior part** is continuous above the inguinal ligament with the **transversalis fascia;** its **posterior part** is continuous with the portion of the **iliac fascia** that lies behind the external iliac vessels (Fig. 18.6). The **lateral boundary** of the femoral sheath is formed by the joining of these two fascial layers around the lateral side of the femoral artery. The femoral sheath can be traced as a distinct structure for only 2.5 cm below the inguinal ligament; beyond this, it blends with the general fascial covering of the vessels. Its chief importance lies in the fact that its anterior and posterior walls do not join immediately on the medial side of the femoral vein but are prolonged farther medially to enclose a compartment of the sheath known as the **femoral canal.** The canal, which lies along the medial side of the uppermost part of the femoral vein, is filled with loose connective tissue, fat, and lymph nodes.

The upper entrance or abdominal end of the femoral canal is known as the **femoral ring.** Insert

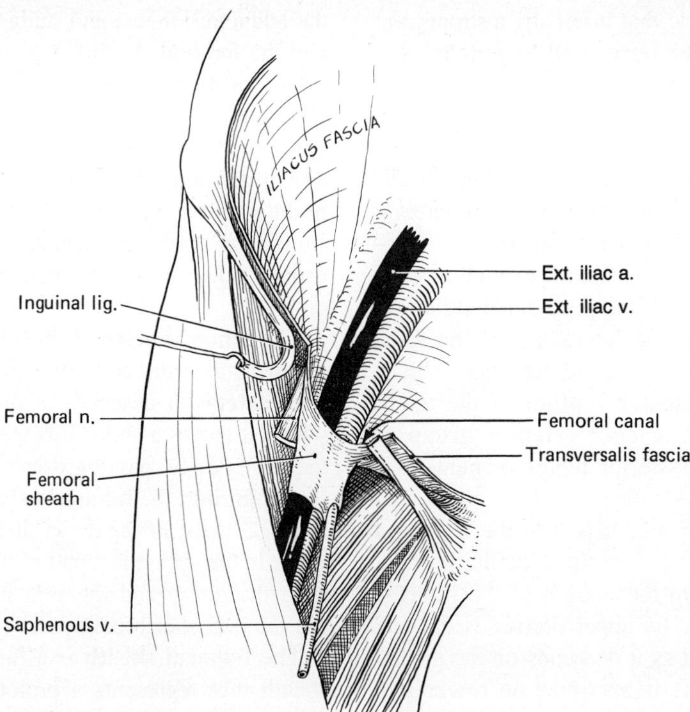

Figure 18.6 The **femoral sheath.**

your finger through the ring into the canal and identify their boundaries. The ring lies posterior to the medial part of the inguinal ligament. It is bounded laterally by the femoral vein, medially by the free margin of the lacunar ligament, and posteriorly by the pecten of the pubis.

Because of its loosely arranged contents, the canal represents a potential weak point in the abdominal wall and therefore is sometimes the seat of a femoral hernia. This type of hernia is more common in women than in men. The herniating mass, which can be a loop of intestine with its covering of peritoneum and extraperitoneal fat, leaves the abdominal cavity at the femoral ring. If left unattended, it may push through the canal and bulge through the saphenous opening in the thigh. Differentiating between an inguinal and a femoral hernia is aided by the relationship of each to the pubic tubercle; an inguinal hernia is anterior and a femoral hernia is posterior to the pubic tubercle. The unsuspecting clinician may mistake swollen inguinal lymph nodes for a femoral hernia or vice versa.

Carefully remove the femoral sheath and, without damaging the femoral artery, the femoral nerve, and their branches, define the borders of the muscles that form the **floor of** the **femoral triangle** (Fig. 18.5). The adductor longus has already been seen to form the medial portion of the floor. The lateral portion of the floor is formed by the **iliopsoas muscle,** which consists of the psoas major tendon and the lower fibers of the iliacus. It enters the thigh by passing behind the lateral part of the inguinal ligament. Its insertion on the **lesser trochanter of** the **femur** is hidden by the sartorius. Between the iliopsoas and the adductor longus, the floor of the femoral triangle is formed by the anterior surface of the **pectineus.** This flat muscle originates from the **outer surface of** the **pubis** below the pecten; its fibers pass downward and laterally to insert into the **pectineal line** behind and below the **lesser trochanter of** the **femur.**

Identify the three large branches that arise from

the **femoral artery** within the femoral triangle. They are the profunda femoris and the medial and lateral femoral circumflex arteries. The **profunda femoris** arises from the posterior aspect of the femoral about 4.0 cm below the inguinal ligament and runs downward through the triangle behind and slightly lateral to the femoral. The arrangement of the femoral circumflex arteries is subject to much variability. In most cases, they are branches of the profunda femoris, but it is very common to find one or both of them arising directly off the femoral a short distance below the origin of the profunda. The **medial femoral circumflex artery** passes medially and posteriorly to leave the femoral triangle between the adjacent borders of the iliopsoas and pectineus muscles; it gives rise to **muscular branches to** the **adductor group** and to branches that anastomose with arteries in the gluteal region and around the hip joint. The **lateral femoral circumflex artery** passes laterally behind the sartorius and rectus muscles. Its branches will be seen later.

The **femoral nerve** enters the femoral triangle by passing downward behind the inguinal ligament anterior to the iliopsoas tendon and lateral to the femoral artery. Notice that the nerve is not enclosed within the femoral sheath. It ends in the upper part of the triangle by dividing into muscular and cutaneous branches. The muscular branches include the **nerve to** the **pectineus,** the **nerve to** the **sartorius,** and **nerves to** the **quadriceps femoris.** The nerve to the pectineus passes medially and downward behind the femoral vessels to reach the anterior surface of the pectineus. The nerve to the sartorius often arises in common with the intermediate cutaneous branch, from which it separates before entering the upper part of the sartorius. The distribution of the **anterior cutaneous branches** has already been studied; the intermediate cutaneous nerve frequently pierces the sartorius before becoming superficial.

As the **femoral artery** leaves the femoral triangle, it enters a space known as the **adductor canal.** To open the canal for study, you will have to reflect the sartorius. Transect it at about its middle and reflect the two segments toward their origin and insertion. The adductor canal is triangular in cross section, having a lateral, a posterior, and an anteromedial wall. The **lateral wall** is formed by the external surface of the **vastus medialis muscle.** The **posterior wall** is formed by portions of the anterior surfaces of the **adductor longus** and **adductor magnus muscles.** The canal is covered **anteromedially** by the **sartorius;** its anteromedial wall is reinforced by an aponeurotic **subsartorial septum** that arches across from the adductors to the vastus medialis under the sartorius. Make a longitudinal incision through the aponeurosis to expose the femoral vessels and the saphenous nerve within the canal.

Observe that within the adductor canal the **femoral vein** lies posterior to the **femoral artery.** Posteriorly, in the upper part of the canal, the vessels rest against the adductor longus and, below the medial border of the adductor longus, against the adductor magnus. Observe the **tendinous opening (adductor hiatus)** in the **adductor magnus** at the side of the medial supracondylar ridge of the femur. As it passes through this opening, the **femoral artery** terminates by becoming the **popliteal artery;** the **femoral vein** begins here as a direct continuation of the **popliteal vein.** In the adductor canal, the femoral artery is crossed anteriorly by the **saphenous nerve.** Trace this nerve proximally and observe that it is one of the deep terminal branches of the **femoral nerve.** Distally, it does not accompany the femoral vessels through the adductor magnus but continues downward under cover of the sartorius to become superficial at the medial side of the knee, between the tendons of the sartorius and the gracilis. Its cutaneous distribution on the leg has been described.

Clean the **descending genicular artery.** It arises from the **femoral artery** just above the tendinous opening in the adductor magnus and almost immediately divides into a saphenous and a musculoarticular branch. The two branches frequently arise separately from the femoral. The **saphenous branch** accompanies the saphenous nerve; the **musculoarticular branch** enters the vastus medialis, giving twigs to it and taking part in the general arterial anastomosis around the knee joint.

Now return to the other **deep branches of** the **femoral nerve.** They are the **saphenous nerve,** which has already been traced, and the **nerves to** the **rectus femoris,** the **vastus lateralis,** the **vastus intermedius,** and the **vastus medialis.** First secure the nerve to the rectus femoris and trace it into the deep surface of the muscle. Then divide the rectus femoris transversely at about its middle and reflect the cut segments toward their origin and insertion. A portion of the vastus intermedius is now visible, and you can more easily study the distribution of the lateral femoral circumflex artery and the nerves to the vasti.

The **lateral femoral circumflex artery** ends behind the upper part of the rectus femoris by dividing into ascending, descending, and transverse branches. Find the **ascending branch** running upward and laterally under the rectus and sartorius, to both of which it gives branches; it ends under cover of the tensor fasciae latae, where it anastomoses with branches of the **gluteal arteries.** The **descending branch** runs downward and laterally deep to the rectus; it provides the main supply to the vastus intermedius and the vastus lateralis. The **transverse branch** courses laterally into the vastus lateralis muscle. It sometimes participates in the anastomosis around the hip joint (Fig. 18.5).

Define the anterior border of the vastus lateralis, raise it from the subjacent vastus intermedius, and study the origins of these two muscles. The **lower fibers of** the **vastus lateralis** arise from the lateral lip of the **linea aspera** and the **lateral intermuscular septum.** Observe that its **upper fibers** arise from the anteroinferior margin of the **greater trochanter** and, below this, from a **line** curving downward and laterally **around** the **femur** to join the lateral lip of the linea aspera. Its nerve passes under the anterior border of the muscle to reach its deep surface. The **vastus intermedius** has a broad origin from the lateral and anterior surfaces of the upper two-thirds of the **shaft of** the **femur.** Passing downward and forward, its fibers join an aponeurosis that lies on the anterior surface of the muscle and inserts, in common with the rectus tendon and the fibers of the other two vasti, into the **proximal border of** the **patella.** The nerve to the vastus intermedius enters the upper part of its anteromedial surface.

The **vastus medialis** arises from the entire length of the medial lip of the **linea aspera.** It is intimately associated above with the vastus intermedius. Distally, its upper fibers join a flat tendon that overlies the medial margin of the tendon of the vastus intermedius and is difficult to separate from it. If you make the proper separation, however, and push the vastus medialis medially, you will see that the broad medial surface of the femur is devoid of muscle attachments and is simply overlain by the deep surface of the vastus medialis.

Adductor Region of the Thigh

In this section, you will dissect the **adductor group of muscles** and the nerves and vessels that supply them. If the anterior surfaces of the adductor longus and pectineus have not been completely cleaned, do it now. At the same time, clean the insertion of the **iliopsoas.** Observe that most of the fibers of the **iliacus** join the **psoas major tendon,** which inserts into the **lesser trochanter,** but that a few of the lowest fibers of the iliacus insert directly into the **femur** along a line extending a short distance below the lesser trochanter.

Trace the **profunda femoris artery** distally and observe that it passes downward behind the adductor longus. Elevate the **adductor longus.** At the same time, secure and preserve the nerve that enters its deep surface; it is a branch of the **obturator nerve.** By elevating the adductor longus, you will expose the lower part of the adductor brevis muscle, which lies behind the lower part of the pectineus and the upper part of the adductor longus. Define the medial border of the adductor brevis and then study the full course of the **profunda femoris artery** (Fig. 18.7).

From its posterior aspect, the **profunda femoris** gives rise to a series of **perforating arteries,** which pass posteriorly through the adductor muscles to reach the back of the thigh. The **first perforating artery** arises at about the level of the

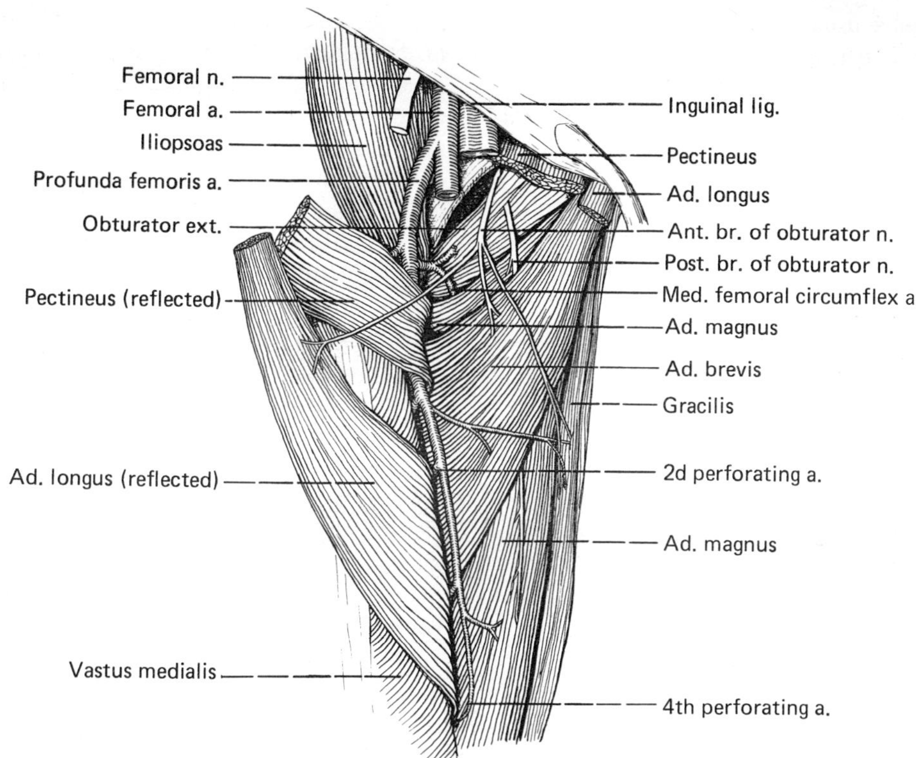

Figure 18.7 The **adductor region.**

upper border of the adductor longus and pierces both the adductor brevis and the adductor magnus. The **second perforating artery** arises somewhat lower and also pierces both of these muscles. The **third perforating artery** arises below the adductor brevis, so it pierces only the adductor magnus. The **fourth perforating artery** is the termination of the profunda itself. From the medial aspect of the profunda, one or two small branches are given to the adductor muscles.

Detach the pectineus from its origin and reflect it to its insertion. Then find the **anterior division of** the **obturator nerve** by tracing proximally the nerve to the adductor longus, which you previously identified. The anterior division descends deep to the pectineus, where it divides into three branches that can be traced into the **adductor longus,** the **adductor brevis,** and the **gracilis.**

Clean the anterior surface of the **adductor brevis.** It has a narrow origin from the outer surface of the **inferior ramus of** the **pubis** under cover of the origins of the pectineus and adductor longus. The fibers diverge laterally, forming a flat triangular muscle that inserts into the upper part of the medial lip of the **linea aspera** immediately lateral to the insertions of the pectineus and adductor longus. Define clearly the upper border of the adductor brevis, and note that the uppermost portion of the adductor magnus extends above it. Find the **posterior division of** the **obturator nerve;** it runs downward on the anterior surface of the adductor magnus and disappears behind the adductor brevis.

Dissect superior to the upper border of the adductor magnus to expose the proximal part of the external surface of the **obturator externus muscle,** which covers the obturator foramen and obturator membrane. The two divisions of the **ob-**

turator nerve usually emerge separately into the upper medial part of the thigh—the **anterior division** running downward over the superior border of the obturator externus, and the **posterior division** piercing the muscle slightly below its superior border (Fig. 18.7).

Retract the adductor brevis anteriorly and laterally, and study the anterior surface of the **adductor magnus.** This muscle has a long origin beginning on the **inferior ramus of** the **pubis** and running backward along the outer surface of the **ramus of** the **ischium** to the **tuberosity.** It has a very extensive linear insertion on the entire length of the **linea aspera** and the **medial supracondylar ridge.** The insertion is interrupted at the tendinous opening already observed, through which you observed the femoral vessels leaving the front of the thigh. The most medial and vertical portion of the **adductor magnus** narrows to a strong rounded **tendon** that inserts on the **adductor tubercle** of the medial epicondyle of the femur.

The nerve to the adductor magnus gives rise to a long, slender twig that pierces the lower part of the muscle to reach the **knee joint.**

The medial femoral circumflex artery has already been seen leaving the femoral triangle between the iliopsoas and the pectineus. Now you can follow it farther toward the back of the thigh above the superior border of the adductor magnus and inferior to the obturator externus.

GLUTEAL REGION

If you have followed the dissection thus far, the external surface of the **gluteus maximus muscle** should already be clean. If not, then do it now so you can clearly define the entire length of its upper and lower borders. Being careful not to damage underlying structures, make an incision through the entire thickness of the muscle running vertically downward from about the middle of the upper border to the lower border. Reflect the lateral segment all the way to its insertion. Observe that while the muscle, for the most part, inserts into the **iliotibial tract,** the deeper fibers of its inferior portion insert directly into the **gluteal tuberosity of** the **femur.** Attempt to identify a closed synovial bursa, which is sometimes very large and is usually interposed between the deep surface of the muscle and the greater trochanter. Next reflect the medial segment of the muscle to its origin. Proceed cautiously and preserve the **inferior gluteal nerve** and the branches of the **superior** and **inferior gluteal arteries,** which ramify on the deep surface of the gluteus maximus and supply it. Observe that some of the lower fibers of the muscle take origin from the outer surface of the **sacrotuberous ligament;** detach these fibers and clean the ligament (Fig. 18.8).

The **sacrotuberous ligament,** which runs downward and laterally from the **sacrum** and **coccyx** to the **ischial tuberosity,** forms the inferomedial boundary of the **lesser sciatic foramen,** the passage through which the **gluteal region communicates with** the ischiorectal fossa of the **perineum.** Both this foramen and the **greater sciatic foramen,** which is more superior and by which the **pelvic cavity** communicates with the **gluteal region,** are covered externally by the gluteus maximus. Now your attention will be directed to structures that emerge from inside the pelvis through the greater sciatic foramen.

Clean first the small **piriformis muscle.** It arises within the pelvis from the **lateral part of** the **sacrum** and also, to some extent, from the upper border of the **greater sciatic notch.** Emerging from the **greater sciatic foramen,** its fibers run downward and laterally, narrowing to a round tendon that inserts on the highest part of the **greater trochanter of** the **femur.** In some cases, the fleshy belly of the muscle is divided by the **common peroneal nerve** passing through it. This nerve is not usually a separate entity in the gluteal region but is bound in a single connective sheath with the **tibial nerve** to form the **ischiadic (sciatic) nerve.** Frequently, however, the ischiadic nerve as a whole is lacking, and its two terminal branches, the **tibial** and the **common peroneal nerves,** arise directly from the sacral plexus. In such cases, the common peroneal nerve usually

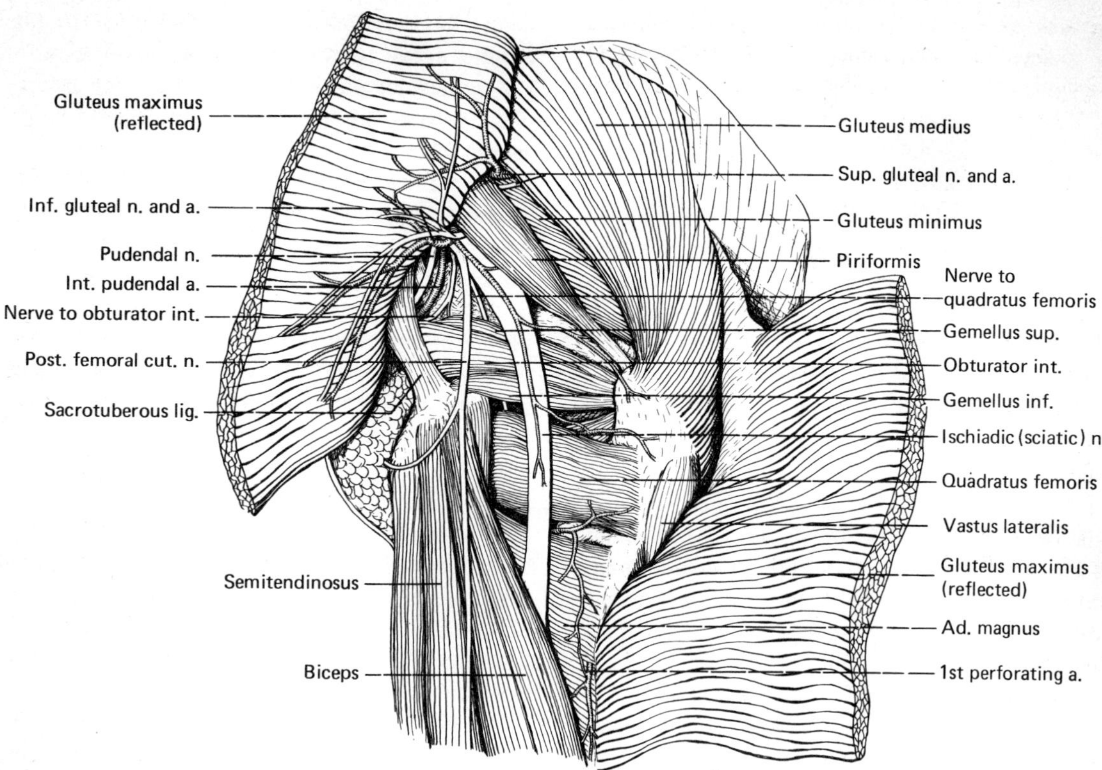

Figure 18.8 The **gluteal region.**

pierces the piriformis, the tibial nerve passing below it.

The **superior gluteal nerve** and **artery** emerge from the **greater sciatic foramen** immediately **above** the **piriformis.** Only a small segment of the superior gluteal nerve is visible at present, since it disappears almost at once under the posterior border of the gluteus medius. The superior gluteal artery lies above the nerve. It gives several large branches to the upper part of the **gluteus maximus** and then accompanies the nerve.

The **inferior gluteal nerve** and **vessels** emerge immediately **below** the **piriformis** (Fig. 18.8). The **inferior gluteal nerve** is distributed entirely to the **gluteus maximus.** The **inferior gluteal artery** divides into numerous branches, the largest of which enter the gluteus maximus. Others pass downward and laterally to take part in the general arterial anastomosis around the greater trochanter, while one long, slender branch accompanies the ischiadic nerve downward into the thigh.

This anastomosis, called the "cruciate anastomosis," is formed by branches of the inferior gluteal, the medial femoral circumflex, the lateral femoral circumflex, and the first perforating arteries. Its importance rests in the fact that it provides collateral circulation between the internal and the external iliac arteries.

The **ischiadic nerve** is the largest nerve in the body. It appears **below** the **piriformis** and runs somewhat laterally and downward into the thigh. It does not have any branches in the gluteal region. Occasionally, as noted above, it is represented by two nerves, the tibial and the common peroneal; the common peroneal is more lateral.

On a surface projection, the ischiadic nerve crosses the midpoint of a line connecting the ischial tuberosity with the greater trochanter. This is important to know, since the buttock is a common site for administering intramuscular injections. In order to avoid injury to the ischiadic nerve and gluteal arteries, the injections should be given in the upper lateral quadrant.

The **posterior femoral cutaneous nerve** emerges from the greater sciatic foramen **below** the **piriformis** and passes downward in close relation to the ischiadic nerve. The remaining structures that pass through the greater sciatic foramen will also be found below the piriformis. Before exposing them, however, identify and clean the obturator internus, the gemelli and the quadratus femoris muscles.

The **obturator internus** has a wide origin on the **internal wall of** the **pelvis** from the inner surface of the **coxal bone** and the **obturator membrane.** Its fibers converge into a flat tendon that curves laterally across the lesser sciatic notch and extends laterally and upward anterior to the ischiadic nerve to insert into the medial surface of the **greater trochanter of** the **femur.** This tendon is overlapped and may be obscured superiorly by the superior gemellus and inferiorly by the inferior gemellus.

The two small **gemelli muscles** insert into and with the **obturator internus.** The **superior gemellus** arises from the outer surface of the **ischial spine.** The **inferior gemellus** arises from the upper part of the **ischial tuberosity** and the **sacrotuberous ligament** near the tuberosity.

The **quadratus femoris** lies below the **inferior gemellus.** It arises from the **outer border of** the **ischial tuberosity.** Its fibers pass almost directly laterally to insert into the **femur** on a vertical ridge that crosses the intertrochanteric crest (Fig. 18.8).

Look in the roughly triangular space bounded by the sacrotuberous ligament, the superior gemellus, and the ischiadic nerve for the **nerve to** the **quadratus femoris,** the **nerve to** the **obturator internus,** the **internal pudendal vessels,** and the **pudendal nerve,** all of which emerge from inside the pelvis through the **greater sciatic foramen below** the **piriformis** and run downward across the outer surface of the ischium. The **pudendal nerve** is most medial; it runs downward and somewhat medially across the outer surface of the **ischial spine** and passes through the **lesser sciatic foramen** to enter the pudendal canal on the lateral wall of the ischiorectal fossa. Immediately lateral to it find the **internal pudendal artery,** which follows a similar course. In some cases, the **inferior rectal nerve,** which is usually a branch of the pudendal, arises separately from the sacral plexus and so will also be found accompanying the pudendal nerve. The **nerve to** the **obturator internus** crosses the ischium lateral to the internal pudendal artery. It gives a branch to supply the **superior gemellus** and then passes through the lesser sciatic foramen to enter the deep surface of the **obturator internus.** The **nerve to** the **quadratus femoris** is farther lateral and often overlapped externally by the ischiadic nerve. It passes downward, anterior to the obturator tendon and the gemelli, gives a branch to supply the **inferior gemellus,** and enters the deep (anterior) surface of the **quadratus femoris.**

Clean and study the **gluteus medius muscle,** which is partly covered by the gluteus maximus. It arises from the **outer lip of** the **iliac crest,** the **external surface of** the **ilium** between the anterior and posterior gluteal lines, and the deep surface of the portion of the **fascia lata** (gluteal fascia) that covers it externally above the gluteus maximus. Its fibers converge downward to a broad, flat tendon that inserts on the external surface of the **greater trochanter** along a diagonal line running from the posterosuperior to the anteroinferior angle of the trochanter. Its insertion is usually intimately connected with the tendon of origin of the uppermost part of the vastus lateralis. Carefully define the posterior border of the **gluteus medius** and observe that, while the **gluteus minimus** lies for the most part under cover of the gluteus medius, a small portion of it is exposed below the posterior border of the medius. To expose the gluteus minimus, carefully detach the gluteus medius from its origin and turn it downward and laterally to its insertion. As you do this, observe the nerve twigs from the **superior gluteal nerve** that enter its deep surface.

Clean and study the **gluteus minimus** and at the same time the superior gluteal nerve and artery. The gluteus minimus arises from the **outer surface of** the **ilium** between the anterior and inferior gluteal lines; its upper anterior part is often partially blended with the gluteus medius. Its fibers converge downward and laterally to a tendon that inserts on the **anterior border of** the **greater trochanter.**

You have already seen the **superior gluteal nerve** emerging from the greater sciatic foramen and disappearing laterally under the gluteus medius. Note that here it divides into a superior and an inferior branch. The **superior branch** passes forward along the upper border of the gluteus minimus and distributes entirely to the **gluteus medius;** the **inferior branch** crosses the middle of the gluteus minimus, supplies both the **medius** and the **minimus,** and ends anteriorly in the deep surface of the **tensor fasciae latae,** which it also supplies.

The **superficial branches of** the **superior gluteal artery** enter the gluteus maximus; the **deep branch** divides into **two branches** that are distributed with the two branches of the superior gluteal nerve. The inferior branch anastomoses with the ascending branch of the **lateral femoral circumflex artery** under cover of the tensor fasciae latae.

The nerves that you have dissected in the gluteal region are derived from the **sacral plexus,** which lies in the pelvis. Direct your attention, therefore, to the interior of the pelvis and attempt to sort out the sacral plexus and its branches. The plexus lies anterior to the lateral part of the sacrum and the piriformis muscle; it is usually buried in pelvic fascia. The pattern of mixing of the nerves that form the plexus is rather complex and difficult to dissect, so concern yourself primarily with its roots and terminal branches.

The **roots of** the **plexus** are the **lumbosacral trunk** and the **ventral rami** of the **first four sacral nerves.** You have already seen that the **lumbosacral trunk** is formed by the junction of a portion of the ventral ramus of the **fourth lumbar nerve** with the entire ventral ramus of the **fifth lumbar nerve.** The trunk descends behind the common iliac artery into the pelvis and there unites with the **first sacral nerve** to form a loop through which the superior gluteal artery usually passes. This loop then joins the **second** and **third** and part of the **fourth sacral nerves** to form a flattened mass of nerves, the sacral plexus. The **terminal branches of** the **plexus** leave the pelvis almost as soon as they are formed. As you come to each branch, you may find it helpful to follow it from the gluteal region, where you have already seen it, back into the pelvis to its derivation.

Before that, attempt to identify the **pelvic parasympathetics,** known as **pelvic splanchnic nerves;** they supply the pelvic viscera with preganglionic fibers whose origins are from the **second, third,** and **fourth sacral nerves.** Now, observe that the **ischiadic (sciatic) nerve** is derived from the lumbosacral trunk and the first three sacral nerves. It passes between the borders of the coccygeus and piriformis muscles and leaves the pelvis through the greater sciatic foramen. The **pudendal nerve** is formed from the second, third, and fourth sacral nerves as well. It follows the same course as the ischiadic nerve. Try to verify that the **nerve to** the **quadratus femoris** and the **superior gluteal nerve** come from the same roots—the fourth and fifth lumbar and the first sacral nerves. Similarly, notice that the **nerve to** the **obturator internus** and the **inferior gluteal nerve** come from the fifth lumbar and first and second sacral nerves. The superior gluteal nerve accompanies the superior gluteal vessels above the piriformis and through the upper part of the greater sciatic foramen.

The first three sacral nerves give rise to the **posterior femoral cutaneous nerve.** Twigs that supply the piriformis are usually derived from the first and second sacral nerves. You may also notice that branches directly off the third and fourth sacral ventral rami supply the levator ani muscle.

Attempt to display the sacral portion of the **sym-**

pathetic trunks and their rami communicantes to the sacral nerves. The trunks lie on the pelvic surface of the sacrum just medial to the anterior sacral foramina. Inferiorly, in front of the first segment of the coccyx, the two trunks end by joining at the **ganglion impar.** There are only three or four small sympathetic ganglia in the sacral region.

FLEXOR REGION OF THE THIGH

Turn to the back of the thigh and clean the surfaces of the three **flexor** or **hamstring muscles.** They are the **biceps femoris,** the **semitendinosus,** and the **semimembranosus** (Fig. 18.4).

The thick, fleshy belly of the **long head of** the **biceps** will be found laterally below the lower border of the gluteus maximus. It arises by a common tendon with the semitendinosus from the medial part of the back of the **ischial tuberosity.** Its fibers run downward and somewhat laterally to join a thick, flat tendon that passes downward along the lateral side of the back of the knee. The inferomedial border of the tendon forms the superolateral boundary of the popliteal fossa, the fat-filled space at the back of the knee. On its lateral side, the long head is joined by the fibers of the **short head,** which arise from the distal part of the lateral lip of the **linea aspera,** from the lateral **supracondylar ridge,** and from the posterior surface of the **lateral intermuscular septum.** Observe that the short head of the biceps is separated from the vastus lateralis only by the lateral intermuscular septum.

The **semitendinosus,** which arises with the long head of the biceps, is medial to the biceps and partly overlapped by it laterally. Its flat belly contracts at about the middle of the thigh into a thick rounded tendon that passes downward behind the medial condyle of the femur. Its insertion will be seen later.

The **semimembranosus** lies immediately in front of the semitendinosus and consequently is partially hidden by it. It arises by a broad, flat tendon from the lateral part of the ischial tuberosity. In the lower part of the thigh, it is considerably wider than the semitendinosus and its posterior surface extends beyond both the medial and lateral borders of the latter. The medial portion of the semimembranosus lies posterior to the gracilis; its lower lateral border forms the superomedial boundary of the popliteal fossa. The flat tendon of insertion of the **semimembranosus** on the **medial condyle of** the **tibia** is covered externally by the tendons of the gracilis and the semitendinosus.

Clean the **branches of** the **ischiadic nerve** that supply the **long head of** the **biceps, semitendinosus,** and **semimembranosus.** They usually arise from the ischiadic nerve under cover of the biceps but may appear at a higher level. Somewhat lower you will find a **branch of** the **ischiadic nerve** that supplies the **short head of** the **biceps.**

Elevate the semimembranosus and semitendinosus muscles to expose the posterior surface of the adductor magnus muscle. You have seen that the **adductor magnus** receives its main nerve supply from the **posterior division of** the **obturator nerve;** now note that it receives an additional branch from the **ischiadic nerve.**

It is convenient at this time to observe the terminal portions of the medial femoral circumflex and the four perforating arteries. The **medial circumflex** reaches the back of the thigh between the upper border of the adductor magnus and the lower border of the quadratus femoris. The **perforating arteries** pierce the adductor magnus in longitudinal series close to the femur. They supply the posterior thigh muscles.

While the hamstring muscles are still in place, dissect the **popliteal fossa.** If the muscles have been partially displaced, restore them to their normal position.

POPLITEAL FOSSA

The **popliteal fossa** is the diamond-shaped space at the back of the knee (Fig. 18.9). Its **apex** is the point at which the **biceps** and **semimembranosus muscles** separate from each other. Its **superolateral boundary** is formed by the medial border of the **biceps,** and its **superomedial boundary** by

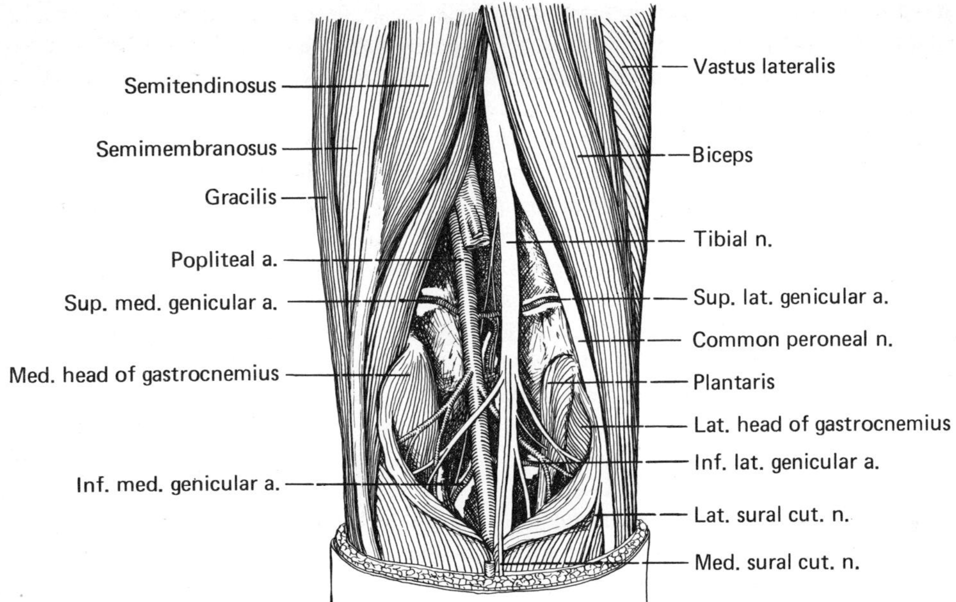

Figure 18.9 The **popliteal fossa.** Its boundaries have been spread apart.

the lateral border of the **semimembranosus.** Its **inferolateral** and **inferomedial boundaries** are formed by the lateral and medial **heads of** the **gastrocnemius** muscle, which arise from the lateral and medial condyles of the femur under cover of the biceps and semimembranosus, respectively. The **roof** or **superficial boundary** of the fossa is formed by **skin** and **fascia;** its **floor** or **deep boundary** is formed from above downward by the popliteal surface of the **femur,** the **oblique popliteal ligament** at the back of the knee joint, and the **fascia covering** the **popliteus muscle.** The fossa is filled with fatty areolar tissue, which you must remove to expose the other contents.

First clean the terminal part of the **small saphenous vein.** It ascends in superficial fascia along the middle of the calf and enters the middle of the popliteal fossa to terminate in the **popliteal vein.** Just lateral to it but on a slightly deeper plane is the **medial sural cutaneous nerve,** which arises from the **tibial nerve** in the upper part of the popliteal fossa and descends on the external surface of the gastrocnemius.

Identify the **common peroneal nerve.** It and the tibial nerve are the two terminal branches of the **ischiadic nerve.** Usually they arise under cover of the biceps, but occasionally not until the apex of the popliteal fossa is reached. At its origin, the common peroneal is lateral to the tibial. It passes downward and laterally, close to the medial margin of the biceps, and leaves the popliteal fossa by crossing the external surface of the lateral head of the gastrocnemius, still closely following the border of the biceps. The common peroneal nerve gives rise to one or two small **articular branches,** which pass deeply into the fossa to reach the **knee joint,** and to the **lateral sural cutaneous nerve,** which descends on the lateral head of the gastrocnemius to supply the lateral side of the leg. The **peroneal communicating branch** is also given off by the common peroneal, but it may arise from the lateral sural cutaneous nerve. It joins the medial sural cutaneous to form the sural nerve. Now clean the upper portions of the two heads of the gastrocnemius muscle, so that the boundaries of the fossa can be clearly defined.

The **tibial nerve** enters the popliteal fossa at its apex and descends almost vertically but does deviate somewhat medially. It lies superficial (posterior) to the popliteal vessels, which it crosses obliquely downward from the lateral to the medial side. It is crossed by the plantaris muscle or its tendon. In the lower part of the fossa, sometimes under cover of the gastrocnemius, the tibial nerve gives rise to a group of **muscular branches.** Spread apart the **two heads of** the **gastrocnemius** and follow one of these branches into the deep surface of each head. A small branch is also given to the **plantaris.** The remaining branches will be seen later supplying the **soleus** and **popliteus muscles.** In addition to the muscular and cutaneous branches, the tibial nerve gives rise to two or three minute **articular branches to** the **knee joint.**

Clean the **plantaris muscle.** It arises from the **lateral part of** the **femur** immediately above the attachment of the lateral head of the gastrocnemius on the lateral condyle. Its small, fleshy belly, which is partially overlapped by the lateral head of the gastrocnemius, runs downward and medially in the popliteal fossa and converges to a long, slender tendon that descends deep to the gastrocnemius.

The **popliteal artery** begins at the tendinous opening in the adductor magnus and descends through the popliteal fossa to the lower border of the popliteus muscle, where it ends by dividing into the **anterior** and **posterior tibial arteries.** It is the most deeply (anteriorly) placed structure in the fossa, being in contact with the floor (anterior wall) of the fossa throughout. Posteriorly, it is covered above by the semimembranosus and below by the gastrocnemius and plantaris. The popliteal vein lies posterior to the artery; remove it if necessary to study the artery and its branches.

The constant, named branches of the **popliteal artery** are its five **genicular branches.** However, the variable muscular branches, which supply the hamstring muscles and the gastrocnemius, soleus, and plantaris, are its largest branches. The two superior genicular arteries arise from each side of the popliteal and wind around the femur immediately above the condyles. The **medial superior genicular** runs medially in front of the semitendinosus and semimembranosus above the medial head of the gastrocnemius and turns forward deep to the tendon of the adductor magnus. The **lateral superior genicular** runs laterally above the lateral condyle and in front of the biceps. The **middle genicular** is a small vessel that pierces the oblique popliteal ligament to enter the knee joint; it may arise by a common stem with one of the superior geniculars. The two inferior genicular arteries arise from the lower part of the popliteal under cover of the upper part of the gastrocnemius. The **medial inferior genicular** runs downward and medially to pass forward below the medial condyle of the tibia. The **lateral inferior genicular** runs straight laterally across the lateral condyle of the tibia above the head of the fibula, and turns forward to reach the front of the knee joint. All these vessels take part in the **arterial anastomosis around** the **knee joint.**

THE LEG

The **muscles of** the **leg** are arranged in **three groups,** each of which occupies a **separate osteofascial compartment.** Superficially, each compartment is limited by the deep fascia that encircles the leg; the deep boundaries of the various compartments are formed by the bones and the fascial septa of the leg (Fig. 18.10). The **anterior group** of muscles, which **dorsiflex** the **foot** and **extend** the **toes,** abut the anterior surfaces of the fibula and the interosseous membrane and the lateral surface of the tibia. The muscles of the **posterior group,** which **plantarflex** the **foot** and **flex** the **toes,** abut the posterior and medial surfaces of the fibula and the posterior surfaces of the interosseous membrane and the tibia. The **lateral group,** which are primarily **evertors of** the **foot,** occupy a narrow compartment that is limited by the lateral surface of the fibula and the short anterior and posterior intermuscular septa. Medially, the subcutaneous medial surface of the tibia intervenes between the muscles of the anterior and pos-

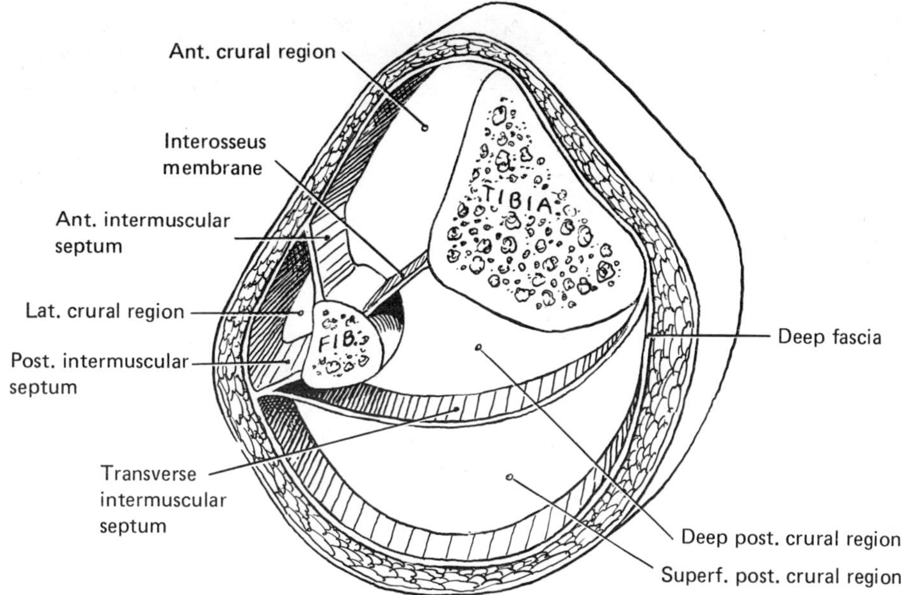

Figure 18.10 Diagrammatic presentation of the **compartments of** the **leg.**

terior groups. The deep fascia covering this surface of the tibia is intimately blended with the periosteum.

Posterior Crural Region

With the cadaver on its stomach, continue now with the **posterior crural region.** The **muscles** of this region are arranged in **three layers** from superficial to deep. Those of the **superficial layer** are the **gastrocnemius, plantaris,** and **soleus,** and they constitute the fleshy prominence known as the calf. The upper part of the gastrocnemius has already been seen. Now clean the entire external surface of the muscle.

The **gastrocnemius** arises by **medial** and **lateral heads** from the upper posterior parts of the **lateral** and **medial condyles of** the **femur;** they join below the popliteal fossa. The muscle is fleshy above and tendinous below. It inserts into the **tuberosity of** the **calcaneus** through the **calcaneal tendon** (Achilles tendon), which is **common to** the **gastrocnemius** and **soleus** (and sometimes to the plantaris).

Before reflecting the gastrocnemius, clean and study the tendon of insertion of the **semimembranosus.** This muscle inserts into a facet on the posterior surface of the **medial condyle of** the **tibia,** medial to the medial head of the gastrocnemius and partially overlapped by it. A **synovial bursa** usually intervenes between the **semimembranosus tendon** and the **medial head of** the **gastrocnemius.** Divide the two heads of the gastrocnemius 1.5 cm below their origins on the femur and reflect the entire muscle downward and backward to its junction with the calcaneal tendon. While doing this, observe the branches that it receives from the **tibial nerve** and the **popliteal artery.** After you have seen them, you can cut them so that the muscle can be completely reflected.

Observe now that the tendon of the **plantaris muscle** passes downward and medially posterior to the popliteal artery and the tibial nerve and between the gastrocnemius and soleus muscles. It joins the **calcaneal tendon** or inserts medial to it into the calcaneus. It is supplied by a twig from the **tibial nerve.** Divide the plantaris just below

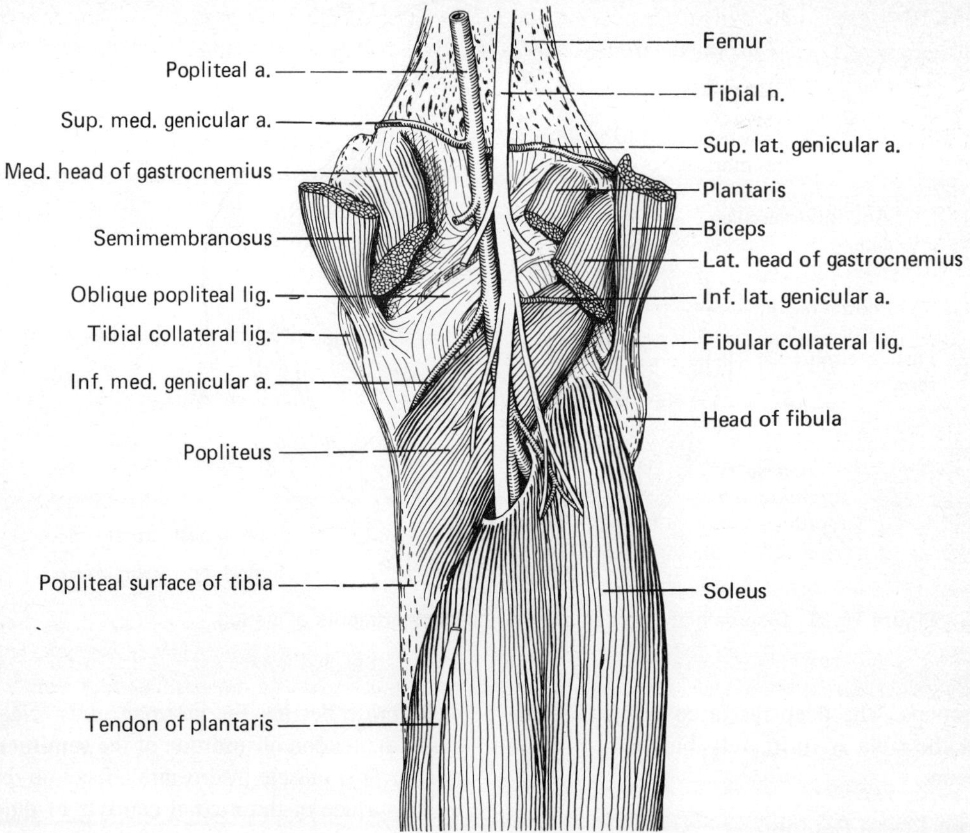

Figure 18.11 The **back of** the **knee** and the upper part of the calf.

its origin and turn it downward. Then clean and study the popliteus and soleus muscles (Fig. 18.11).

The **soleus** is a thick, fleshy muscle whose long linear origin has roughly the outline of an inverted V. It arises from the middle third of the **medial border of** the **tibia,** from the **soleal line** on the back **of** the **tibia,** from a strong **fibrous band** that bridges the interval between the upper end of the tibia and the head of the fibula, from the posterior surface of the **head of** the **fibula,** and from the upper third of the **posterior surface of** the **fibula.** It inserts, together with the gastrocnemius, into the **tuberosity of** the **calcaneus** by means of the **calcaneal tendon.** Find and clean its nerve supply, which arises from the **tibial nerve** in the popliteal fossa and enters the proximal part of the external surface of the soleus.

The terminal part of the popliteal artery can now be seen better than was possible when the popliteal fossa was dissected. The **popliteal artery** ends, usually opposite the lower border of the popliteus, by dividing into the **anterior** and **posterior tibial arteries.** Observe that these two vessels and the tibial nerve descend into the leg by passing anterior to the fibrous band between the tibia and fibula, from which the soleus partly takes origin.

Detach the **soleus** entirely from its origin and reflect it downward and backward toward the calcaneus. As you do this, observe that its deep surface receives an additional nerve supply from the **tibial nerve** and several branches from the **pos-**

terior tibial artery. Cut the nerves and arteries so that the muscle can be completely reflected. Observe the considerable amount of fatty areolar tissue that lies between the calcaneal tendon and the posterior aspect of the ankle joint.

The **deep** posterior crural compartment consists of four muscles, the **popliteus,** the **flexor hallucis longus,** the **flexor digitorum longus,** and the **tibialis posterior.** Before cleaning them, define the **flexor retinaculum,** a thickened portion of the deep crural fascia at the medial side of the heel. This strong fascial band stretches downward and backward from the **medial malleolus** to the prominence on the posterior part of the **medial surface of** the **calcaneus.** It retains the tendons of the tibialis posterior, the flexor digitorum longus, and the flexor hallucis longus and the terminal portions of the tibial nerve and the posterior tibial artery in position against the talus and the calcaneus. You will find some small medial **calcaneal branches of** the **tibial nerve,** which supply the skin on the medial side of the heel piercing the retinaculum; they are accompanied by the medial **calcaneal branches of** the **posterior tibial artery.** Do not remove the flexor retinaculum, but proceed to clean and study the flexor digitorum longus and the flexor hallucis longus. You will find the posterior tibial artery and the tibial nerve descending through the posterior crural compartment in the groove between the borders of these two muscles (Fig. 18.12).

The **flexor digitorum longus** arises from the distal part of the **soleal line** and the middle half of the medial side of the **posterior surface of** the **tibia;** its fibers pass obliquely downward to join a tendon that passes behind the medial malleolus, deep to the flexor retinaculum.

The **flexor hallucis longus** arises from the distal two-thirds of the **posterior surface of** the **fibula.** Its tendon also passes deep to the flexor retinaculum, lying a short distance behind the tendon of the flexor digitorum longus.

The **popliteus** is a flat triangular muscle that lies in front of the lower part of the popliteal artery in relation to the popliteal surface of the tibia; it is covered by a fairly dense layer of fascia. It arises within the cavity of the knee joint from the lower lateral part of the **lateral condyle of** the **femur.** Now you will find it emerging from the lateral side of the posterior aspect of the joint capsule. The muscle fibers expand downward and medially to cover the **popliteal surface of** the **tibia,** upon which they insert. The popliteus is supplied by a branch of the **tibial nerve** that arises in the popliteal fossa and winds around the lower border of the muscle to reach its deep surface.

Clean the posterior tibial artery and the tibial nerve. The **posterior tibial artery** begins at the lower border of the popliteus as a terminal branch of the popliteal artery and descends anterior to the soleus, between the flexor digitorum longus and the flexor hallucis longus. Anteriorly, it is related, from above downward, to the tibialis posterior, the posterior surface of the tibia, and the capsule of the ankle joint. Its largest branch is the **peroneal artery;** this vessel arises about 2.5 cm below the origin of the posterior tibial and runs laterally and distally across the tibialis posterior to pass from view under the flexor hallucis longus. The posterior tibial artery gives **muscular branches** to the soleus and the deeper posterior crural muscles, several small **medial calcaneal branches,** and a **posterior medial malleolar branch,** which runs forward across the medial malleolus to anastomose with the anterior medial malleolar branch of the anterior tibial artery. It ends under the flexor retinaculum by dividing into the **medial** and **lateral plantar arteries.**

The **tibial nerve** is at first medial to the posterior tibial artery but then crosses behind it and for the rest of its course lies lateral to the artery. It gives a branch to the deep surface of the **soleus** and **branches** that supply the **flexor digitorum longus,** the **flexor hallucis longus,** and the **tibialis posterior.** It terminates under the flexor retinaculum by dividing into the **medial** and **lateral plantar nerves.** Just proximal to its termination, it gives a **small articular twig to** the **ankle joint** and the **medial calcaneal cutaneous branches.**

The deepest muscle of the posterior crural com-

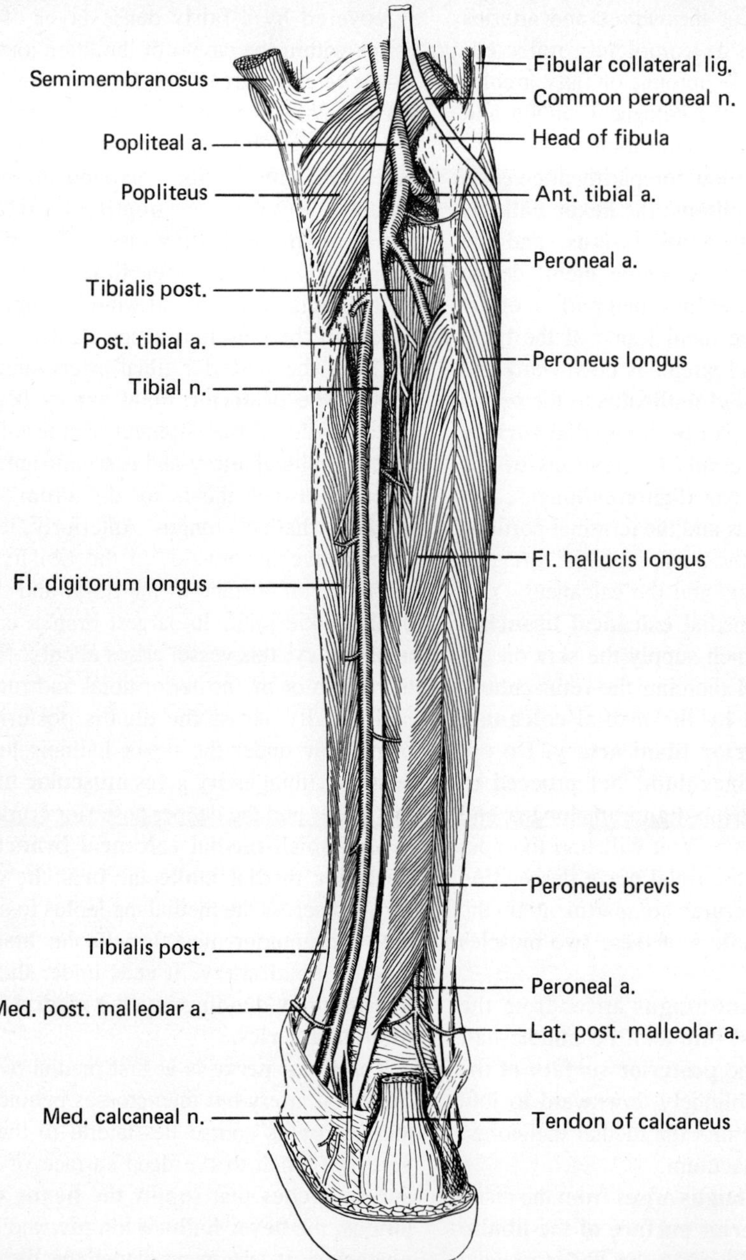

Figure 18.12 The **posterior** aspect of the **leg** after removal of the gastrocnemius and soleus muscles.

partment is the **tibialis posterior.** Except for its most proximal portion, it is completely covered by the flexor hallucis longus and the flexor digitorum longus muscles; spread them laterally and medially.

The **tibialis posterior** arises from the upper two-thirds of the lateral part of the **posterior surface of** the **tibia** below the soleal line, from the entire **medial surface of** the **fibula,** and from the posterior surface of the upper two-thirds of the **interosseous membrane.** Its tendon passes distally and medially deep to the flexor digitorum longus, behind the medial malleolus, and deep to the flexor retinaculum, where it lies immediately anterior to the flexor digitorum longus.

While the flexor hallucis longus is displaced laterally, trace the course of the **peroneal artery.** It descends adjacent to the fibula, between the **tibialis posterior** and the **flexor hallucis longus,** giving branches to these muscles and to the **peroneus longus** and **brevis muscles.** In the distal part of the leg, it lies on the interosseous membrane, and here it gives rise to a **perforating branch** that courses to the anterolateral side of the ankle and foot. Behind the lateral malleolus, the peroneal artery gives rise to the **posterior lateral malleolar branch** that passes forward across the lateral malleolus to anastomose with the anterior lateral malleolar branch of the anterior tibial artery. The peroneal artery terminates as small **lateral calcaneal branches** that ramify on the lateral side of the heel.

The course of the **anterior tibial artery** in the posterior crural region is very short. From its origin, it runs downward and forward to pierce the proximal part of the interosseous membrane above the tibialis posterior. Before piercing the membrane, however, it gives rise to a **posterior tibial recurrent branch,** which ascends deep to the popliteus muscle to reach the knee joint.

Now reflect the flexor retinaculum to expose the terminations of the tibial nerve and the posterior tibial artery and the relative positions of these structures and the three flexor tendons. Observe that, under the **flexor retinaculum,** these structures are arranged in the following order from anterior to posterior (or, as sometimes described, from medial to lateral): the tendon of the **tibialis posterior,** the tendon of the **flexor digitorum longus,** the **posterior tibial artery,** the **tibial nerve,** and the tendon of the **flexor hallucis longus.** The three tendons and the medial and lateral plantar nerves and arteries, which arise here, all pass distally into the sole of the foot.

Lateral Crural Region

The lateral crural region or compartment is bounded by the anterior and posterior intermuscular septa on the anterolateral aspect of the leg. First clean and study the insertion of the **biceps femoris** into the highest part of the **head of** the **fibula;** it also gives a tendinous expansion to the fascia covering the lateral part of the leg. Observe that the insertion is split into two parts just above its attachment to the fibula by the **fibular (lateral) collateral ligament.** This is a strong, rounded cord that extends from the **lateral condyle of** the **femur** downward to the **head of** the **fibula.** The upper part of the ligament is covered externally by the biceps (Fig. 18.13).

The lateral crural compartment contains two muscles, the **peroneus longus** and **brevis.** Before cleaning them, attempt to locate and define the **peroneal retinacula.** They are similar to ligaments and represent thickenings of the deep fascia that serve to hold the tendons of the peroneal muscles in place against the calcaneus. Note that the **superior retinaculum** passes from the posterior distal part of the **lateral malleolus** downward and backward to the upper lateral part of the **calcaneus.** The **inferior retinaculum,** which inclines downward and backward, also attaches to the upper anterior part of the **calcaneus,** where it is continuous with the lateral end of the inferior extensor retinaculum, and to the **trochlear process of** the **calcaneus.** Retain the retinacula but clean the remaining portions of deep fascia as completely as possible from the outer surface of the peroneus longus.

The **peroneus longus** arises from the proximal

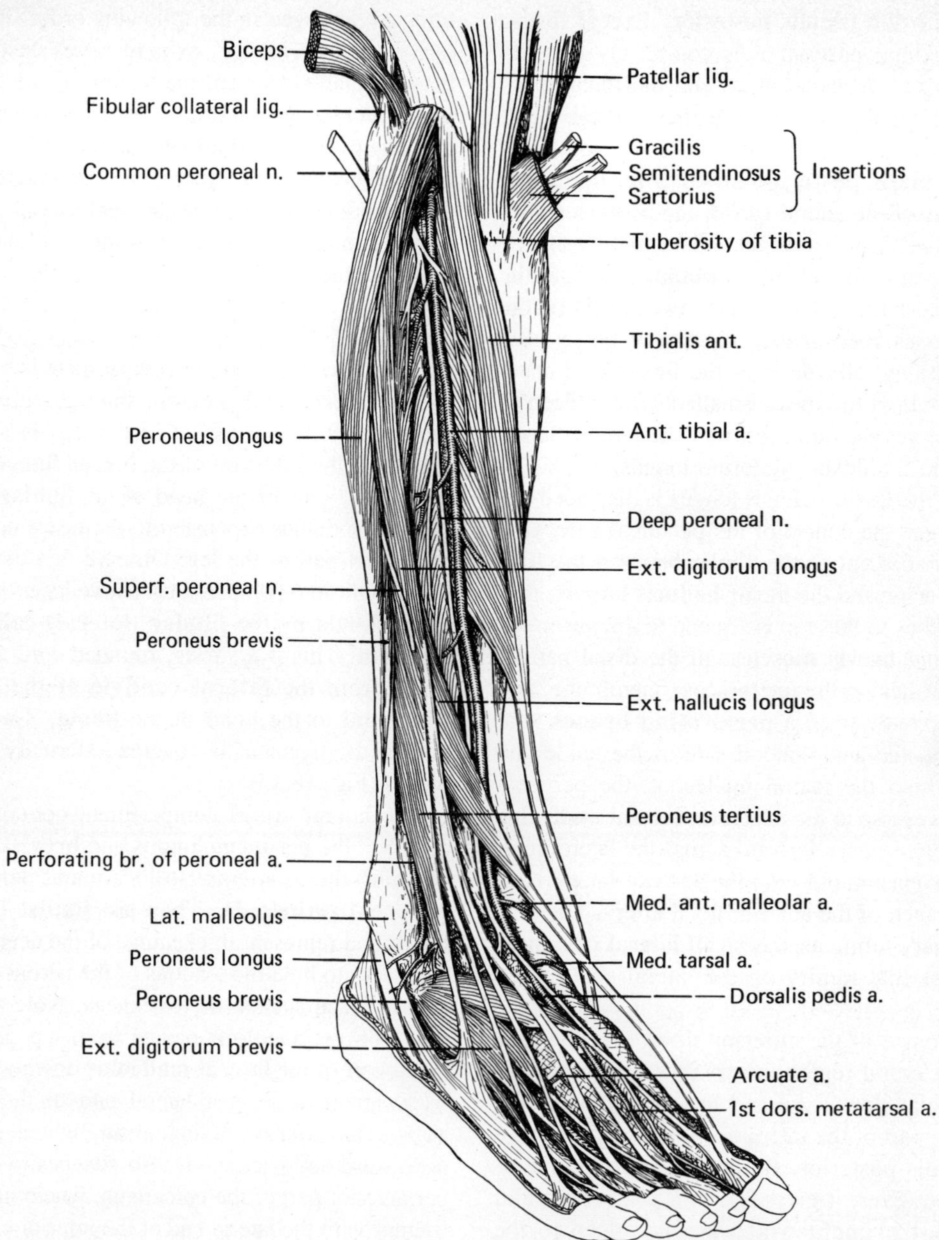

Figure 18.13 The anterior and lateral **crural regions** and the **dorsum of** the **foot.**

half of the **lateral surface of** the **fibula,** from the **anterior** and **posterior intermuscular septa,** and, to some extent, from the deep fascia that covers it. Its tendon passes distally and crosses the lateral surface of the calcaneus posterior to the lateral malleolus and posterior to the peroneus brevis. As it lies deep to the peroneal retinacula against the calcaneus, its tendon is enclosed in a synovial sheath that is common to it and the peroneus brevis. From here the tendon is guided by a groove in the **cuboid bone** into the **sole of** the **foot,** where its further course will be seen later.

Draw the lower part of the peroneus longus laterally and posteriorly and delineate the **peroneus brevis muscle.** It arises from the distal half of the **lateral surface of** the **fibula** and from the **intermuscular septa.** Its tendon is at first covered by the tendon of the peroneus longus; however, as it turns forward behind the lateral malleolus, it lies anterior to the latter tendon. It inserts into the **tuberosity** at the **base of** the **fifth metatarsal bone** (Fig. 18.13).

The **common peroneal nerve** has been followed downward and laterally along the border of the biceps femoris to the head of the fibula. At the posterior border of the peroneus longus, the nerve disappears from view by passing deep to the muscle. Now cut carefully through the peroneus longus in order to expose the further course of the nerve. Observe that as it crosses the neck of the fibula, the common peroneal nerve gives off a small **recurrent articular branch to** the **knee joint** and then divides into the deep and superficial peroneal nerves. Note that the **deep peroneal nerve** passes through the upper part of the extensor digitorum longus, from which point its further course will be traced. The **superficial peroneal nerve** passes distally in the interval between the **peroneus longus** and **brevis muscles,** both of which it supplies. In the distal part of the leg, it pierces the deep fascia, from which point its distribution is cutaneous to the lower leg and foot.

Trauma to the head and neck region of the fibula jeopardizes the integrity of the common peroneal nerve, which is quite superficial and close to the bone. Injury to the nerve results in ''foot drop,'' or inability to dorsiflex the foot.

Anterior Crural Region

Now you are ready to clean and study the patellar ligament and the insertions of the sartorius, gracilis, and semitendinosus muscles.

The **patellar ligament** is a strong, flat fibrous band that extends from the **distal border of** the **patella** to the **tuberosity of** the **tibia;** it is actually the insertion of the four parts of the **quadriceps femoris.** It is an integral part of the capsule of the knee joint, as will be apparent when you dissect the joint tendons. The **sartorius, gracilis,** and **semitendinosus tendons** insert close together on the upper part of the **medial surface of** the **tibia.** Observe that at its insertion, the flat tendon of the sartorius covers the other two tendons externally, and that the gracilis tendon lies immediately above the semitendinosus, partially overlapping it.

Before cleaning the muscles in the anterior crural compartment, define the extensor retinacula at the ankle. They are merely thickened portions of the deep fascia of the leg. The **superior extensor retinaculum** stretches across the front of the leg just proximal to the malleoli; laterally, it blends with the periosteum of the subcutaneous surface of the **fibula,** and medially, with the **tibia.** The **inferior extensor retinaculum** is larger. Laterally, it is a single band that stretches from the **anterior part of** the **calcaneus** medially across the front of the ankle joint; here it divides into two limbs. The upper one passes proximally to the **medial malleolus,** and the lower one passes distally around the medial margin of the foot to join the **plantar aponeurosis.**

Now clean the muscles in the anterior compartment. You will find that the deep fascia of the leg is not easily separated from the underlying muscles. This is because the muscles take origin partly from its deep surface. This compartment also contains the anterior tibial artery, its accompanying veins, and the deep peroneal nerve.

The **tibialis anterior** arises from the proximal half of the **lateral surface** of the **tibia,** the medial side of the anterior surface of the **interosseous membrane,** and the **deep fascia** that covers it. Its strong tendon passes over the front of the ankle joint, deep to the retinacula, and onto the dorsum of the foot. It inserts into the medial part of the **first cuneiform bone** and the **base of** the **first metatarsal.**

The **extensor digitorum longus** arises from the anterior part of the **head of** the **fibula** and the proximal two-thirds of the anterior surface of its **shaft,** from the anterior surface of the **anterior intermuscular septum,** which separates it from the lateral crural compartment, and from the **deep fascia** covering it. Its tendon descends in front of the ankle joint, and on the dorsum of the foot, it divides into **four slips** that reach the dorsal surfaces of the **four lateral toes.** Remove the skin from the dorsum of the toes and investigate the manner of insertion of the extensor tendons. Observe that each slip expands on the dorsal aspect of the proximal phalanx and then divides into a **central** and **two collateral parts.** The **central part** inserts into the **base of** the **middle phalanx;** the **collateral parts** insert together into the **base of** the **terminal phalanx.**

The **peroneus tertius,** while described as a separate muscle, usually has more the appearance of an additional **slip of** the **extensor digitorum longus** (Fig. 18.13). It arises distally from the anterior surface of the fibula. Its slender tendon inserts into the dorsal side of the **base of** the **fifth metatarsal.**

The **extensor hallucis longus** lies between and is covered by the tibialis anterior and the extensor digitorum longus. It arises from the middle half of the **anterior surface of** the **fibula,** medial to the attachment of the extensor digitorum longus, and from the anterior surface of the adjacent part of the **interosseous membrane.** Its tendon crosses the front of the ankle joint just lateral to the tibialis anterior and passes distally onto the dorsum of the foot to insert into the **terminal phalanx of** the **great toe.**

Three closed tendon **synovial sheaths** surround the tendons of these muscles as they course deep to the retinacula in front of the ankle and onto the dorsum of the foot. The sheaths cannot usually be very satisfactorily demonstrated in the ordinary anatomical specimen. The most **medial sheath** encircles the tendon of the **tibialis anterior** and extends from about the proximal border of the superior extensor retinaculum to within a short distance of the insertion of the muscle. A **second sheath** encloses the tendon of the **extensor hallucis longus** and extends from about the distal border of the superior extensor retinaculum to the base of the proximal phalanx of the great toe. The **third sheath** is common to the tendons of the **extensor digitorum longus** and the **peroneus tertius;** it extends from the distal border of the superior extensor retinaculum to about the middle of the dorsum of the foot.

Cut the superior extensor retinaculum and displace the tibialis anterior medially and the remaining muscles of the anterior compartment laterally; clean and study the anterior tibial artery and the deep peroneal nerve (Figs. 18.13 and 18.14). The **anterior tibial artery** is one of the terminal branches of the **popliteal artery.** It enters the anterior compartment by piercing the proximal part of the interosseous membrane close to the neck of the fibula. It descends in the anterior compartment on the interosseous membrane, lying first between the tibialis anterior and the extensor digitorum longus, and then between the tibialis anterior and the extensor hallucis longus. In the distal part of the leg, it rests on the anterior surface of the tibia and is crossed anteriorly by the tendon of the extensor hallucis longus. It becomes superficial just proximal to the ankle, where it lies between the tendons of the last-named muscle and the extensor digitorum longus. It ends in front of the ankle joint, after which its continuation is known as the **dorsalis pedis artery.** In addition to numerous muscular branches in the anterior compartment, the anterior tibial gives rise to the anterior tibial recurrent and the medial and lateral anterior malleolar arteries. The **anterior tibial recurrent** arises from the proximal part of the anterior tibial and ascends through the substance of the upper part of the tibialis anterior to reach the front of the knee joint. The **anterior malleolar arteries** are small vessels that arise from either side of the anterior tibial just proximal to the ankle. The **lateral anterior malleolar** runs laterally deep to the tendons of the extensor digitorum longus and peroneus tertius and then turns posteriorly on the lateral surface of the lateral malleolus. The **medial anterior malleolar artery** crosses the distal portion of the tibia deep to the tendons of the extensor hallucis longus and the tibialis anterior.

Locate the **perforating branch of** the **peroneal**

artery. It enters the anterior compartment by piercing the interosseous membrane about 4 cm above the lateral malleolus. Descending in front of the distal part of the fibula, it anastomoses with the **lateral anterior malleolar artery.** It is usually a small vessel but in some cases is greatly enlarged and continues onto the dorsum of the foot as the **dorsalis pedis artery;** in such cases, the anterior tibial, which normally gives rise to the dorsalis pedis, ends in small twigs to the ankle joint.

Finally, follow the **deep peroneal nerve,** one of the terminal branches of the **common peroneal nerve.** It enters the anterior compartment by piercing the upper part of the extensor digitorum longus. It accompanies the anterior tibial artery distally to the front of the ankle joint, from which point it accompanies the dorsalis pedis artery onto the dorsum of the foot. It lies to the lateral side of the anterior tibial throughout, except in the middle third of the leg, where it may lie in front of the artery. It supplies all the **muscles of** the **anterior compartment.**

DORSAL REGION OF THE FOOT

In order to display the structures on the dorsum of the foot effectively, you are advised to cut the **inferior extensor retinaculum** and to displace the tendons of the extensor digitorum longus and the peroneus tertius laterally.

Clean the **extensor digitorum brevis.** It arises from the lateral and superior surfaces of the **body of** the **calcaneus.** As its fibers pass distally, they divide into **four fleshy bellies,** each of which gives rise to a separate **small tendon.** The **most medial** muscular **belly** is sometimes described as a separate muscle, the **extensor hallucis brevis.** Its tendon inserts into the dorsum of the **proximal phalanx of** the **great toe.** The other three **tendons** are given to the **second, third,** and **fourth toes.** They do not, however, insert directly into the phalanges of these toes, but each joins the lateral side of the corresponding **tendon of** the **long extensor** near the base of the proximal phalanx (Fig. 18.13).

Clean the **dorsalis pedis artery** and its branches. You have seen that the dorsalis pedis begins in front of the ankle joint as a continuation of the **anterior tibial** and extends to the base of the first interosseous space, where it ends by dividing into the **deep plantar** and **first dorsal metatarsal arteries** (Fig. 18.14). It rests successively on the talus, the navicular, the second cuneiform, and the base of the second metatarsal bones. As it crosses the tarsal bones, it gives rise to a lateral tarsal and (usually) two medial tarsal branches. The **lateral**

Figure 18.14 The **arterial system of** the **anterior leg** region and the **dorsum of** the **foot.**

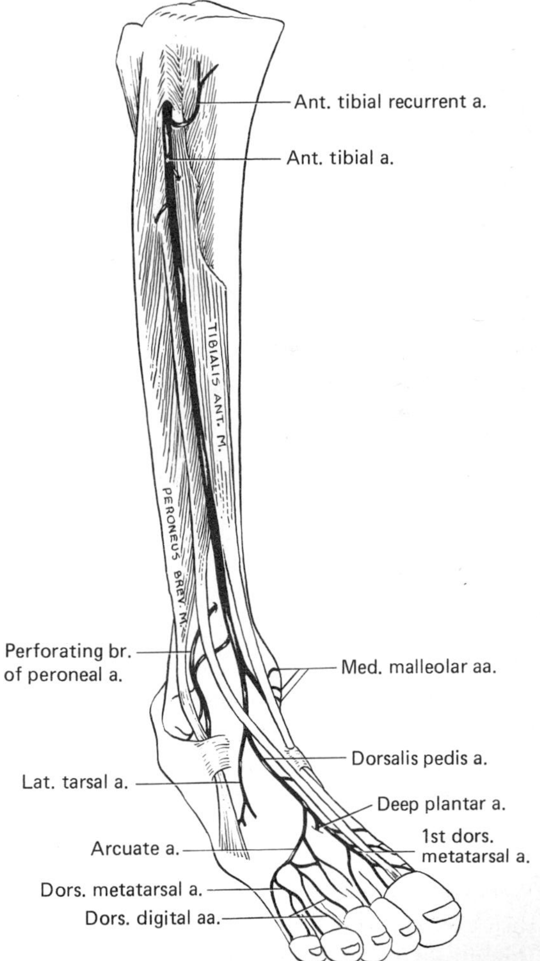

tarsal courses laterally deep to the extensor digitorum brevis and supplies this muscle and the bones and articulations of the region. The **medial tarsals** are small twigs that supply the skin and bones in the medial tarsal region. Near its termination, the dorsalis pedis gives rise to the **arcuate artery.** This vessel runs laterally across the bases of the metatarsal bones; from it arise the **second, third,** and **fourth dorsal metatarsal arteries.** Each one passes forward along the corresponding interosseous space and divides into two **dorsal digital branches** that are distributed to the adjacent sides of two toes. The first dorsal metatarsal artery is, as has been seen, one of the terminal branches of the dorsalis pedis; it usually gives rise to a branch that supplies the medial side of the great toe. The other terminal branch, the **deep plantar artery,** passes downward through the base of the first interosseous space into the sole of the foot, where, as will be seen later, it takes part in the formation of the **plantar arch.**

Finally, the **deep peroneal nerve** lies lateral to the first part of the dorsalis pedis artery. Just after crossing the ankle joint, it terminates by dividing into a lateral and a medial branch. The **lateral branch** passes deep to the **extensor digitorum brevis** and supplies it and the **tarsal joints.** The **medial branch** passes forward with the dorsalis pedis artery; its distribution to the **skin** on the adjacent sides of the great and second toes has already been seen.

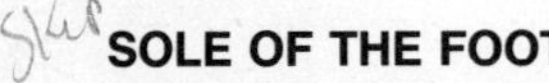

SOLE OF THE FOOT

Remove the superficial fascia and clean the **plantar fascia.** It is continuous with the fascia on the dorsum of the foot and covers the superficial muscles on the plantar aspect of the foot. It is subdivided into narrow **medial** and **lateral portions,** which are relatively thin and cover the muscles of the great and little toes, respectively. Centrally, the fascia is greatly thickened to form the **plantar aponeurosis.** It stretches forward from the calcaneus, to which it is firmly attached, widens, and toward the bases of the toes divides into **digital slips.** Each slip ends anteriorly by blending with the fibrous sheaths that bind the flexor tendons down to the plantar surfaces of the metatarsophalangeal joints and the phalanges.

Carefully remove the aponeurosis so you can study the muscles of the sole; its posterior portion cannot, however, be successfully removed, since some muscles take origin in part from its deep surface. Preserve the **medial plantar nerve,** which emerges between the abductor hallucis and the flexor digitorum brevis, and the superficial branch of the **lateral plantar nerve,** which appears at the lateral side of the flexor digitorum brevis (Fig. 18.15).

Customarily, the muscles of the sole are easier to learn and dissect if they are arranged in four layers. Begin the **first layer** with the **abductor hallucis muscle.** It arises from the medial process of the **tuberosity of** the **calcaneus** and from the portion of the **plantar aponeurosis** that covers it. Its tendon inserts into the medial side of the **base of** the **proximal phalanx of** the **great toe;** as you will see later, this insertion is common to the abductor hallucis and the medial belly of the flexor hallucis brevis.

The **abductor digiti minimi** arises from the lateral process of the **tuberosity of** the **calcaneus.** Its fibers extend forward along the lateral side of the sole and join a tendon that inserts into the lateral side of the **base of** the **proximal phalanx of** the **fifth toe;** often a secondary slip inserts into the tuberosity at the base of the fifth metatarsal.

The **flexor digitorum brevis** arises from the medial process of the **tuberosity of** the **calcaneus** and from the deep surface of the **plantar aponeurosis.** As it passes distally, it divides into **four** separate tendons that pass to the **second, third, fourth,** and **fifth toes;** the slip to the fifth toe is frequently lacking. Their insertions will be examined later; for the present, clean only as far forward as the heads of the metatarsal bones, where they enter the fibrous sheaths of the flexor tendons.

The **medial plantar nerve** emerges between the abductor hallucis and the flexor digitorum brevis,

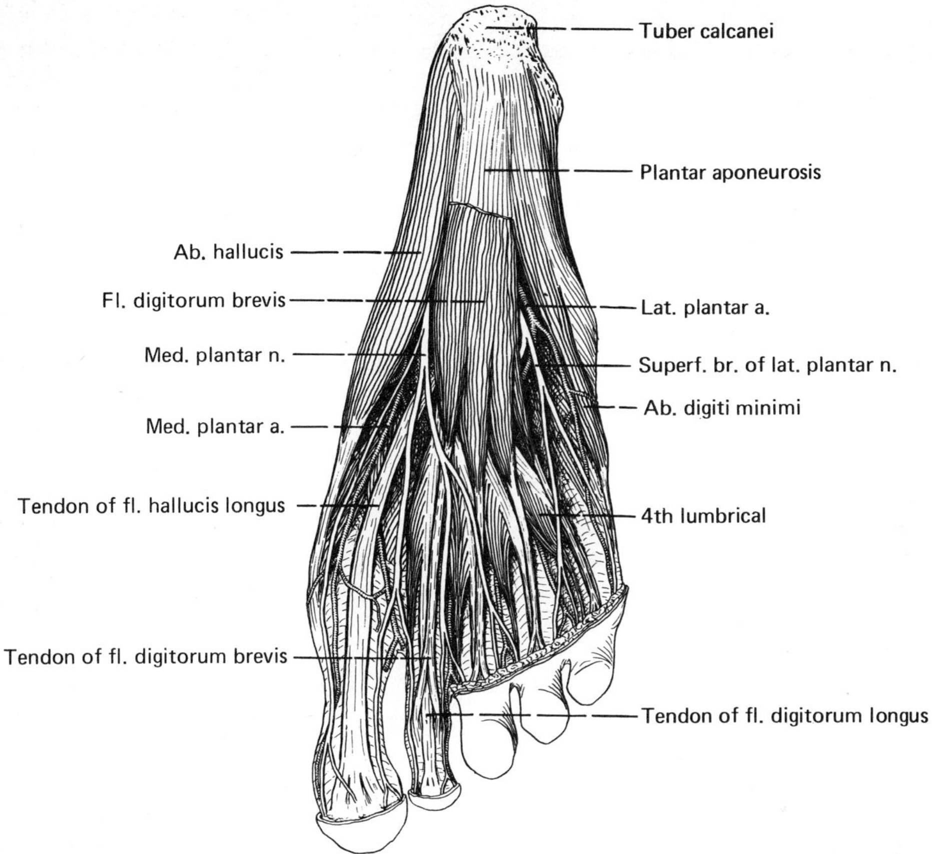

Figure 18.15 The **first layer of** the **sole** of the foot.

both of which it supplies, and runs forward to divide into **four cutaneous branches.** Of these, the most medial is a proper digital branch that passes to the skin on the medial side of the plantar aspect of the great toe. The remaining three, which are known as **common plantar digital nerves,** each divide near the heads of the metatarsal bones into **two proper plantar digital nerves** that supply the adjacent sides of the first, second, third, and fourth toes. The superficial branch of the **lateral plantar nerve** emerges from under cover of the lateral side of the flexor digitorum brevis and divides into **two branches;** the more **medial** one gives rise to two proper digital branches that supply the adjacent sides of the fourth and fifth toes, and the more **lateral** one supplies the lateral side of the fifth toe. These cutaneous nerves supply the entire plantar surface and also the nail bed of the toes.

The **second layer of muscles** in the sole of the foot includes the tendons of the **flexor hallucis longus** and the **flexor digitorum longus,** the **quadratus plantae** (sometimes called the accessory flexor, which is more descriptive of the muscle's function), and the four **lumbrical muscles.** At this level you will also find the trunks of the medial plantar nerve and artery, which cross deep to (above) the abductor hallucis, and the lateral plantar nerve and artery, which cross deep to both the abductor hallucis and the flexor digitorum brevis (Fig. 18.16).

Divide the **abductor hallucis** and the **flexor**

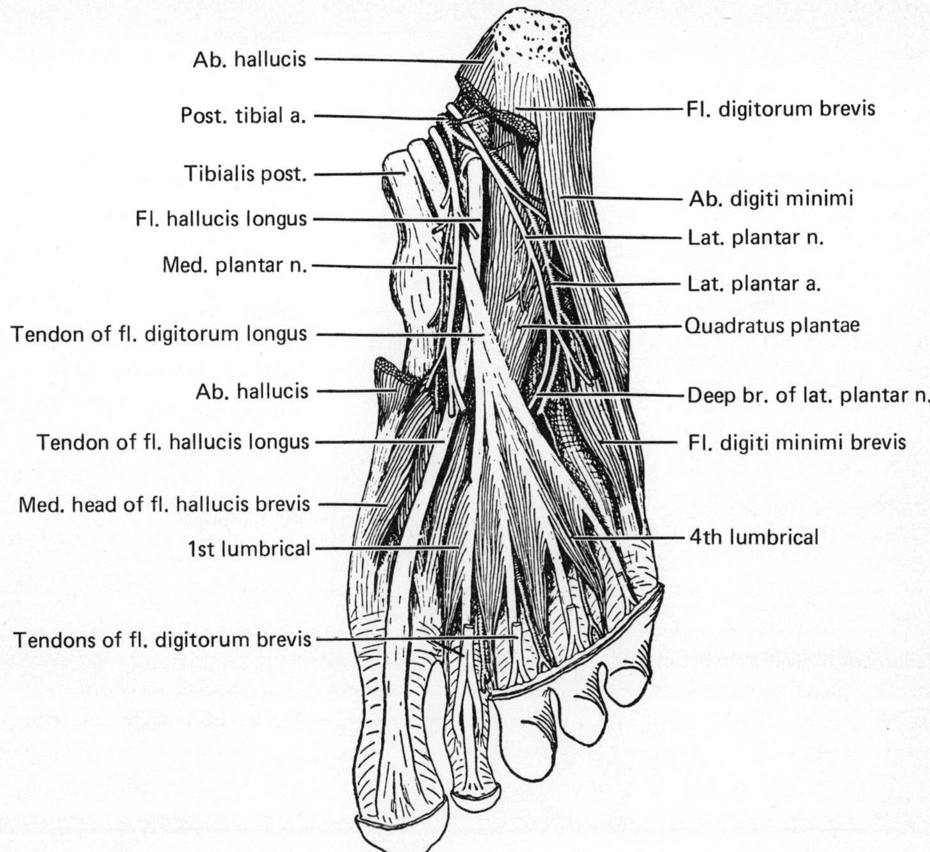

Figure 18.16 The **second layer of** the **sole** of the foot.

digitorum brevis close to their origins and reflect them forward. As you do this, secure their nerve supply, which they receive from the **medial plantar nerve.** Trace the full course of the medial plantar nerve and artery. In addition to the branches already described, the **medial plantar nerve** gives twigs of supply, usually from its two medial common digital branches, to the **flexor hallucis brevis** and the **first lumbrical muscles.** The **medial plantar artery,** which is usually much smaller than the lateral plantar artery, accompanies the medial plantar nerve. It gives rise to numerous small arteries that, for the most part, correspond to the branches of the nerve.

The **lateral plantar nerve** runs forward and laterally across the sole to about the base of the fourth interosseous space, where it ends by dividing into a deep and a superficial branch. From the **nerve trunk,** twigs are given to the **abductor digiti minimi** and the **quadratus plantae.** Near its beginning, the **superficial branch** supplies twigs to the **flexor digiti minimi brevis** and the **interosseous muscles of** the **fourth space;** its further course has been traced. The **deep branch** turns medially, deep to the **quadratus plantae,** where it will be followed later. The **lateral plantar artery** accompanies the lateral plantar nerve to the base of the fourth interosseous space, where it turns medially and deeply into the foot with the deep branch of the nerve. From the part of its course now visible, small twigs are given to the various neighboring muscles.

Trace the tendon of the **flexor digitorum longus** forward into the sole. Observe that it divides into **four tendons** that pass into the fibrous sheaths of the **four lateral toes,** where they lie deep to the corresponding tendons of the flexor digitorum brevis. Clean the **quadratus plantae.** This short, flat muscle arises by two heads from the lower parts of the **lateral** and **medial surfaces of** the **calcaneus.** Its fibers pass forward to insert into the lateral aspect of the **tendon of** the **flexor digitorum longus.** The lateral plantar nerve and artery rest directly on this muscle as they cross the sole.

There are four small **lumbrical muscles** in the foot. The **first lumbrical** arises from the medial side of the first tendon of the flexor digitorum longus; the **remaining three** each arise from the adjacent sides of two long flexor tendons. Each lumbrical gives rise to a slender tendon that passes around the medial side of its own digit to join the extensor expansion of that digit on the **dorsal side of** the **proximal phalanx.** By virtue of their attachments, the lumbrical muscles make it possible to flex the metatarsophalangeal joints and, to a small degree, to extend the interphalangeal joints.

Now study the manner of insertion of the **flexor tendons.** First observe that these tendons are held in place on the plantar aspects of the phalanges by **fibrous bands,** which, with the plantar surfaces of the phalanges, form an **osteofibrous canal** on each digit. Within each of these canals, the tendons of the long and short **flexors** are enclosed in a **common synovial sheath.** Open the fibrous sheaths by a longitudinal incision. Observe that the tendon of the flexor longus splits the tendon of the flexor brevis and passes forward to insert onto the **base of** the **terminal phalanx.** The **flexor brevis tendon** inserts onto the **base of** the **middle phalanx.**

Trace the tendon of the **flexor hallucis longus** into the foot. Observe that as it enters the sole, it rests in a groove on the undersurface of the **sustentaculum tali,** to which it is bound by a strong fibrous band. It then passes forward, crosses deep to the tendon of the flexor digitorum longus, to which it often gives a tendinous slip, and enters the fibrous sheath on the plantar aspect of the great toe. It inserts into the **terminal phalanx.**

Divide the tendon of the flexor digitorum longus at the point where it enters the foot and detach the quadratus plantae from its origin. Turn the divided portion of the tendon forward, together with the quadratus and the lumbrical muscles. At the same time, attempt to find the twigs that the **three lateral lumbricals** receive from the deep branch of the **lateral plantar nerve.**

Then clean and study the **muscles of** the **third layer.** They are the **flexor hallucis brevis,** the **adductor hallucis,** and the **flexor digiti minimi brevis.** The **flexor hallucis brevis** arises from the **third cuneiform** and **cuboid bones.** As its fibers pass forward, they divide into two fleshy bellies that lie on each side of the tendon of the flexor hallucis longus. The **medial belly** inserts with the abductor hallucis into the **medial side of** the **base of** the **proximal phalanx;** the **lateral belly** inserts with the adductor hallucis into the **lateral side of** the **base of** the **proximal phalanx.**

The **adductor hallucis** arises by two heads, an oblique and a transverse. The **oblique head** is large and fleshy. It arises from the **bases of** the second, third, and fourth **metatarsal bones,** and inserts, together with the lateral belly of the flexor hallucis brevis, into the **base of** the **proximal phalanx.** The **transverse head** is small and thin. It arises from the **capsules of** the third, fourth, and fifth **metatarsophalangeal joints** and inserts medially with the oblique head.

The **flexor digiti minimi brevis** is a fleshy slip that arises on the **base of** the **fifth metatarsal** and runs straight forward to insert into the lateral side of the base of the **proximal phalanx of** the **little toe.**

To display the **plantar arch,** you must detach the flexor hallucis brevis and the oblique head of the adductor hallucis from their origins and turn them forward. The **plantar arch** is formed by the medial continuation of the **lateral plantar artery,** deep to the quadratus plantae and the oblique head of the adductor hallucis, and by its junction with the **deep plantar branch of** the **dorsalis pedis**

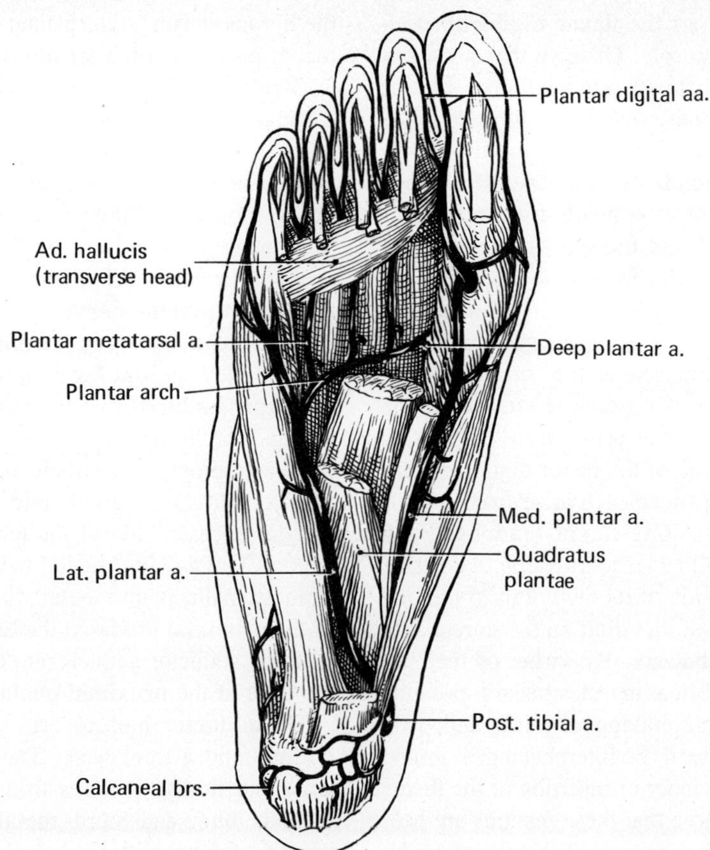

Figure 18.17 The **arteries of** the **sole** of the foot.

artery, which appears in the sole at the base of the first interosseous space (Fig. 18.17). It rests upon the bases of the second, third, and fourth metatarsal bones and gives rise to four **plantar metatarsal arteries.** They pass forward in the interosseous spaces, and each divides into two **plantar digital arteries,** which supply the adjacent sides of two toes. The deep branch of the **lateral plantar nerve** accompanies the lateral part of the deep plantar arch. This nerve is distributed to the **adductor hallucis,** the **lateral three lumbrical muscles,** and the **interosseous muscles** of the first, second, and third spaces (Fig. 18.18).

To display the seven interosseous muscles, which make up the **fourth layer,** it is advisable to remove the transverse head of the adductor hallucis and to cut the deep transverse ligaments that bind the heads of the adjacent metatarsal bones together. The **interossei** occupy the **interosseous spaces.** They are arranged in two groups consisting of **three plantar** and **four dorsal interosseous muscles.** The **first, second,** and **third plantar interosseous muscles** arise from the proximal thirds of the medial plantar surfaces of the third, fourth, and fifth metatarsal bones, respectively. Their fibers pass obliquely forward to insert into the medial sides of the bases of the proximal phalanges of the third, fourth, and fifth toes. One **dorsal interosseous muscle** is found in each space. Each arises from the adjacent **sides** of the **two metatarsal bones** bounding the space in which it lies. The **first dorsal interosseous muscle** inserts onto

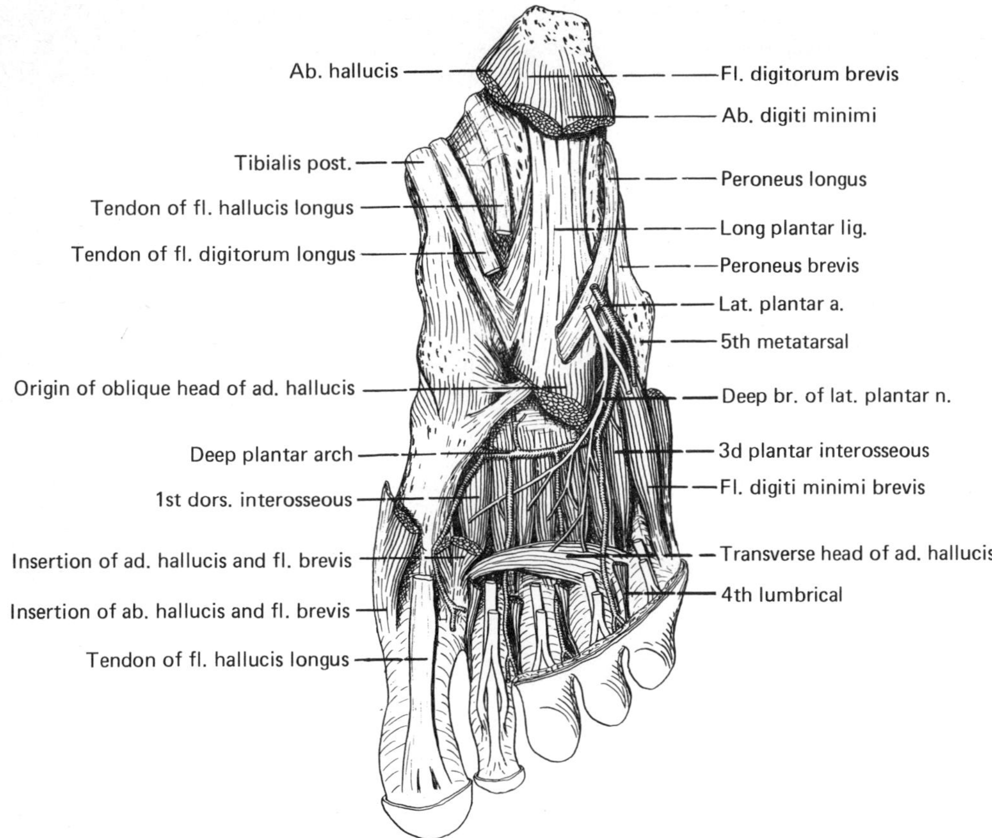

Figure 18.18 The **fourth layer of** the **sole** of the foot.

the medial side of the base of the **proximal phalanx** of the second toe. The **second, third,** and **fourth** insert on the lateral side of the bases of the **proximal phalanges** of the second, third, and fourth toes.

The **tendon of** the **tibialis posterior** can now be traced to its insertion. Observe that while its principal attachment is onto the **tuberosity of** the **navicular,** it gives off a secondary slip that spreads over the sole of the foot to attach to the **second** and **third cuneiform,** the **cuboid,** and the **fourth metatarsal bones.** The **tendon of** the **peroneus longus** has been traced to the lateral border of the **cuboid bone;** follow it now across the sole to its insertion on the inferior surface of the **first cuneiform** and the adjacent part of the base of **first metatarsal.** Observe that as it crosses the cuboid bone, it is partially ensheathed by the **long plantar ligament.** This ligament is a strong fibrous band that is attached posteriorly to the entire **inferior surface of** the **calcaneus** and passes forward to the **tuberosity of** the **cuboid,** from which its fibers spread out to reach the **bases of** the four lateral **metatarsal bones.** It is of considerable importance in preserving the **longitudinal arch of** the **foot.**

JOINTS

Dissect the joints only in one extremity; save the other one for a review of the entire dissected limb and for the relationships of the various structures to the joints. As you clean the muscles and other structures from the joints, note the course of the **collateral vessels** and the **nerves to** the **joints** since they could not be dissected adequately in the preceding sections.

Hip Joint

Clean the posterior aspect of the **capsule of** the **hip joint** (Fig. 18.19). First, transect the ischiadic nerve about 2.5 cm below the greater sciatic foramen and turn the distal portion downward. Then sever the tendons of the piriformis, the obturator internus, and the gemelli about 2 cm proximal to their insertions, and turn their cut ends laterally and medially. Observe that as they approach their insertions, all of these muscles lie immediately posterior to the joint capsule. Observe the **synovial bursa** that intervenes between the anterior surface of the **obturator internus** and the **lesser sciatic notch.** Detach the quadratus femoris from its insertion on the femur and turn it medially. Anterior to the quadratus, you will expose the **tendon of** the **obturator externus;** it winds laterally and superiorly across the lower posterior part of the joint capsule to insert into the **trochanteric fossa.** The upper posterior part of the joint capsule is covered by the gluteus minimus. First, cut the **tensor fasciae latae** from its origin, if this has not already been done, and turn it downward; then detach the **gluteus minimus** from its origin and reflect it completely to its insertion. As you do this, note that some of its deeper fibers insert on the **joint capsule;** detach them.

The **fibrous capsule** of the hip joint is attached

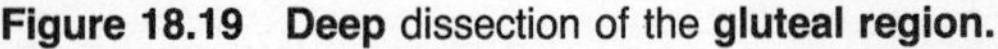

Figure 18.19 Deep dissection of the **gluteal region.**

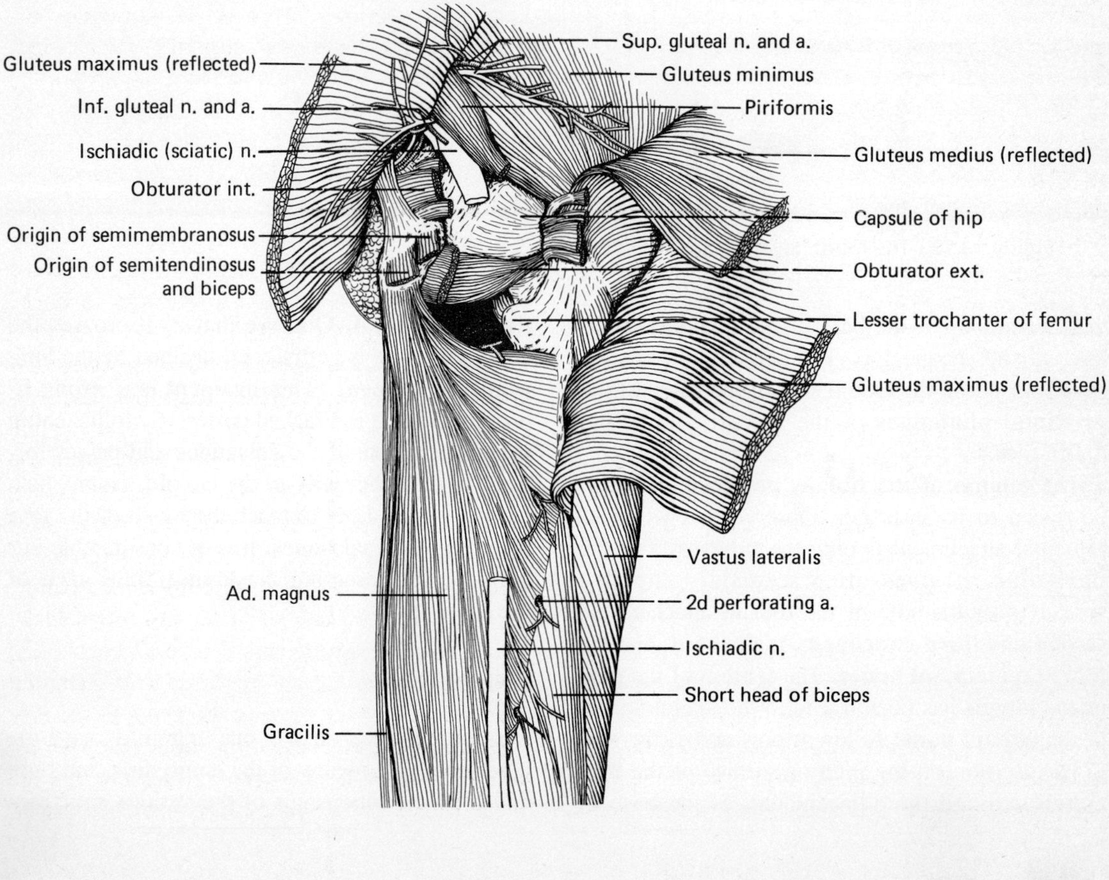

posteriorly to the **ilium** and the **ischium** about 1 cm medial to the acetabular rim; from here, it stretches laterally and downward to attach to the posterior surface of the **neck of** the **femur.** The thickened upper portion of the capsule is known as the **ischiofemoral ligament;** it stretches horizontally to the upper part of the greater trochanter and is closely associated with the insertions of the piriformis, obturator internus, and gemelli muscles.

Turn next to the anterior aspect of the hip. Take the opportunity now to study the origin of the **rectus femoris muscle.** Its **straight head** runs downward from the anterior inferior iliac spine; the **reflected head** arises from the posterosuperior surface of the rim of the acetabulum, closely related to the capsule of the hip joint, and goes forward under cover of the gluteus minimus and tensor fasciae latae to join the straight head (Fig. 18.20).

Review the origins of the pectineus, gracilis, and adductor muscles. Sever the gracilis close to its origin and turn it downward. Then define clearly the upper border of the **adductor magnus,** taking care to distinguish it from the **obturator externus,** which lies posterosuperior to the magnus. Then divide the adductor magnus along its entire origin and reflect it backward and laterally toward its insertion. The origin of the obturator externus is now exposed and should be cleaned.

The **obturator externus** arises, under cover of the origins of the adductors brevis and magnus, from the ischium and pubis along the anterior margin of the obturator foramen and, to a slight extent, from the external surface of the **obturator membrane.** Its fibers converge laterally and posteriorly into a tendon that winds around the lower part of the joint capsule, as already noted.

The anterior aspect of the hip joint is covered by the **iliopsoas muscle.** Sever it just above its insertion into the lesser trochanter and turn it upward to expose the anterior surface of the capsule. Observe the large **psoas bursa** that intervenes between the deep surface of the muscle and the anterior surface of the capsule; this bursa frequently communicates with the synovial sac of the joint cavity. For a better field of vision, you may have to remove the iliopsoas muscle up to the inguinal ligament.

Anteriorly, the **capsule** is attached to the **ilium** and the **pubis** close to the rim of the acetabulum, from which it stretches downward and laterally to attach to the **intertrochanteric line of** the **femur.** Two thickened portions of the capsule are described as ligaments. The stronger one is the **iliofemoral ligament.** It is attached superiorly to the **ilium** immediately below the anterior inferior iliac spine and widens inferiorly to reach the upper two-thirds of the **intertrochanteric line.** The **pubofemoral ligament** is less marked; it stretches from the outer surface of the **pubis,** near its junction with the ilium, to the lower part of the **intertrochanteric line** (Fig. 18.20).

Before you open the joint cavity, reflect the obturator externus to expose the **obturator membrane** and the distribution of the **obturator artery.** Cut through the entire breadth of the obturator externus close to its origin and turn the cut portion toward its insertion. As you do this, observe the twigs of the **obturator nerve** that supply it. Then clean the outer surface of the obturator membrane. The **obturator artery** emerges from the pelvis at the obturator canal in company with the obturator nerve. It divides almost at once into an **anterior** and a **posterior branch.** The **anterior branch,** which is usually smaller than the posterior branch, is distributed to the **adductor muscles,** near their origins, and to the **obturator externus.** The **posterior branch** gives rise to an **acetabular branch** that pierces the joint capsule in the region of the acetabular notch to reach the **head of** the **femur** by way of the **ligamentum capitis femoris.** Also from the posterior branch, arteries are given to the various muscles that arise from the ischial ramus.

Now study the **interior of** the **hip joint.** Make an incision through the entire circumference of the articular capsule 1.5 cm proximal to the femoral attachment; note the extreme thickness of the **iliofemoral ligament.** Then draw the head of the femur away from the acetabulum. Observe that the bones cannot be drawn entirely apart because of

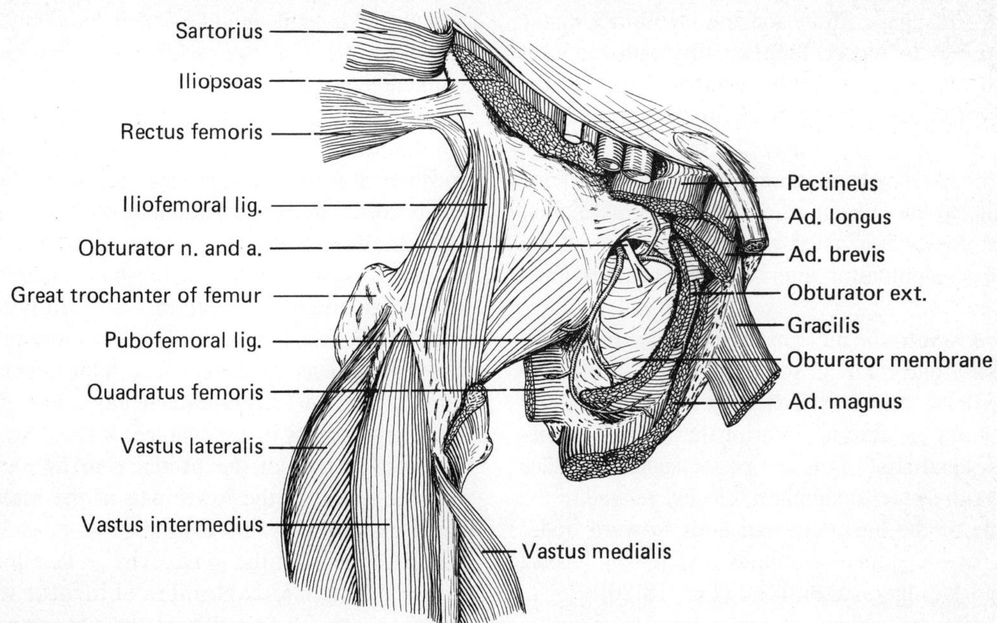

Figure 18.20 The anterior aspect of the **capsule of** the **hip joint.**

the presence of the **ligamentum capitis femoris,** a strong fibrous band that stretches between the **head of** the **femur** and the **acetabular fossa.** Observe that the **head of** the **femur,** except at the attachment of the ligamentum capitis femoris, and the **articular surface of** the **acetabulum** are each covered with **hyaline cartilage.** All other portions of the internal surface of the **joint cavity** are lined by the **synovial membrane.**

The **ligaments of** the **internal aspect of** the **hip joint** are the **ligamentum capitis femoris,** the **transverse acetabular ligament,** and the **glenoid lip.** The **transverse acetabular ligament** is a fibrous band that bridges the **acetabular notch** and converts it into a foramen; the acetabular branch of the obturator artery reaches the acetabular fossa through the foramen. The **glenoid lip** is a **fibrocartilaginous ring** that surmounts the rim of the acetabulum and the transverse ligament and thus deepens the acetabulum.

Although not frequent, dislocation of the hip joint does occur. When the thigh is flexed, medially rotated, and adducted, a traumatic blow against the knee can dislodge the head of the femur posteriorly, thus endangering the ischiadic nerve. Striking the knee against the dashboard in an auto accident is a common cause.

Knee Joint

Define clearly the inferior margins of the distal parts of the **vasti muscles.** Observe that these muscles for the most part attach either directly or by means of the tendon of the quadriceps to the proximal border of the patella. On either side of the patella, aponeurotic extensions of the vasti fuse with the crural fascia to form tendinous expansions known as **medial** and **lateral patellar retinacula;** these pass distally to join the articular capsule and the condyles of the tibia. The capsule is covered on its lateral side by the **biceps femoris;** detach the short head from its origin on the femur and remove the entire muscle, except for its insertion, which may be left attached to the head of the fibula. Also remove the **semimembranosus** from the capsule, except for about 1.5 cm proximal to its attachment to the tibia. The

fibular (lateral) collateral ligament, whose distal end was already seen piercing the tendon of the biceps, will be clearly exposed and should be cleaned (Fig. 18.21). It is the only external ligament of the knee joint that is not intimately blended with the articular capsule. Make a longitudinal incision through the middle of the **quadriceps tendon** a short distance above the patella to open the **suprapatellar bursa.** This bursa lies between the deep surface of the quadriceps tendon and the anterior surface of the distal part of the shaft of the femur; it is continuous distally with the synovial sac of the knee joint.

Attempt to demonstrate the **arterial anastomosis** that is found on the anterior aspect of the knee joint encircling the patella. The terminal portions of **six arteries,** the proximal portions of which have already been cleaned, take part in this anastomosis. They are the musculoarticular branches of the **descending genicular** from the **femoral,** the **medial** and **lateral superior** and **inferior genicular branches** from the **popliteal,** and the **anterior tibial recurrent** from the **anterior tibial.**

Of the **external ligaments of** the **knee joint,** the fibular collateral and patellar ligaments have already been cleaned. The **tibial (medial) collateral ligament** is a strong flat band lying on the medial side of the joint under cover of the tendons of the sartorius, gracilis, and semitendinosus. It extends from the **medial condyle of** the **femur** to the uppermost portion of the **medial surface of** the **tibia,** below the medial condyle. The **oblique** and **arcuate popliteal ligaments** are thickenings in the posterior part of the capsule. The **oblique popliteal ligament** lies in front of the middle portion of the popliteal artery; it is a tendinous expansion of the tendon of the semimembranosus that extends upward and laterally across the **back of** the **joint** from the posterior aspect of the medial condyle of the tibia. The **arcuate popliteal ligament** lies at the posterolateral side of the knee, extending from the apex of the **head of** the **fibula** upward to the back of the **lateral condyle of** the **femur;** the tendon of the popliteus muscle emerges from the joint cavity deep to the medial border of this ligament.

Divide the quadriceps femoris transversely about 5 cm above the patella and turn the distal segment of the muscle downward and forward. Then open the knee joint anteriorly by incising the articular capsule close to its line of attachment to the distal portion of the anterior surface of the femur. Flex the knee completely, draw the distal portion of the quadriceps with the attached patella downward and forward, and study the **interior of** the **joint** (Fig. 18.21).

The bony **articular surfaces of** the **knee joint** include the **condyles** and the **patellar surface of** the **femur,** the **superior articular surface of** the **tibia,** and the **internal surface of** the **patella.** Observe that each of these surfaces is covered by a layer of **hyaline cartilage.** The joint cavity is lined by the **synovial membrane** and elsewhere is packed with fat. Observe the **patellar synovial fold;** this is a fat-filled fold of the synovial membrane that runs from the lower border of the **patella** back to the **intercondyloid fossa of** the **femur.**

The **menisci** may be seen without dissection. They are **two** semilunar **fibrocartilaginous disks** that rest upon the outer portions of the **articular surfaces of** the **condyles of** the **tibia** and partially separate these surfaces from the corresponding articular surfaces of the condyles of the femur. Their inner margins are sharp and free; their outer margins are thicker and attached to the fibrous capsule of the joint. The **medial meniscus** is oval and is the larger of the two. It is attached medially to the tibial collateral ligament. The **lateral meniscus** is circular and is not attached to either collateral ligament.

In knee injuries, the medial meniscus is more frequently torn than the lateral meniscus, probably because of its attachment to the tibial collateral ligament, which restricts its movement.

The internal ligaments of the knee joint include the transverse ligament and the anterior and posterior cruciate ligaments. To expose them, you

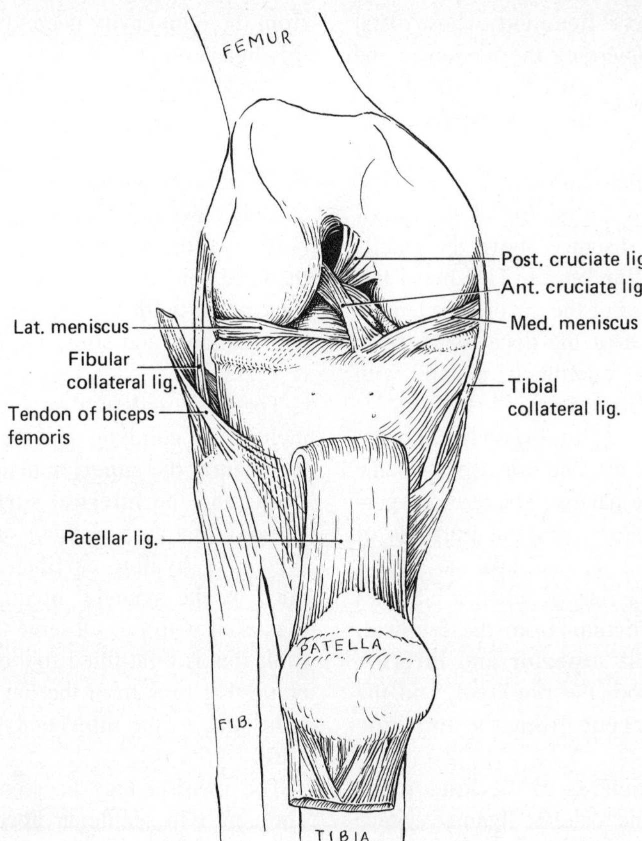

Figure 18.21 An anterior view into the **knee joint.**

will have to clear away the patellar synovial fold and the fat contained in it. The **transverse ligament** is a fibrous cord that extends across the anterior margin of the upper surface of the tibia from the rounded anterior margin of the **lateral meniscus** to the sharp anterior extremity or cornu of the **medial meniscus.** The cruciate ligaments are strong fibrous bands that occupy the intercondyloid fossa of the femur. The **anterior cruciate ligament** extends upward, backward, and laterally from the **anterior intercondyloid fossa of** the **tibia** to the medial surface of the **lateral condyle of** the **femur.** The **posterior cruciate ligament** is partly covered anteriorly by the anterior ligament. It extends upward and medially from the **posterior intercondyloid fossa of** the **tibia** to the lateral surface of the **medial condyle of** the **femur.**

The cruciate ligaments check anterior-posterior displacement of the tibia on the femur. A tear of the anterior cruciate will result in anterior movement of the tibia, whereas a tear of the posterior cruciate will allow the tibia to slip posteriorly.

Extend the knee, divide the posterior portion of the capsule of the joint, and observe the origin of the popliteus muscle from the lower lateral part of the lateral condyle of the femur, within the cavity of the joint.

Ankle Joint

Clean the capsule of the **ankle joint.** At this joint the **talus** articulates with the **distal end** and **medial malleolus of** the **tibia** and the **lateral malleolus of** the **fibula.** Its capsule is very thin anteriorly and posteriorly but is thickened laterally and medially. The thickened medial portion is known as the **deltoid ligament.** It is attached above to the **medial malleolus** and spreads out inferiorly to attach to the **navicular,** the **talus,** the **sustentaculum tali of** the **calcaneus,** and the **posterior part of** the **talus.** The thickened lateral portion of the capsule consists of three distinct slips, the **anterior talofibular ligament,** the **calcaneofibular ligament,** and the **posterior talofibular ligament.**

Motion at the ankle is purely dorsiflexion and plantar flexion. Ankle sprain, the most common ankle injury, usually is caused by sudden and forceful inversion of the foot. The weaker lateral ligaments are involved.

Tarsal and Metatarsal Joints

The **articulations of** the **foot** include the **intertarsal,** the **tarsometatarsal,** the **intermetatarsal,** the **metatarsophalangeal,** and the **interphalangeal** joints. While studying these joints, you should constantly refer to the foot of a mounted skeleton.

The **tarsal** and **metatarsal bones** are arranged in the form of **two arches,** a **longitudinal** and a **transverse arch,** the concavities of which face toward the sole. The **longitudinal arch** rests posteriorly on the tuberosity of the **calcaneus** and anteriorly on the heads of the **metatarsal bones.** It is supported principally by the **long plantar ligament** (the **calcaneocuneiform ligament**), the **short plantar (calcaneocuboid) ligament,** and the **spring (plantar calcaneonavicular) ligament.**

The **tarsal** and **metatarsal bones** are connected to one another by **dorsal, plantar,** and **interosseous ligaments.** There are **six** separate **articular cavities** for the various intertarsal, tarsometatarsal, and intermetatarsal articulations. The **talus,** through which the entire weight of the body is transmitted to the foot, takes part in **two of these;** one articulation is between the **body of** the **talus** and the **posterior facet of** the **calcaneus,** and the other one is between the **head of** the **talus** and the **navicular** and the **sustentaculum tali** of the calcaneus.

Disarticulate the talus to open these two articular cavities. Observe that in order to disarticulate the talus, a very strong ligament that fills the tarsal canal must be cut. This is the interosseous **talocalcaneal ligament,** which binds the **talus** and the **calcaneus** firmly together and separates the two articular cavities in which the talus takes part. Observe also that the articular surface of the head of the talus is not completely taken up by its articulations with the navicular and the calcaneus but rests also upon a strong ligament that stretches between the plantar surfaces of the two latter bones. This is the **plantar calcaneonavicular (spring) ligament;** it rests inferiorly on the tendon of the tibialis posterior.

Of the remaining **four articular cavities of** the **tarsus, one** is for the articulation between the **calcaneus** and the **cuboid.** A **second** single large articular **cavity** includes the articulations between the **navicular,** the three **cuneiforms,** the **cuboid,** and the **second** and **third metatarsals.** The **third cavity** includes the articulations between the **cuboid** and the **fourth** and **fifth metatarsals.** The **fourth cavity** is for the articulation of the **first cuneiform** with the **first metatarsal.** These cavities may be opened and the bones spread apart for observation of the articular surfaces by cutting through the dorsal ligaments.

Functional inversion and eversion of the foot are produced at the transverse tarsal joint. It is a plane that stretches across the foot between the talus and navicular bones medially, and the calcaneus and cuboid bones laterally.

The intermetatarsal, metatarsophalangeal, and interphalangeal joints are similar to those of the hand.

Sacroiliac Joint

The sacroiliac joint is formed between the auricular surfaces of the sacrum and ilium. This joint is held together by the **anterior sacroiliac, posterior sacroiliac,** and **interosseous ligaments.** An attempt should be made to identify these ligaments since they are important in maintaining the sacrum between the two ilia.

Index

Index